Atlas of Anatomic Pathology

Series Editor

Liang Cheng

More information about this series at http://www.springer.com/series/10144

Bryan H. Schmitt
Editor

Atlas of Infectious Disease Pathology

Springer

Editor
Bryan H. Schmitt
Department of Pathology and Laboratory Medicine
Indiana University School of Medicine
Indianapolis, IN, USA

Atlas of Anatomic Pathology
ISBN 978-3-319-54701-5 ISBN 978-3-319-54702-2 (eBook)
DOI 10.1007/978-3-319-54702-2

Library of Congress Control Number: 2017936053

Printed on acid-free paper

This Springer imprint is published by Springer Nature
The registered company is Springer International Publishing AG
The registered company address is: Gewerbestrasse 11, 6330 Cham, Switzerland

To my wife, Ingrid, who has been there from the beginning. Thank you for all of your love and support.

Series Preface

One Picture Is Worth Ten Thousand Words
—Frederick Barnard, 1927

Remarkable progress has been made in anatomic and surgical pathology during the last 10 years. The ability of surgical pathologists to reach a definite diagnosis is now enhanced by immunohistochemical and molecular techniques. Many new clinically important histopathologic entities and variants have been described using these techniques. Established diagnostic entities are more fully defined for virtually every organ system. The emergence of personalized medicine has also created a paradigm shift in surgical pathology. Both promptness and precision are required of modern pathologists. Newer diagnostic tests in anatomic pathology, however, cannot benefit the patient unless the pathologist recognizes the lesion and requests the necessary special studies. An up-to-date atlas encompassing the full spectrum of benign and malignant lesions, their variants, and evidence-based diagnostic criteria for each organ system is needed. This atlas is not intended as a comprehensive source of detailed clinical information concerning the entities shown. Clinical and therapeutic guidelines are served admirably by a large number of excellent textbooks. This atlas, however, is intended as a "first knowledge base" in the quest for definitive and efficient diagnosis of both usual and unusual diseases.

The *Atlas of Anatomic Pathology* is presented to the reader as a quick reference guide for diagnosis and classification of benign, congenital, inflammatory, nonneoplastic, and neoplastic lesions organized by organ systems. Normal and variations of "normal" histology are illustrated for each organ. The atlas focuses on visual diagnostic criteria and differential diagnosis. The organization is intended to provide quick access to images and confirmatory tests for each specific organ or site. The atlas adopts the well-known and widely accepted terminology, nomenclature, classification schemes, and staging algorithms.

This book series is intended chiefly for use by pathologists in training and practicing surgical pathologists in their daily practice. It is also a useful resource for medical students, cytotechnologists, pathologist assistants, and other medical professionals with special interest in anatomic pathology. We hope that our trainees, students, and readers at all levels of expertise will learn, understand, and gain insight into the pathophysiology of disease processes through this comprehensive resource. Macroscopic and histological images are aesthetically pleasing in many ways. We hope that the new series will serve as a virtual pathology museum for the edification of our readers.

Indianapolis, IN, USA Liang Cheng

Preface

Infectious disease pathology is a wide encompassing special interest within anatomic pathology, aided by various ancillary testing methods that often fall into the clinical/molecular microbiology realm. Infectious agents can be encountered in any subspecialty of pathology, and while large academic practices may confront them more frequently, smaller community practices are certainly not exempt. While many wonderful general and subspecialty volumes have been written on the subject, the aim of this publication is to provide primarily image-based educational content, geared toward the most frequently encountered infectious entities. It is my hope that this volume will prove to be an easy-to-use reference guide for daily anatomic pathology sign-out in a wide variety of practice settings as well as an educational collection for those interested in learning more about the histopathological manifestations of various infections.

The focus of the images will be on the hematoxylin and eosin (H&E) stained appearances of infectious agents and will highlight common special stains that can be used to aid in diagnoses. Where appropriate, commentary regarding additional testing such as immunohistochemistry and molecular-based testing is supplied. The atlas is organized primarily by pathogen type, followed by a discussion of the various manifestations that may occur in individual organ systems.

As infectious disease pathology is not an emphasis of a typical residency or fellowship curriculum, those pursuing advanced education must often seek the experience of others. As such, I would especially like to thank Dr. Bobbi Pritt for being instrumental in furthering my interest in the subject during my microbiology fellowship training at Mayo Clinic and beyond. I would also like to thank my colleagues Dr. Ryan F. Relich, Dr. Thomas E. Davis, and Dr. James W. Smith from the Indiana University School of Medicine for their insights and access to their extensive archival material. Special thanks also to Lee Klein, senior editor at Springer, for keeping me (mostly) on track during the year and a half development and writing process. I greatly appreciate the assistance. Lastly, I need to thank my wonderful wife, Ingrid, for putting up with the late nights and lost weekends and for her support not only on this project but over my entire career.

For the readers, I hope you enjoy the atlas and that it is a valuable contribution to your medical knowledge.

Indianapolis, IN, USA Bryan H. Schmitt

Contents

Contributors

Ryan F. Relich Department of Pathology and Laboratory Medicine, Indiana University School of Medicine, Indianapolis, IN, USA

Bryan H. Schmitt Department of Pathology and Laboratory Medicine, Indiana University School of Medicine, Indianapolis, IN, USA

An Introduction to Infectious Disease Pathology

1

Bryan H. Schmitt

Infectious diseases may be encountered in every subspecialty of pathology and can often present difficulties in identification and proper diagnosis. Most anatomic pathology microscopes and workstations are geared toward generally low-magnification diagnoses based primarily on patterns of tissue growth or inflammation. The microscopic diagnosis of many infectious diseases, however, requires much higher magnification, preferably up to at least 1000× total. Therefore, as the initial chapter in this atlas, we will first suggest some basic concepts to help achieve your optimal approach for high-magnification histologic and cytologic microscopy. Readers are of course encouraged to adapt these suggestions to their own practices as they see fit.

1.1 Microscope Setup

Although the setup of microscope objectives is largely a matter of personal preference, the pathologist or clinical microbiologist dealing with frequent infectious disease cases does benefit from proper positioning of oil immersion objectives in particular in order to avoid exposing low-lying objectives (such as a typical 40×) to the oil on the slide. While most surgical pathologists would prefer a 2× scanning objective for daily anatomic pathology work, the author has substituted a 60× "high and dry" objective because this provides additional magnification above a typical 40× without the need for oil immersion.

A stage clip, while eschewed by most anatomic pathologists, is essential here for fine adjustment of the viewing field, especially at higher magnifications. A stage

B.H. Schmitt (✉)
Department of Pathology and Laboratory Medicine, Indiana University School of Medicine, Indianapolis, IN, USA
e-mail: bhschmit@iupui.edu

B.H. Schmitt (ed.), *Atlas of Infectious Disease Pathology*,
Atlas of Anatomic Pathology, DOI 10.1007/978-3-319-54702-2_1

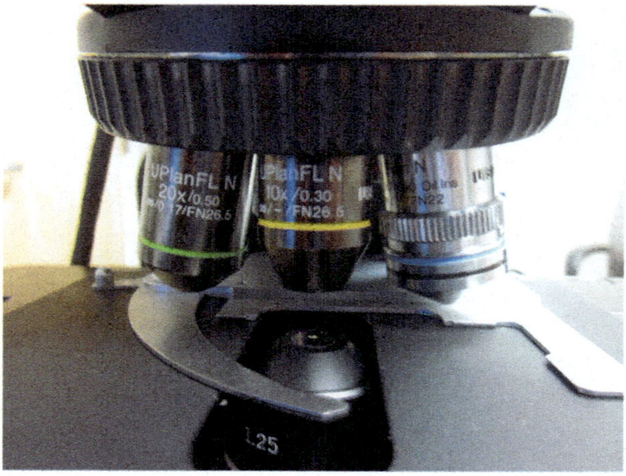

Fig. 1.1 Example image of a microscope nosepiece or "turret" with a 50× oil objective (*blue band*) installed adjacent to a 10× dry objective. This setup allows for switching back and forth between higher magnification oil immersion objectives and lower magnification dry objectives appropriate for scanning without running the risk of exposing non-oil objectives to oil

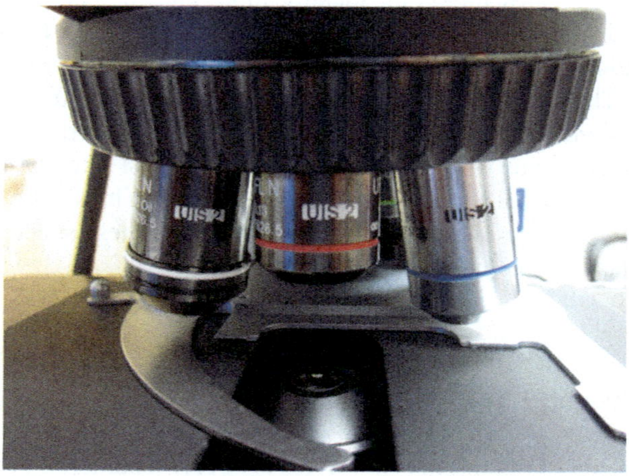

Fig. 1.2 Opposite side of the turret. Note the 4× objective installed adjacent to the 100× oil objective. The author has also opted for a 60× dry objective seen here, which could be swapped out for a 2× scanning objective depending on user preference and mechanics of the microscope. Importantly, the objectives adjacent to the oil immersion objectives are both of a shorter length so as to not allow for submersion into oil, but are also of lower magnification to allow for low power scanning on either side of the higher magnification objectives

clip is also very helpful when taking images for publication, obtaining remote second opinions, or sharing with colleagues.

Several of the microorganisms that will be discussed have components that are birefringent when observed under polarized light. If your microscope setup does not have integrated polarizing capabilities, several low-cost options for external filters are available. Additionally, as the size of microorganisms is often diagnostically helpful, access to a properly calibrated ocular micrometer is very important (Figs. 1.1, 1.2 and 1.3).

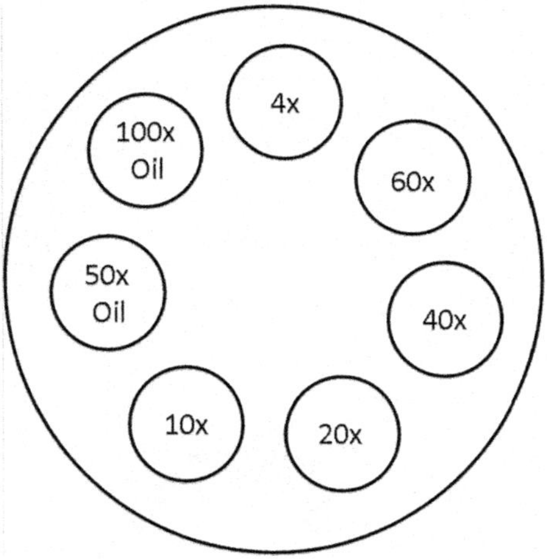

Fig. 1.3 Example layout for a seven objective turret viewed from the stage up. This setup allows for quick switching between high and low magnification objectives, while keeping distance between oil and longer, dry objectives

1.2 Caveats Regarding Histologic Sectioning and the Appearance of Microorganisms

Since histopathology involves sectioning through three-dimensional objects in a flat plane, the appearance of tissues and even cells is significantly altered, depending on orientation. This problem is no more pronounced than in infectious disease cases in which infectious agents, such as parasites, are often comparatively large and folded, resulting in multiple cross-sections through single or multiple organisms; this produces difficulties in reconstructing what is seen under the microscope versus most fine-tuned and ideal images seen in publications or online. While this atlas makes an effort to provide ideal images, "real-world" images are also included to reflect what is more likely to be encountered in clinical practice.

Also of note is that most infectious agents are living organisms, and as such appearances may change depending on the environment, exposure to antimicrobials, or other factors. A good example illustrating this point is found in filamentous fungi, in which the classic "acute angle branching" such as that described in *Aspergillus* species culture specimens may be disrupted. In many cases, this classically described appearance may not be perfectly maintained in histologic sectioning because the organisms grow through different environments, as well as into and around tissues or around themselves. Therefore examination of multiple sections to achieve an overall "consensus" in organism appearance is often required to come to a probable differential diagnosis, with culture results required for a definitive diagnosis (Figs. 1.4, 1.5 and 1.6).

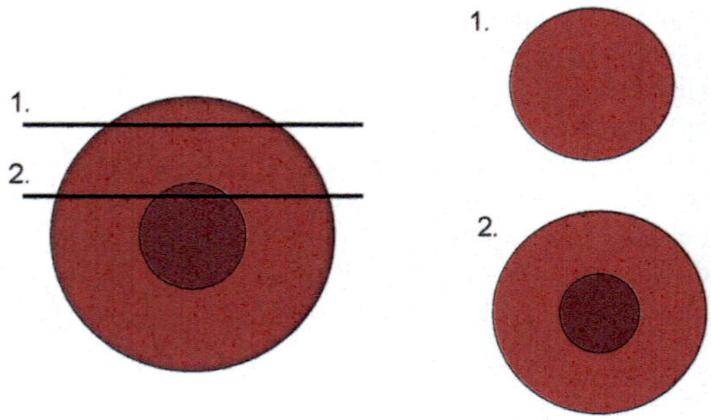

Fig. 1.4 In histopathology, three-dimensional objects are cut along a two dimensional plane. In this simple example, a cell cut along the top, as in plane 1, will only demonstrate cytoplasm, however when cut in plane 2, it will demonstrate the nucleus

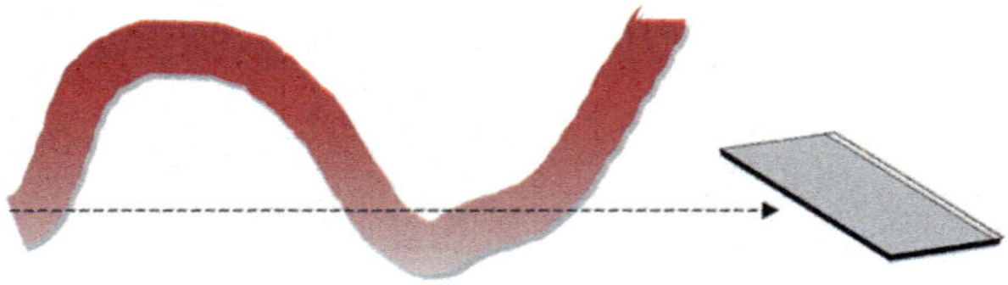

Fig. 1.5 Taking this concept one step further, you can see that if a large organism, such as a worm, were cut in perfect coronal or sagittal section, the overall appearance of the organism as a worm would be maintained, however, we are much more likely to receive cuts in an off-plane, such as the facing of the cartoon microtome blade in this illustration

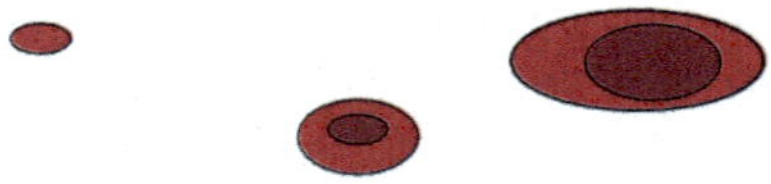

Fig. 1.6 The end result of the illustration in Fig. 1.5, may therefore end up looking like something more akin to what is seen here, with apparently differently sized and shaped sections as well as evidence of internal structures (*dark red dots*) in some sections and not others

1.3 Special Stains and Immunohistochemistry

Many infectious agents, particularly those of larger size, can be easily visualized using hematoxylin and eosin (H&E) staining alone. Often, however, inflammatory patterns are seen that are suggestive of an infectious process without showing readily identifiable organisms. In these cases, the use of special stains may be necessary to provide a diagnosis.

While evidence of bacterial processes can be suggested by an abundance of acute inflammatory cells or even in some cases visualized by clumps of bacteria, a tissue Gram stain may be helpful in delineating the nature of the infection. The most popular tissue Gram stains are Brown and Hopps and Brown and Brenn. Brown and Hopps stains are traditionally thought to more reliably stain Gram-negative bacteria their intended red color, whereas Brown and Brenn stains are thought to more reliably stain Gram-positive bacteria their intended blue color. Regardless, it is unlikely that most laboratories maintain access to both stains, and there are many additional variables that affect staining of bacteria, particularly within fixed tissues. However, if tissue Gram stain results do not appear to correlate with other available information, the respective characteristics of the stains may be a factor to take into account when considering the morphologies of the bacteria observed.

One of the most commonly encountered tissue manifestations of infectious agents seen in the pathology laboratory is the presence of granulomas. Particularly in cases where necrotizing granulomas are found and an infectious disease is part of the differential diagnosis, it may be prudent to order a stain for acid-fast bacilli (AFB) and fungi together in order to minimize turnaround time, since these tests are often only performed once per day.

Typically AFB consists of a Ziehl-Neelsen or Kinyoun stain, although Fite stains may also be used. The Fite technique was developed as a gentler method specifically for the identification of the very weakly acid-fast *Mycobacterium leprae*, but it generally performs well for the identification of most acid-fast bacilli and is the preferred staining method for suggesting an identification of *Nocardia* species (often called partially acid-fast) in tissue when seen in the author's laboratory.

The most frequently utilized stain for the visualization of fungi in most laboratories is the Gomori methenamine silver (GMS) stain or a variant thereof. Fungi are frequently encountered infectious agents in dermatopathology, and many dermatopathologists prefer the use of periodic acid–Schiff (PAS) staining formulated for fungi, since GMS stains can be very nonspecific. This issue is particularly problematic when examining skin tissue, which often has an abundance of cracks and crevices that can retain silver particles. Additionally, GMS has a predilection for staining intracellular granules, elastin, and various other nonhuman materials. However, in general GMS staining provides much better contrast for the examination of fungi than PAS staining.

Most institutions have immunohistochemistry (IHC) techniques available for commonly identified viruses in histopathologic sections such as cytomegalovirus, herpes simplex virus, and adenoviruses and may provide stains for some bacteria of frequently identifiable significance such as *Helicobacter pylori*. In general, however, unless in a research setting, most infectious agents are either not frequently encountered enough or are more easily identifiable by other methods such that the development and provision of IHC for these organisms is not viable. A variety of IHC stains for more esoteric organisms are available at some larger reference laboratories or used as part of consulting services such as those located at the Centers for Disease Control and Prevention.

Suggested Reading

Ash LR, Orihel TC. Ash and Orihel's atlas of human parasitology. 5th ed. Chicago: ASCP Press; 2015.
Cooke RA. Infectious diseases, atlas, cases, text. Sydney: McGraw-Hill; 2008.
Garcia LS. Diagnostic medical parasitology. 5th ed. Washington, DC: ASM Press; 2007.
Larone DH. Medically important fungi: a guide to identification. 5th ed. Washington, DC: ASM Press; 2011.
Procop GW, Pritt BS, editors. Pathology of infectious diseases. Philadelphia: WB Saunders; 2015.

Bacterial Infections

2

Bryan H. Schmitt

Infections caused by bacteria are varied and can affect every organ system. As such, this chapter initially focuses on specific types of infections such as pneumonias and endocarditis and later discusses typical presentations associated with specific bacteria. In most cases, the definitive identification of the bacterial entity causing disease will require additional testing. At the basic level this consists of submission of tissue, blood, or fluid for culture. If a specific disease entity such as cat scratch disease is suspected, the microbiology laboratory should be informed so that proper media and culture conditions can be utilized. Specimens obtained from patients with certain bacterial infections, including tularemia, tuberculosis, brucellosis, anthrax, and melioidosis, pose a risk of transmission to laboratory professionals. As such, if specimens suspected of harboring the causative agents are to be submitted to the laboratory, prior notification must be given so that proper precautions may be taken by laboratory personnel in all areas of the clinical laboratory.

Obtaining a proper culture specimen is of utmost importance. Definitive identification of the organism and subsequent proper antimicrobial susceptibility testing depend on the state of the initial specimen received by the laboratory. Ideally, material submitted for culture should be collected in as sterile a manner as possible and submitted directly to the microbiology laboratory from the surgical suite or office. If material is submitted from the pathology gross room, all care should be taken to divide the tissue using sterile technique, sterile gloves, petri dishes, and instrumentation. In addition to sterile technique, issues

B.H. Schmitt (✉)
Department of Pathology and Laboratory Medicine, Indiana University School of Medicine, Indianapolis, IN, USA
e-mail: bhschmit@iupui.edu

B.H. Schmitt (ed.), *Atlas of Infectious Disease Pathology*,
Atlas of Anatomic Pathology, DOI 10.1007/978-3-319-54702-2_2

of safety in the gross room should also be addressed. All gross rooms should have a biological safety cabinet available for the dissection of specimens demonstrating necrotizing or caseating granulomas as well as for cases of suspected aerosol-transmissible infections. The primary concern regarding granulomas is that they may be harboring tuberculosis, although other conditions such as tularemia may present similarly and may also pose a significant risk of transmission if grossed on the open bench. Often an infectious disease is not considered as part of the top differential diagnosis, and tissue or fluid is submitted only for histopathologic or cytopathologic examination. In such cases, the material submitted for examination has likely been placed in formalin or another fixative, rendering bacterial culture useless. In some cases, molecular techniques such as 16S sequencing may be successful in identifying pathogenic microorganisms from formalin-fixed and paraffin-embedded tissue, but if organisms cannot be correlated with microscopy findings, the results obtained by 16S sequencing may be dubious. The inherent nonsterile nature of gross room practice can present multiple sources for contamination of tissues, and these factors need to be accounted for as well.

2.1 Typical Appearances of Common Pathogenic Bacteria

In anatomic pathology, the definitive identity of cultured bacteria may not be available at the time of initial interpretation. As such, it is important to be able to identify in a general fashion the morphologic appearance of common bacterial pathogens; this increases the chances that a possible culprit may be identified at the time of microscopic examination or reasonably tied to culture results if obtained. The following general bacterial morphotypes are discussed with the caveat that antimicrobial treatment may at times significantly alter the appearance of bacteria (Figs. 2.1, 2.2, 2.3, 2.4, 2.5, 2.6, 2.7, 2.8, 2.9, 2.10, 2.11, 2.12, 2.13 and 2.14).

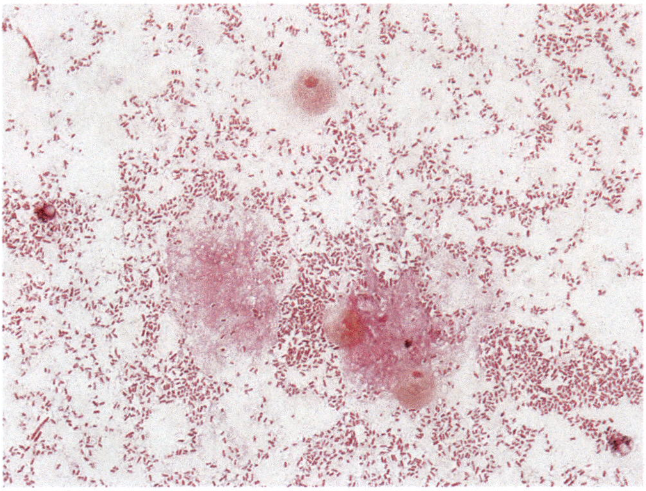

Fig. 2.1 Enterobacteriaceae such as *Escherichia coli* and *Klebsiella pneumoniae* are Gram-negative rods, typically having a "short and fat" morphologic appearance. Many also demonstrate a capsule which presents as a "clearing" or "halo" around the organism. Bronchoalveolar lavage, Gram stain, 1000× magnification

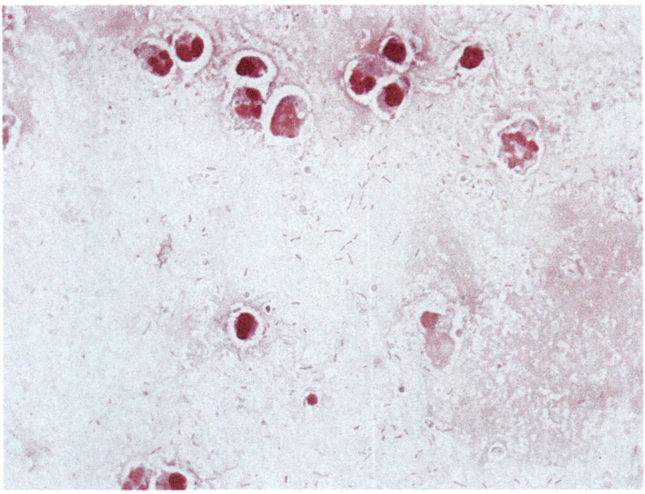

Fig. 2.2 *Pseudomonas* species typically appear as thin Gram-negative rods. This general appearance is also shared by *Stenotrophomonas* species, which are increasingly recognized as a cause of hospital-acquired infections. Capsules may be prominent, especially in respiratory specimens obtained from patients with cystic fibrosis. Bronchoalveolar lavage, Gram stain, 1000× magnification

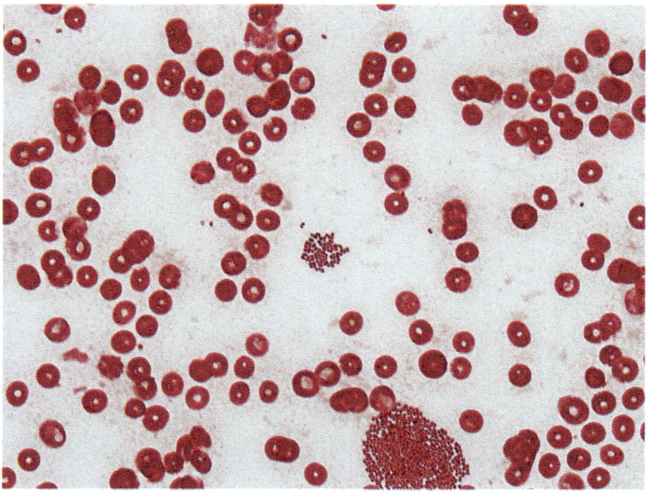

Fig. 2.3 Gram-negative diplococci include *Neisseria* and *Moraxella* species, although each genus has members that may take on more "rod-like" forms. These diplococci are generally morphologically indistinguishable, presenting as Gram-negative cocci in pairs, with a "kidney" or "coffee bean" shaped appearance. *Moraxella* and *Neisseria* species do tend to cause infections of different organ systems with *Moraxella catarrhalis*, being a common culprit in lower respiratory tract disease, sinusitis, and middle ear infections. *Neisseria gonorrhea* and *Neisseria meningitidis* are implicated in genitourinary and joint infections and infections of the central nervous system and bloodstream. Blood culture demonstrating *N. meningitidis*, Gram stain, 1000× magnification

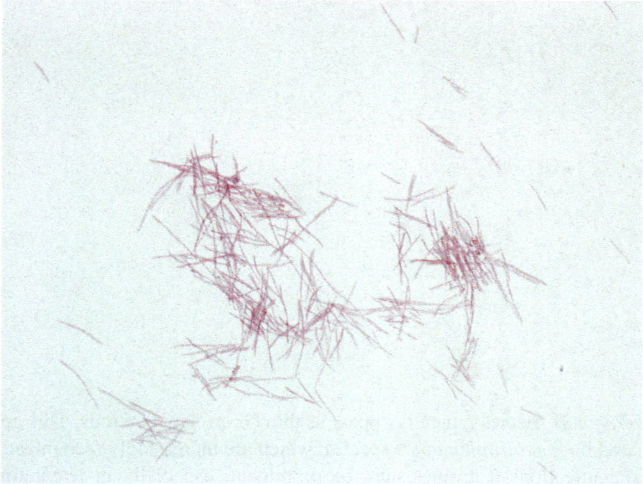

Fig. 2.4 *Fusobacterium* species usually appear as very long and spindled Gram-negative bacteria. *Fusobacterium* species can be involved in anaerobic infections, including brain abscesses and Lemierre syndrome, which is typically caused by *Fusobacterium necrophorum*. Pictured here is a direct from colony smear of *Fusobacterium nucleatum*. *Fusobacterium necrophorum* may also exhibit shorter, rod-like forms. Gram stain, 1000× magnification

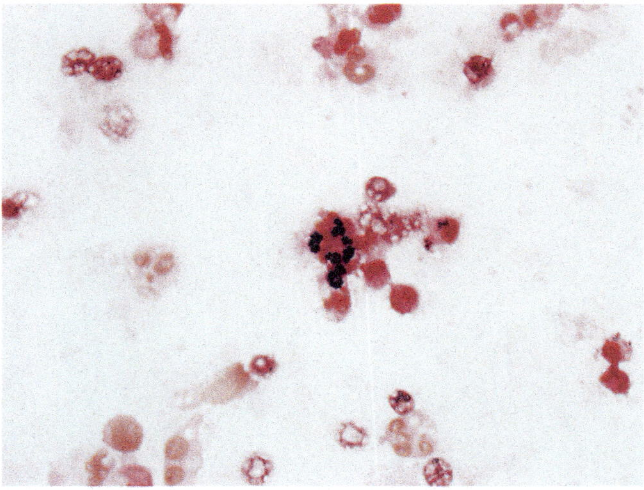

Fig. 2.5 Gram-positive cocci appearing in clusters suggesting *Staphylococcus* species. The most common pathogen is *S. aureus*, which is often broadly categorized as coagulase-positive *Staphylococcus*. It is important to note that coagulase-negative staphylococci are most often contaminants when identified within anatomic pathology specimens but may also be implicated in disease, particularly in non-native valve endocarditis. Bronchoalveolar lavage, Gram stain, 1000× magnification

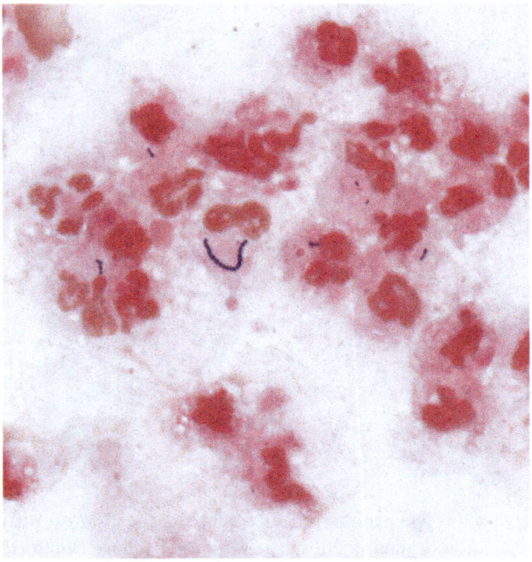

Fig. 2.6 Gram-positive cocci in chains suggest *Streptococcus* or *Enterococcus* species. Liver abscess aspirate, Gram stain, 1000× magnification

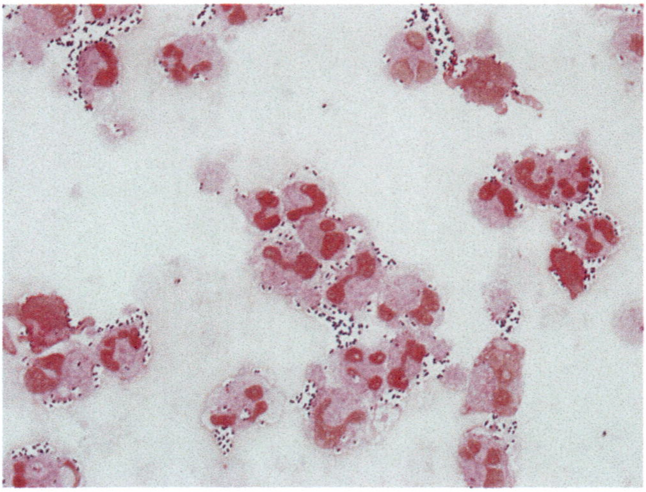

Fig. 2.7 Gram-positive cocci in pairs, particularly from respiratory specimens, including sputum and BAL, are strongly suggestive of *Streptococcus pneumoniae*. These streptococci very often demonstrate an "American football" or "lancet-shaped" morphology. A clear halo can often be seen with common stains, representing the capsule associated with *S. pneumoniae*. Bronchoalveolar lavage, Gram stain, 1000× magnification

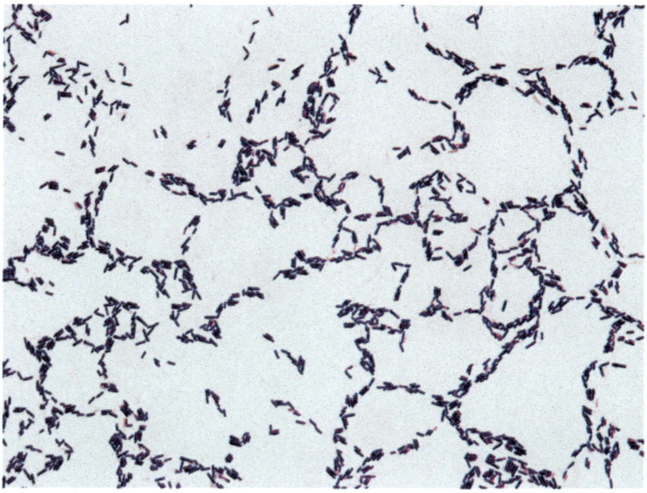

Fig. 2.8 Gram-positive rods. The primary differential for large Gram-positive rods is *Bacillus* or *Clostridium* species. Location of the infection is paramount because *Bacillus* species tend to cause respiratory or cutaneous disease (with the exception of *B. cereus*), whereas infections with clostridia, particularly *Clostridium difficile*, tend to be gastrointestinally oriented. Importantly, other clostridia such as *C. septicum* or *C. perfringens* may cause soft-tissue or solid organ infections. As demonstrated here, Gram-positive rods may appear to stain "Gram-variable," with some staining Gram-positive and others Gram-negative. Gram stain, *Clostridium* species, direct from culture, 1000× magnification

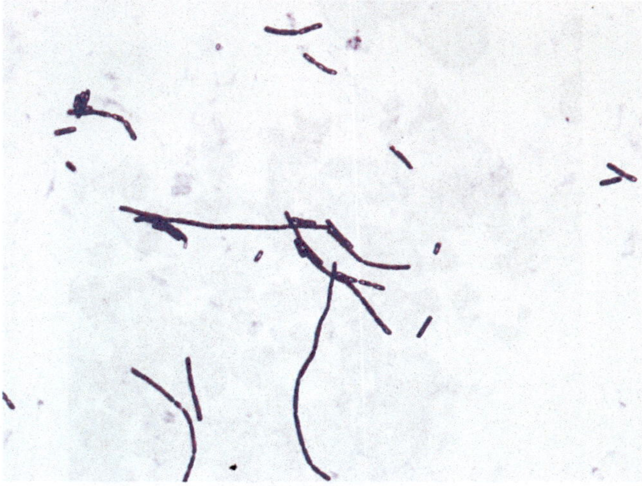

Fig. 2.9 Spores can be produced by many Gram-positive rods and may at times be visualized. Shown here is a Gram stain of cultured *Bacillus anthracis*. Note the intracellular inclusions, which represent spore formation. The location of the spores within the bacterial cells may help to speciate the organism. Direct from culture, 1000× magnification

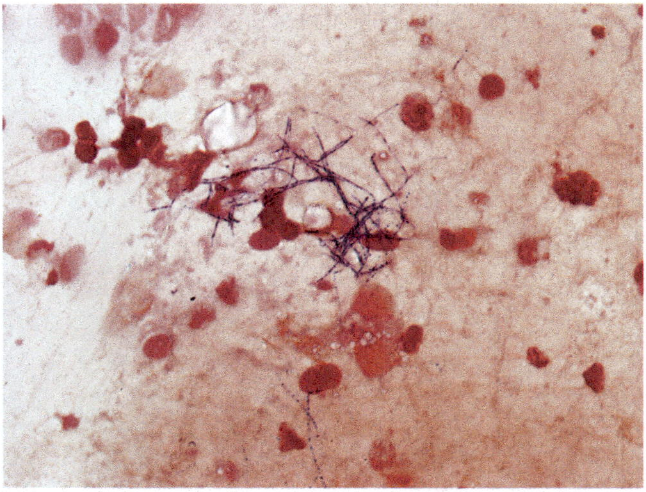

Fig. 2.10 Filamentous, branching, Gram-positive bacteria. The primary differentials of bacteria with this appearance are *Actinomyces* and *Nocardia* species. It should be noted that other Actinomycetes such as *Streptomyces* species have also been identified in human infections, although less commonly. *Nocardia*, in particular, has been identified as an agent of primary respiratory infection that can spread in a metastatic fashion. Because of this, nocardial infections can easily be mistaken for a mycobacterial infection or infections with dimorphic fungi, most notably *Histoplasma capsulatum*. It should be noted that Actinomycetes often retain the crystal-violet stain in a beaded fashion. Bronchoalveolar lavage, Gram stain, 1000× magnification

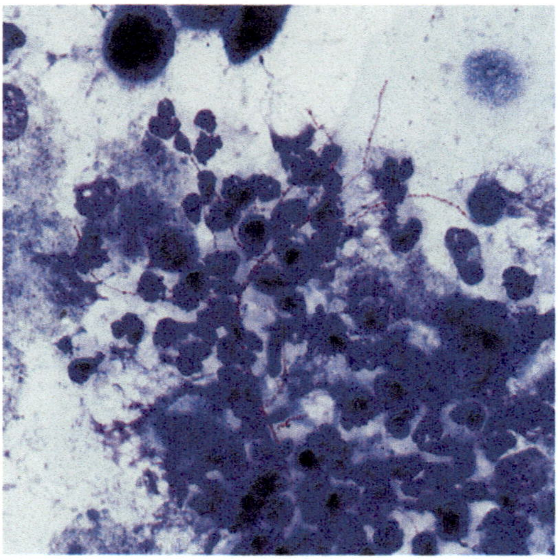

Fig. 2.11 In distinguishing *Nocardia* from *Actinomyces* species, a modified acid-fast stain may be useful, since *Actinomyces* species are negative and *Nocardia* species are considered partially acid-fast. In practice, however, *Nocardia* species are often negative with acid-fast staining. Therefore, acid-fast staining, if positive, is good evidence of a nocardial infection, but a negative result should not be interpreted as definitive for a non-nocardial infection, and culture results should be relied upon for final identification. Bronchoalveolar lavage, modified Kinyoun stain, 1000× magnification

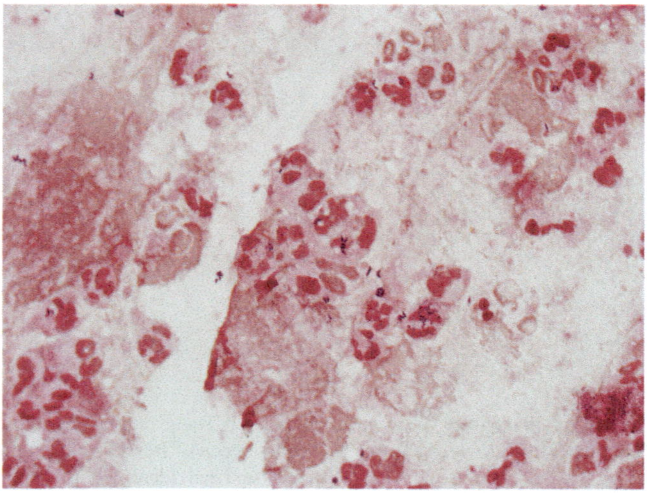

Fig. 2.12 "Diphtheroid" Gram-positive rods such as *Corynebacterium* species are smaller than *Clostridium* or *Bacillus* species and do not branch like Actinomycetes, although overlapping bacteria may appear to be doing so. These bacteria are often "club-shaped," being larger on one end and often demonstrate "pallisading" or "picket-fence" formations. Bronchoalveolar lavage, Gram stain, 1000× magnification

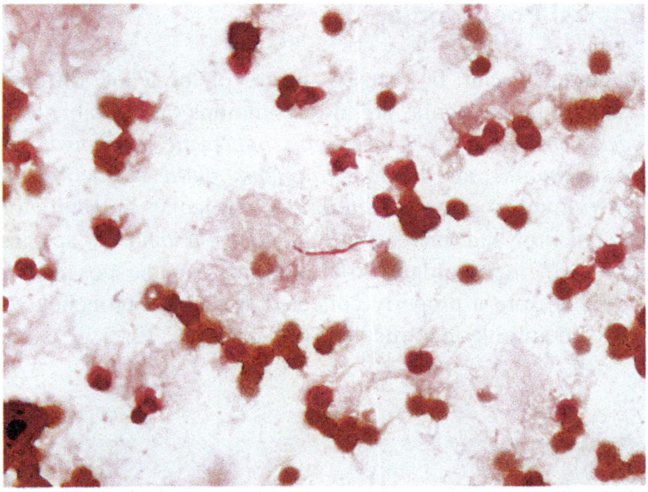

Fig. 2.13 Bacteria exposed to antimicrobials may take on bizarre shapes. Gram-positives will tend to swell, appearing larger than normal. Gram-negative rods, as shown here, will tend to show elongate forms, sometimes with a centrally located swelling or bubble. Gram stain, 1000× magnification

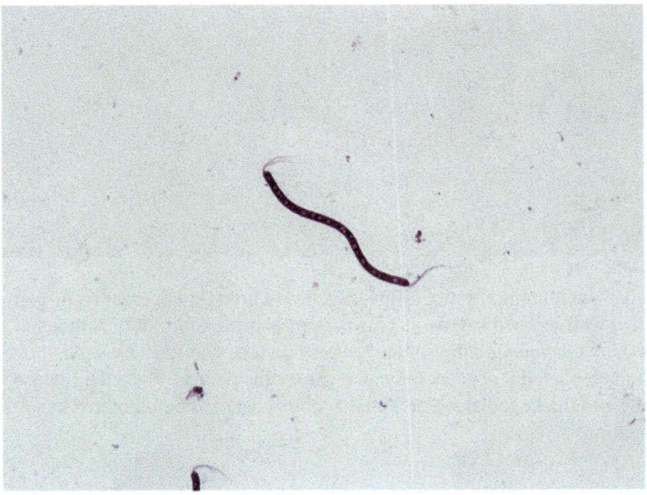

Fig. 2.14 The vast majority of bacterial morphologies that are involved in human disease are covered in this section. However, it is important to note that rare human bacterial pathogens may have other forms, such as that of *Spirillum* species. Pictured here is *Spirillum volutans*. A related and morphologically similar species, *Spirillum minus* is a causative agent of rat-bite fever. Note that it is much larger and longer than typical bacterial human pathogens and demonstrates easily identifiable bipolar flagellar tufts. Gram stain, direct from colony, 1000× magnification

2.2 Bacterial Pneumonia

Bacterial pneumonias can be caused by a plethora of different bacteria. Community-acquired pneumonias are most commonly attributable to species such as *Streptococcus pneumoniae, Haemophilus influenzae, Chlamydia pneumoniae, Mycoplasma pneumoniae,* and *Legionella pneumophila.* Nosocomial pneumonias more frequently involve enteric bacteria. In particular in ventilator-associated patients *Pseudomonas* and increasingly *Stenoptrophomonas* species are seen. As discussed above, morphologic differentiation may be possible to a limited extent, but cultures from a properly collected sputum or bronchoalveolar lavage are important for definitive identification (Figs. 2.15, 2.16, 2.17, 2.18, 2.19, 2.20 and 2.21).

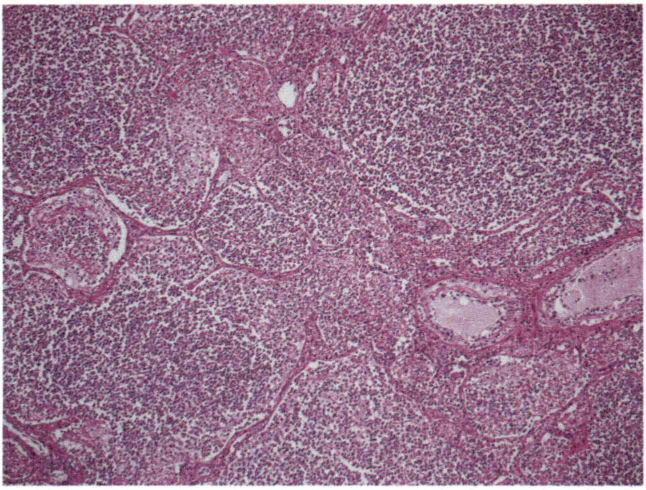

Fig. 2.15 Lobar pneumonia, by definition, has the radiologic appearance of consolidation of a lung lobe or of a well-defined segment. This pattern is most commonly associated with infection with *Streptococcus pneumoniae*, but other bacteria such as *Klebsiella pneumoniae*, *Haemophilus influenza,* and mycobacterial species may also cause this pattern. Note the intense, acute inflammatory infiltrate and thickened alveolar walls, which appear to be obliterated in some areas. H&E, 100× magnification

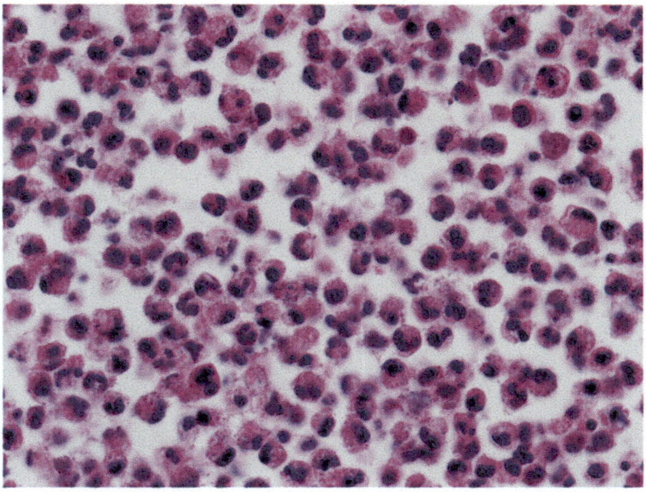

Fig. 2.16 Higher magnification demonstrating acute inflammatory infiltrate. Fragments of bacterial cells are evident inside some of the neutrophils. H&E, 1000× magnification

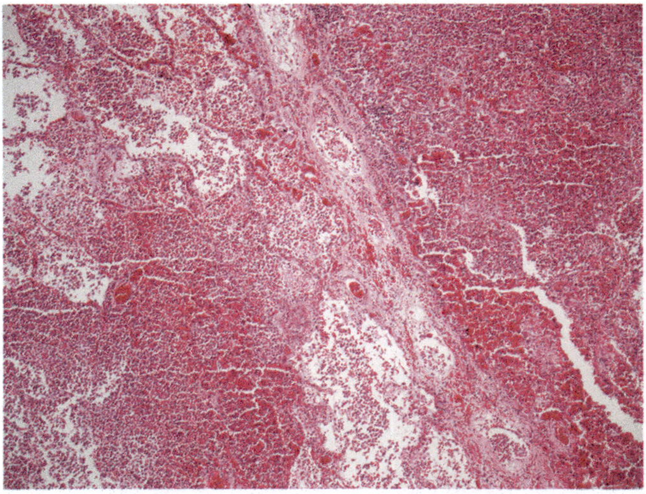

Fig. 2.17 Late stage lobar pneumonia demonstrating abscess formation on the *right half* of the image. H&E, 100× magnification

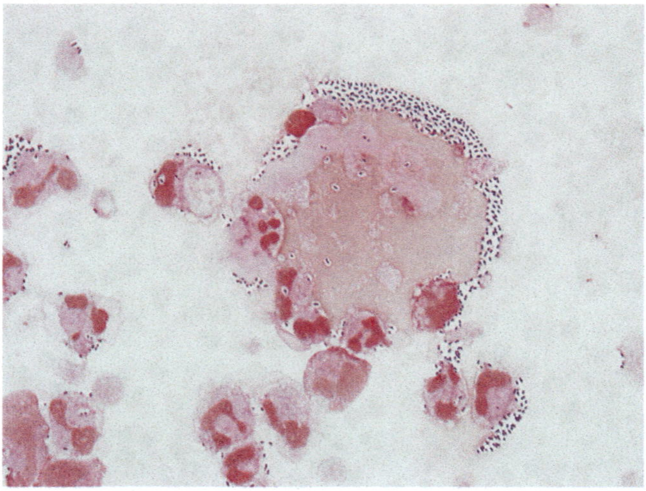

Fig. 2.18 Classic appearance of *Streptococcus pneumoniae* in bronchoalveolar lavage fluid. Note that most of the bacteria are in pairs, with a "lancet-shaped" morphology surrounded by a clear capsule. Gram stain, 1000× magnification

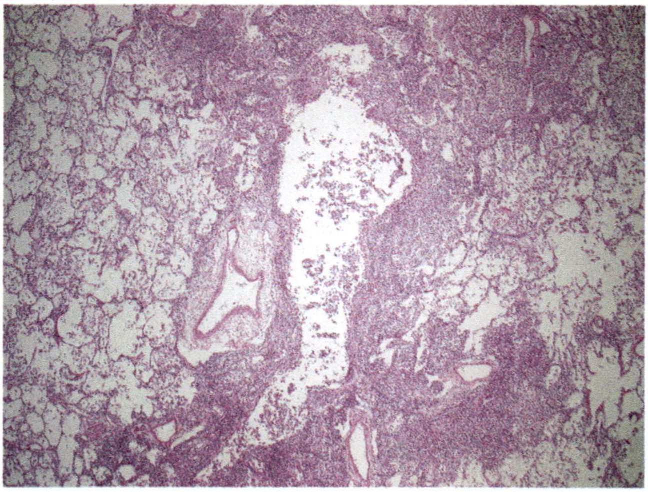

Fig. 2.19 In a typical bronchopneumonia pattern, smaller foci of inflammation are seen. Note that the inflammation is centered around the bronchioles and becomes less intense as the distance from the bronchioles increases. Common bacterial infections causing this pattern include *Staphylococcus aureus*, *Klebsiella pneumoniae*, *Haemophilus influenzae*, *Pseudomonas aeruginosa*, *Escherichia coli*, and anaerobic bacteria. H&E, 40× magnification

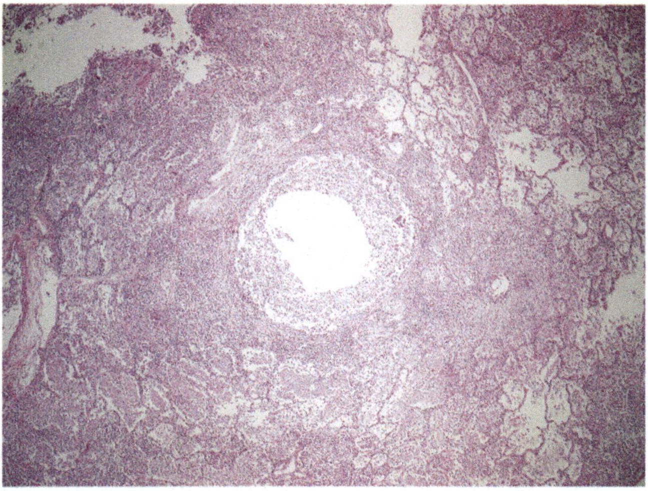

Fig. 2.20 An additional image demonstrating bronchopneumonia with a more intense neutrophilic infiltrate in a peribronchiolar pattern. H&E, 40× magnification

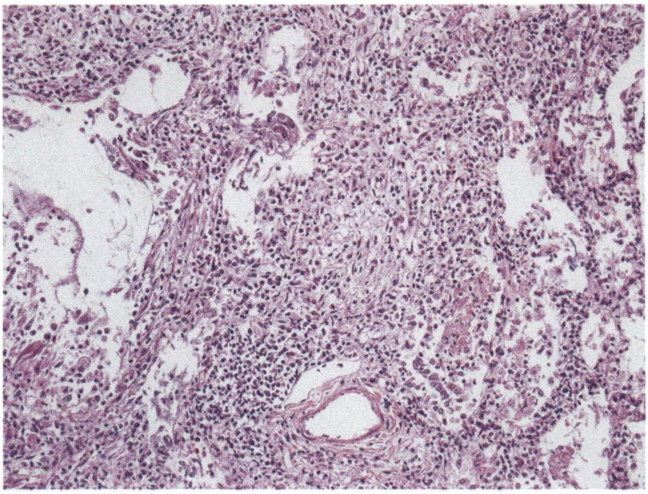

Fig. 2.21 Areas of organization may be present, particularly with longstanding disease. H&E, 200× magnification

2.3 Diphtheria

The causative agent of this disease is the Gram-positive bacillus, *Corynebacterium diptheriae*. While this disease is now rarely seen in the developed world as a result of widespread vaccination, diphtheria is still common in medically underserved

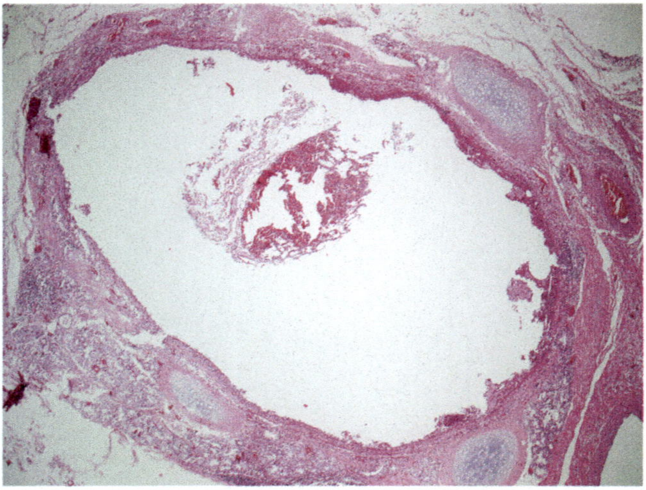

Fig. 2.22 Intrapulmonary bronchus circumferentially coated with a pseudomembrane associated with *C. diptheriae* infection. H&E, 40× magnification

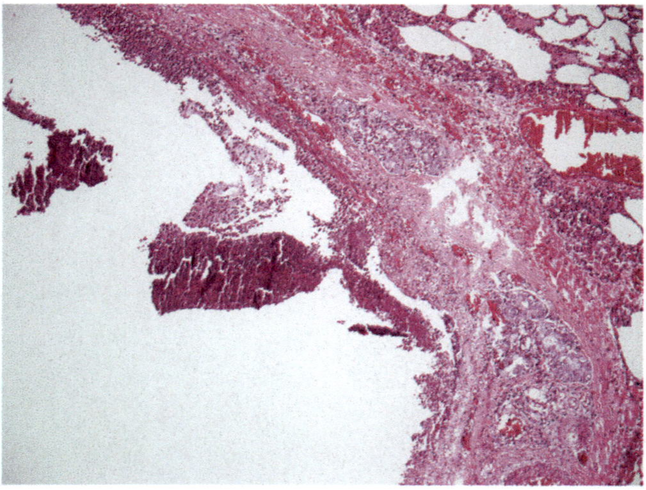

Fig. 2.23 Pseudomembrane associated with *C. diptheriae* infection consisting of fibrin, necrotic cells, and bacteria. Patchy acute inflammatory cells are also present. H&E, 200× magnification

regions. Other more commonly encountered upper respiratory illnesses, most notably streptococcal pharyngitis, may produce pseudomembranes mimicking those of diphtheria. As such, the disease remains an infrequent part of the differential diagnosis (Figs. 2.22, 2.23 and 2.24).

2.4 Bacterial Endocarditis (Figs. 2.25, 2.26, 2.27, 2.28, 2.29,2.30, 2.31 and 2.32)

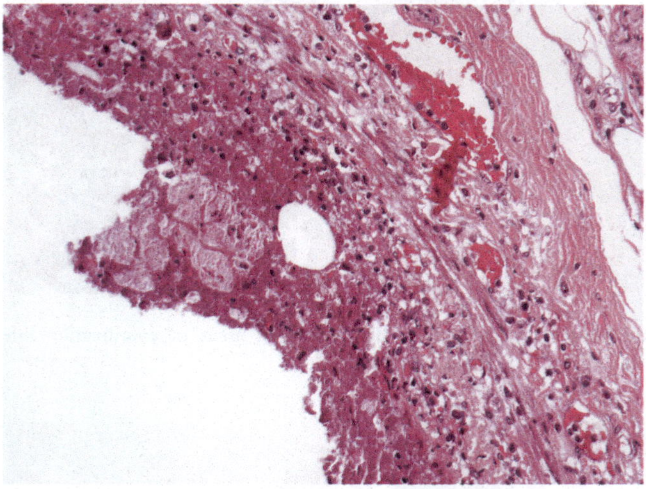

Fig. 2.24 Higher magnification demonstrating a pseudomembrane consisting of fibrin and acute inflammatory and necrotic cells. H&E 400× magnification

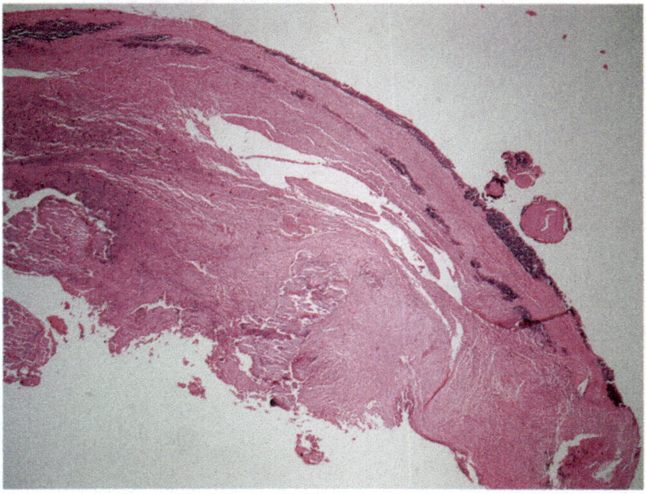

Fig. 2.25 Low-power view of a heart valve leaflet. Areas of necrosis are present, along with visible clusters of bacteria and calcification. H&E, 40× magnification

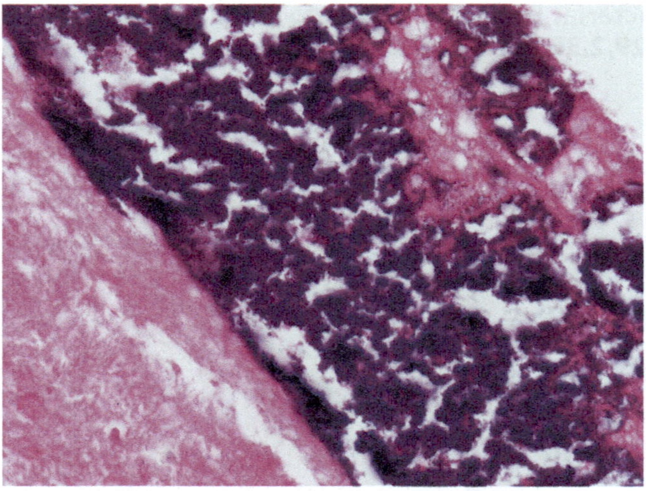

Fig. 2.26 Higher power magnification demonstrating areas of calcification intermixed with clumped bacteria. H&E, 1000× magnification

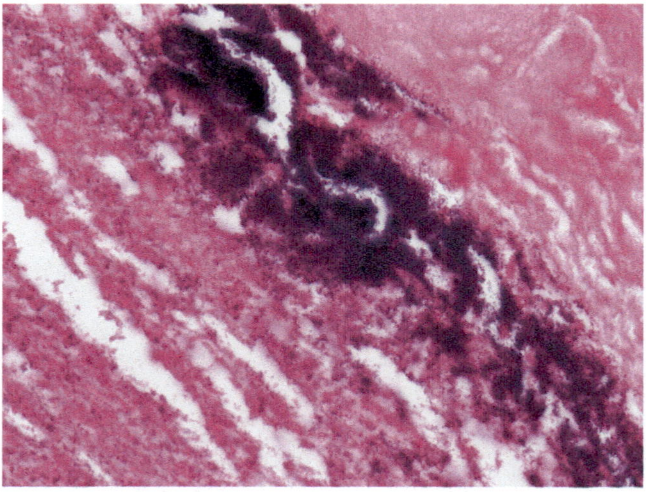

Fig. 2.27 Clumps of bacteria near the surface of the valve leaflet. While these forms are clearly suggestive of endocarditis caused by Gram-positive cocci, H&E staining does not differentiate bacteria by Gram reaction. H&E, 1000× magnification

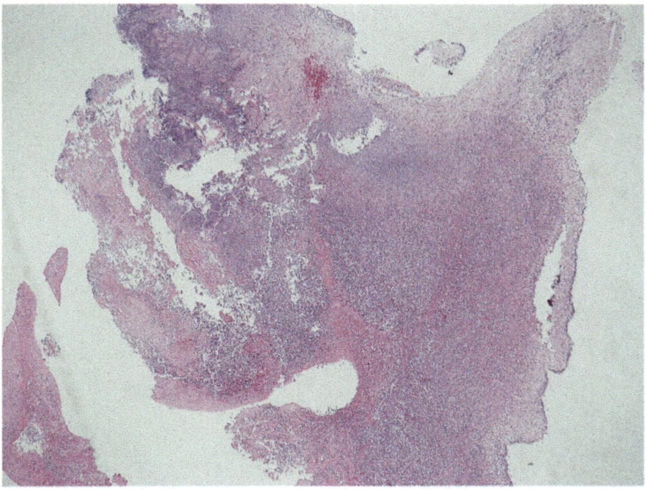

Fig. 2.28 Acute endocarditis in which *S. aureus* was later identified by culture. The image is a section through the vegetation demonstrating acute inflammation and clumps of bacteria. H&E, 40× magnification

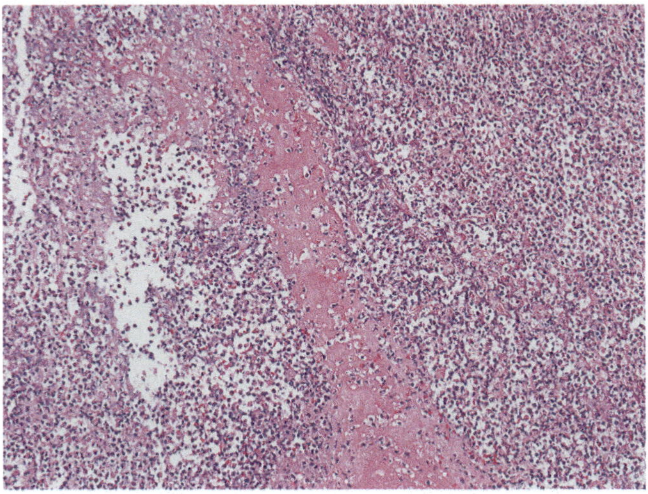

Fig. 2.29 Higher power magnification demonstrating diffuse predominantly acute inflammation and bands of fibrin-like material. H&E, 200× magnification

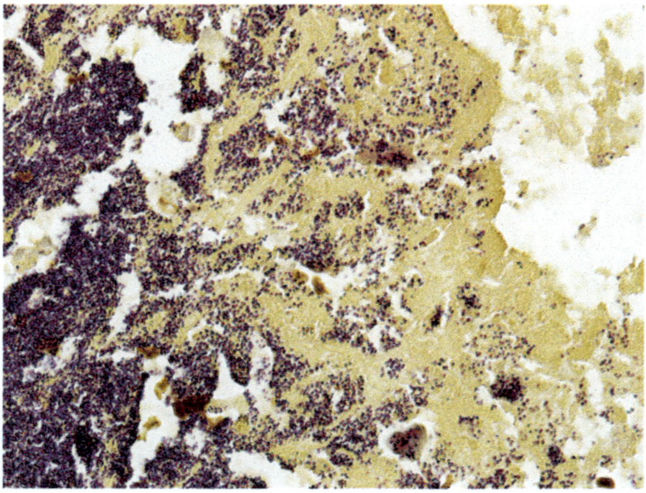

Fig. 2.30 Gram stain demonstrating clumped Gram-positive cocci consistent with *S. aureus*. Brown and Hopps, 1000× magnification

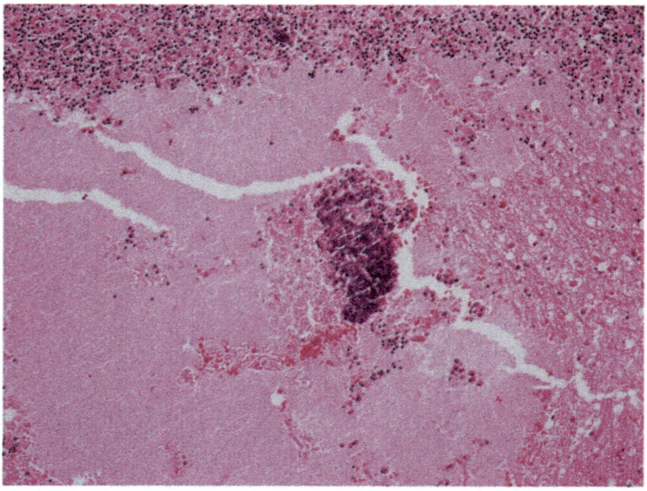

Fig. 2.31 One danger of bacterial endocarditis is that clumps of bacteria may break off and embolize throughout the body. This is of particular concern when bacteria embolize to the brain, as shown here. Note the clumps of purple staining bacteria with surrounding liquefactive necrosis. H&E, 200× magnification

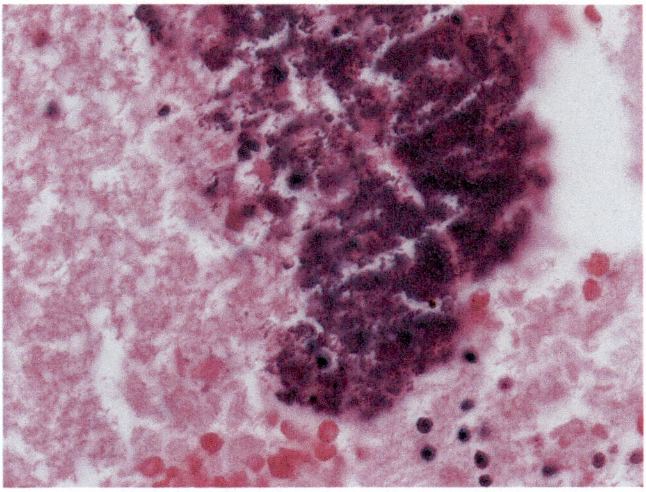

Fig. 2.32 Higher magnification of the embolized bacteria, again suggesting likely Gram-positive cocci. Cultures from this autopsy case later grew *Staphylococcus aureus*. H&E, 1000× magnification

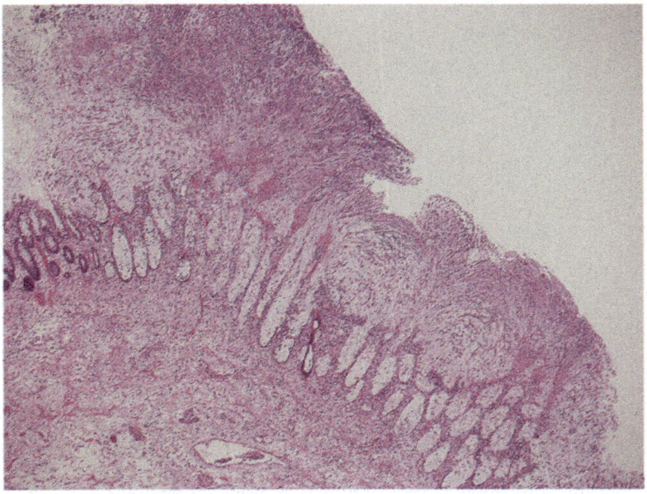

Fig. 2.33 Membranous colitis caused by *Clostridium difficile* infection. H&E, 40× magnification

2.5 Gastrointestinal Bacterial Infections (Figs. 2.33, 2.34, 2.35, 2.36, 2.37, 2.38, 2.39, 2.40, 2.41, 2.42, 2.43, 2.44, 2.45, 2.46 and 2.47)

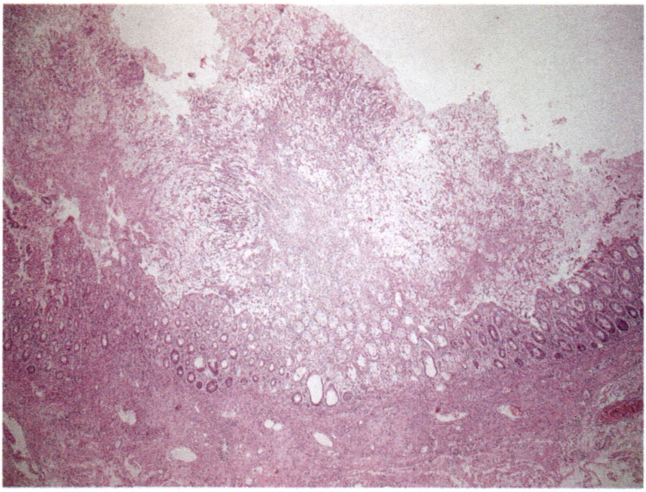

Fig. 2.34 Membranous colitis caused by *Clostridium difficile* infection. H&E, 40× magnification

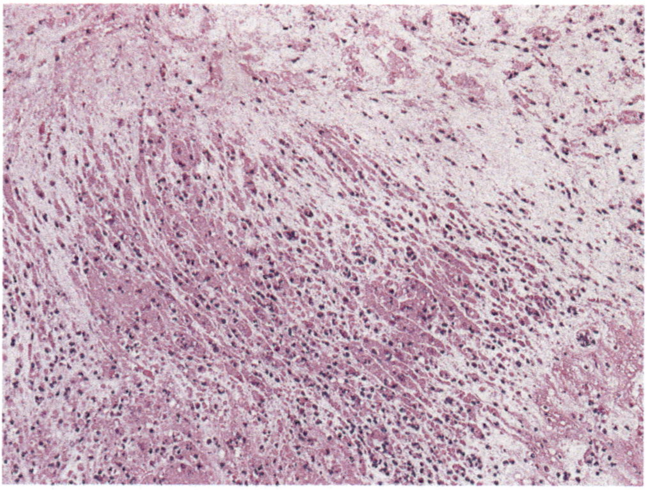

Fig. 2.35 Higher magnification demonstrating the pseudomembrane contents. H&E, 200× magnification

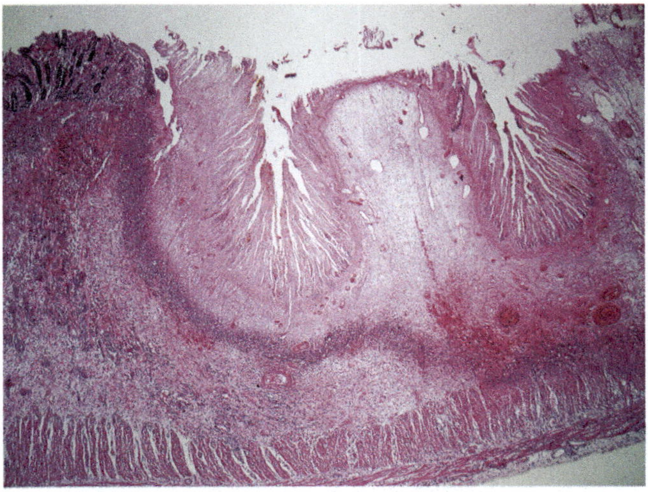

Fig. 2.36 Clostridial necrotizing enteritis (pig-bel) caused by *Clostridium perfringens* type C, producing beta toxin. Note areas of deep ulceration with a distinct band of neutrophilic infiltrate. Tissue on the left side of the image is relatively well preserved. H&E, 40× magnification

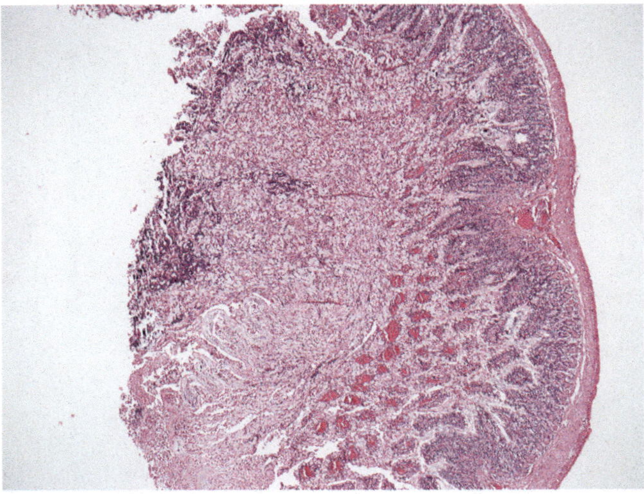

Fig. 2.37 Cases of necrotizing enteritis may demonstrate pseudomembrane formation similar to that seen in *C. difficile* infections. H&E, 40× magnification

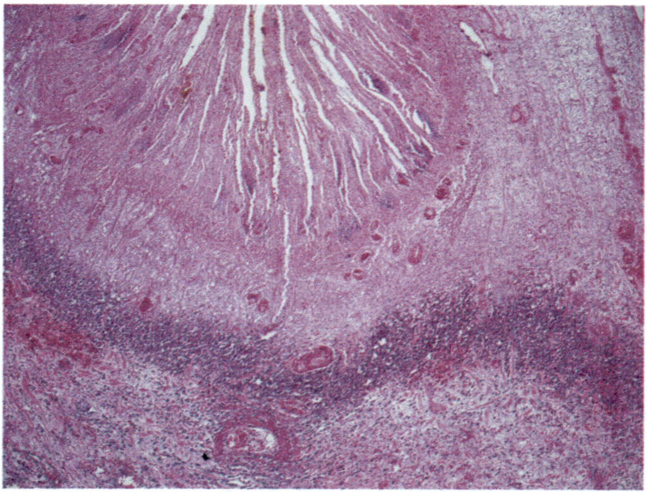

Fig. 2.38 Higher magnification image of the same area in Fig. 2.36 demonstrating thrombosis of blood vessels at the base of the lesion and a sharply demarcated neutrophilic infiltrate. H&E, 100× magnification

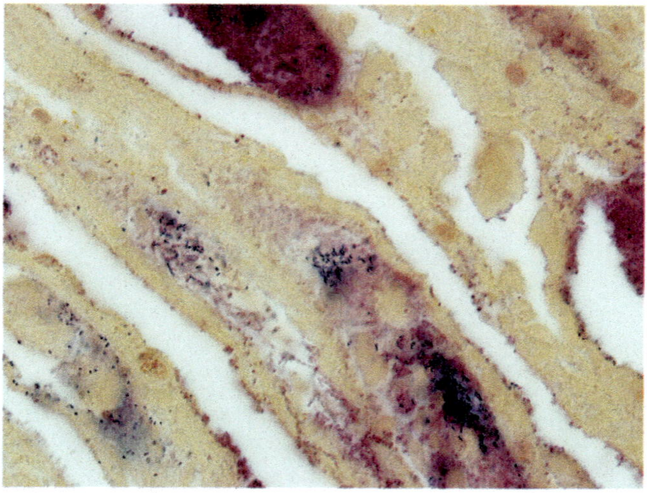

Fig. 2.39 Tissue Gram stain demonstrating bacteria of various Gram reactions and morphologies. While Gram-positive rods consistent with *Clostridium* species are prominent, it would be impossible to differentiate between pathogenic bacteria and intestinal microbiota using microscopy alone. Brown and Hopps, 1000× magnification

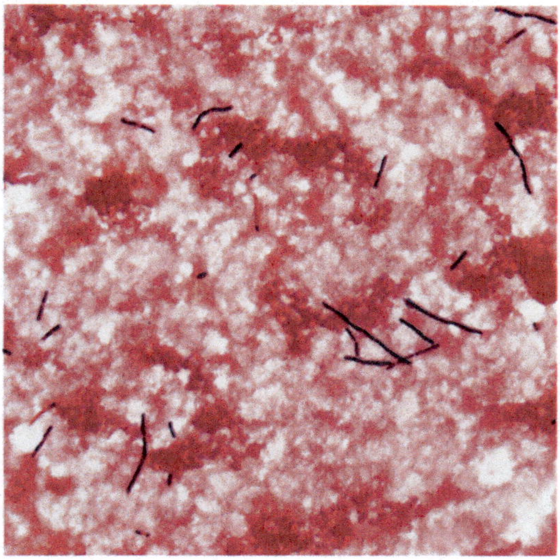

Fig. 2.40 Aspirate obtained from a brain abscess in an apparently healthy child. The aspirate contained Gram variable bacilli in a background of blood, necrotic debris, and predominantly acute inflammation. The organism was identified as *Clostridium septicum* and is included here owing to strong associations (along with *Streptococcus gallolyticus* subspecies *gallolyticus* (*S. bovis* biotype I) with gastrointestinal neoplasms. The child had been complaining of severe abdominal pain for several days prior to undergoing rapid mental status changes. Autopsy was declined by the parents, and no definitive gastrointestinal association was identified. Gram stain 1000× magnification

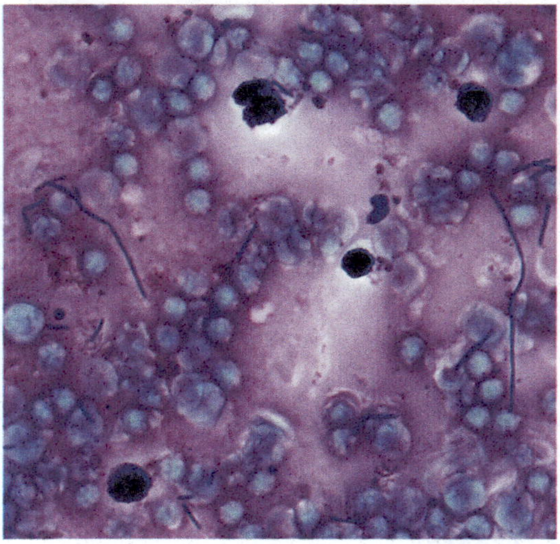

Fig. 2.41 Giemsa stained slide of the same case from Fig. 2.40. 1000× magnification

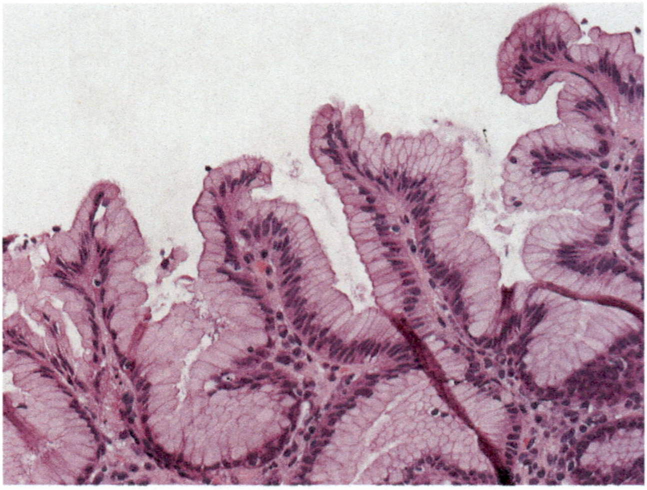

Fig. 2.42 *Helicobacter pylori* in the gastric antrum. Note the pale staining curved to spindle-shaped bacteria that appear at the luminal surface. Often minimal to no gastric atrophy is seen, and any associated inflammatory cells are chronic in nature. Focal areas of ulceration and a predominant neutrophilic infiltrate can be seen in active cases. H&E, 400× magnification

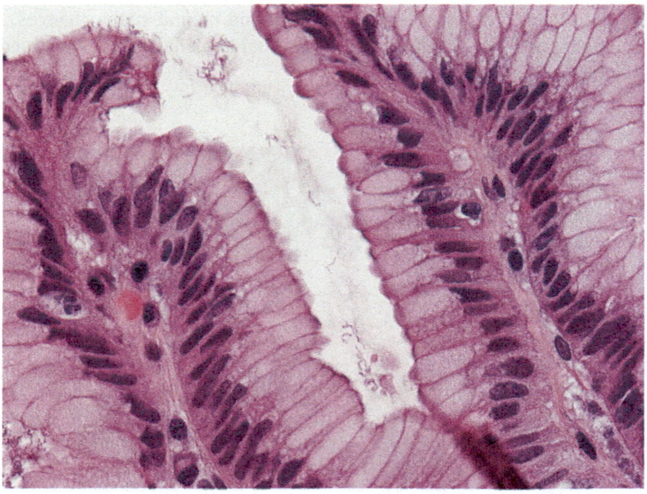

Fig. 2.43 Higher magnification better demonstrating the morphology of the bacteria. A related species, *Helicobacter heilmannii,* infrequently infects humans and will present as longer bacteria with a tight "corkscrew" appearance. 1000× magnification

2.5.1 Whipple Disease

Whipple disease is caused by infection with the bacterium *Tropherema whipplei*. It primarily causes a malabsorption syndrome in the small intestine, which is the usual route of identification, but the disease can also be systemic, causing arthritis,

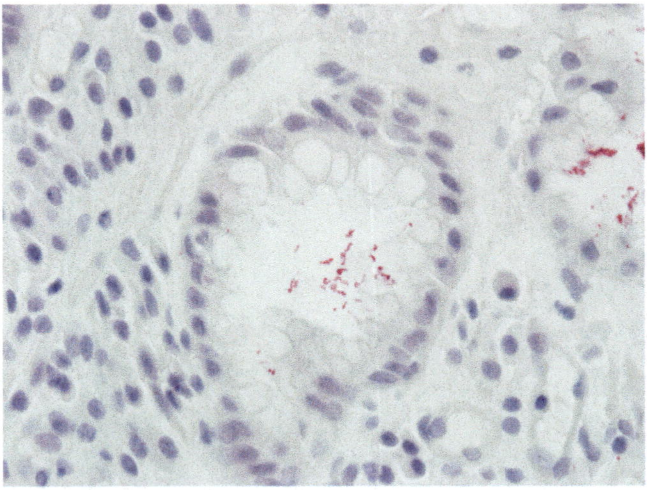

Fig. 2.44 Many laboratories offer immunohistochemical staining for *H. pylori*, which may make identification of the organism, particularly in light infections, an easier task. 1000× magnification

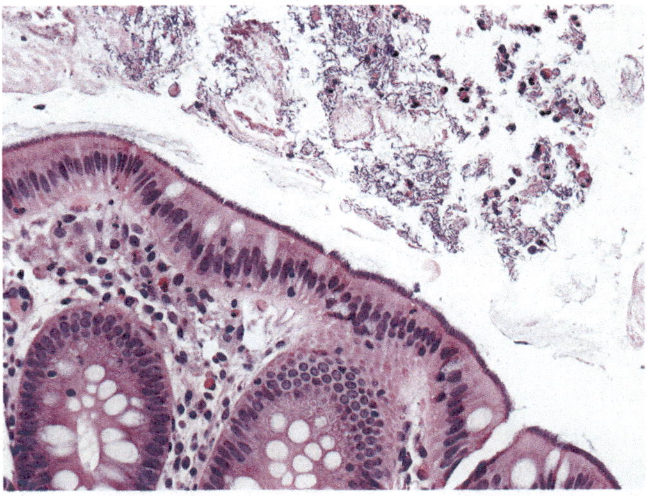

Fig. 2.45 Intestinal spirochetosis demonstrated in a biopsy taken from the ascending colon. This entity appears as a hair or brush-like fringed basophilic collection of spirochetes projecting from the luminal border, typically in the colonic mucosa. The organisms can sometimes only be focally present. Inflammation is usually absent or mild, with no associated endoscopic changes. Therefore these findings are often incidental, and association with gastrointestinal symptoms is controversial. H&E, 400× magnification

diarrhea, weight loss, skin hyperpigmentation, and uveitis. As a member of the Actinomycetes, this organism is considered Gram-positive but may stain poorly, Gram-negative, or not at all under laboratory conditions. The organism is also very difficult and laborious to grow. Polymerase chain reaction methods have been

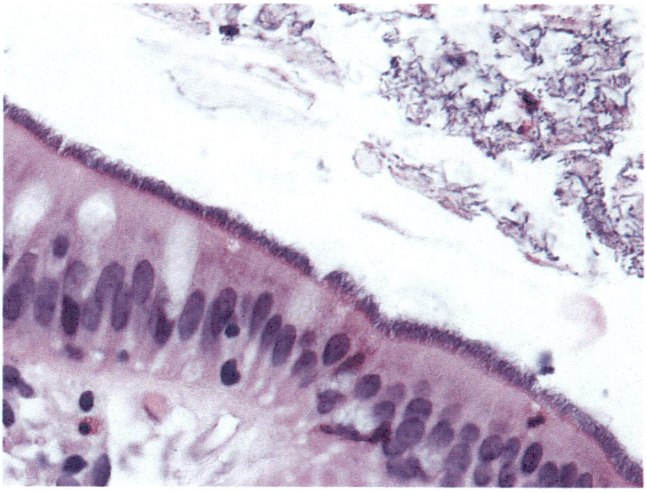

Fig. 2.46 Higher magnification demonstrating the organisms more clearly. Note the uniform, upright appearance of the spirochetes, somewhat resembling cilia. The spirochetes do not invade and are usually associated with no or mild inflammation. H&E, 1000× magnification

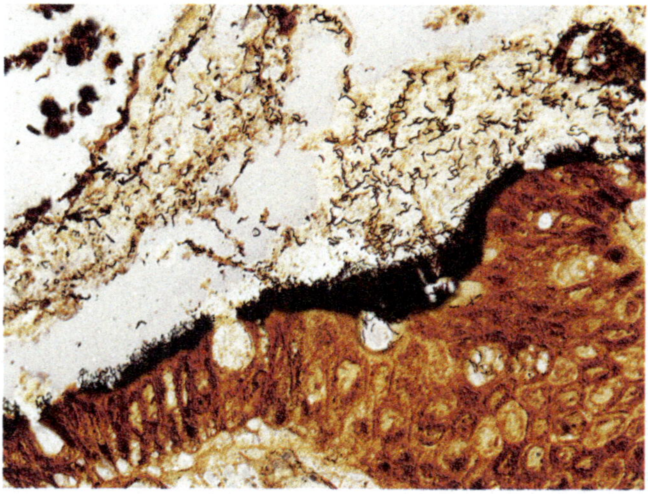

Fig. 2.47 A Warthin-Starry stain may be used to highlight the spirochetes, usually resulting in a dense black border. Note that some of the spirochetes may break off during histologic preparation and artifactually appear to have invaded the tissue. 1000× magnification

relatively recently developed to directly diagnose this infection from tissue. The disease is most often initially identified in the small intestine; however, it can be present throughout the body, including in bone marrow, lymph nodes, and the central nervous system as collections of pale, blue-gray to light pink staining foamy macrophages by hematoxylin and eosin (H&E). This appearance alone may invoke the presence of other entities such as infection with *Mycobacterium-avium* complex (MAC) or, depending on location, a glycogen storage disorder. The former, in particular can be ruled in or out with an acid-fast stain (MAC should be positive). An additional caveat in the identification of Whipple disease is that MAC is also positive with periodic acid Schiff (PAS) staining but retains its typical rod-like structure as opposed to the appearance of typical Whipple disease granules (*see* Fig. 2.51) (Figs. 2.48, 2.49, 2.50 and 2.51).

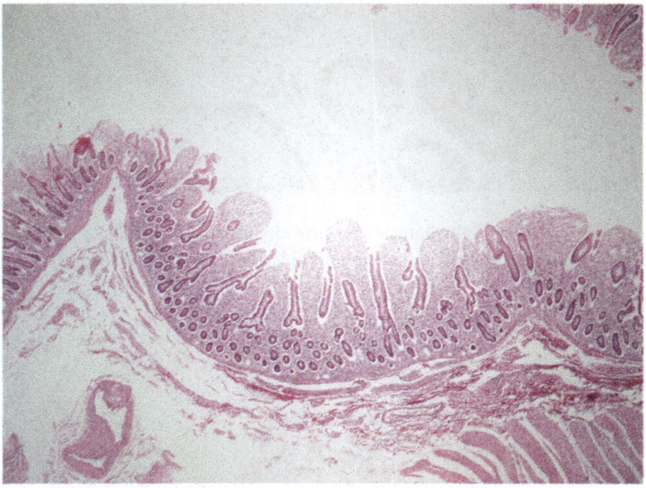

Fig. 2.48 Whipple disease of the small intestine. Note the diffuse infiltration of large foamy macrophages into the lamina propria with swollen appearing villi. H&E, 40× magnification

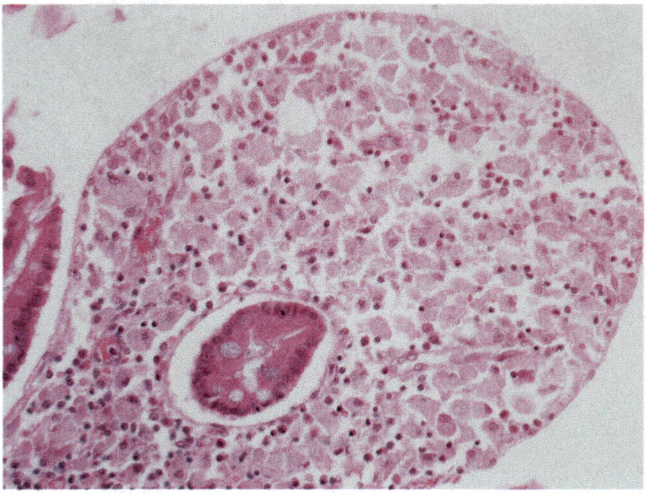

Fig. 2.49 Higher magnification image demonstrating diffuse infiltration by foamy macrophages into the lamina propria. H&E, 400× magnification

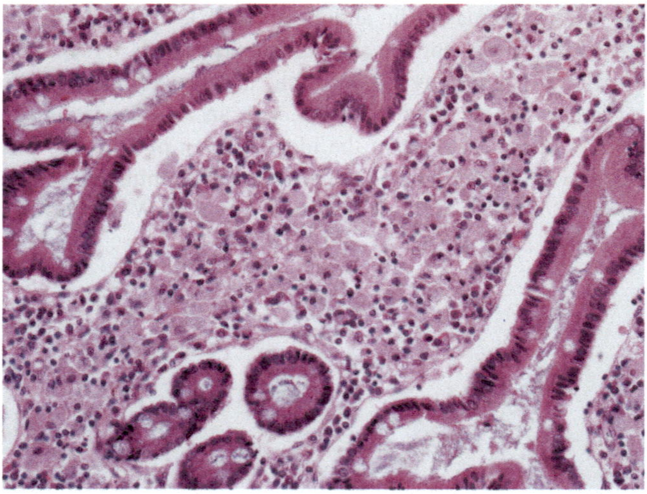

Fig. 2.50 A deeper portion of the lamina propria demonstrating diffuse infiltration by foamy macrophages. Scattered eosinophils are also seen. H&E, 400× magnification

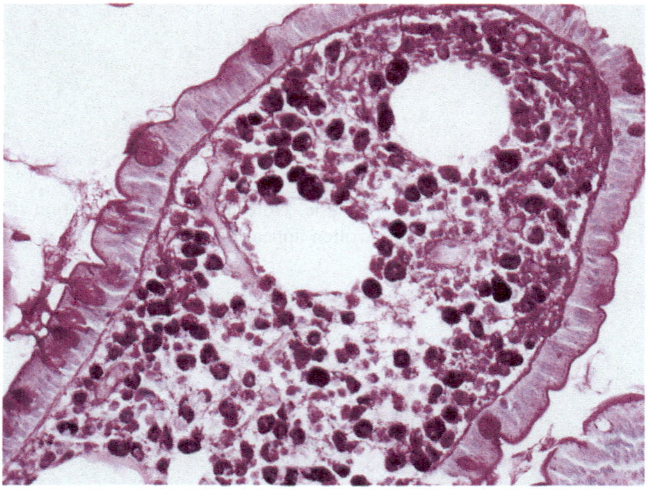

Fig. 2.51 PAS staining of macrophages within the lamina propria. They are characteristically filled with PAS-positive granular material. 400× magnification

2.6 Bacterial Infections of Skin and Soft Tissue

2.6.1 Bacillary Angiomatosis

Bacillary angiomatosis is associated with infection with the *Bartonella* species *B. henselae*, also the infectious agent of cat scratch disease (transmitted primarily by cat scratches or bites) as well as *B. quintana*, which is the causative agent of trench fever (transmitted by the human body louse). This entity is characterized by a proliferation of blood vessels often presenting as a tumor-like mass, primarily in the skin, but other organs may be affected as well (Figs. 2.52, 2.53, 2.54 and 2.55).

2.6.2 Rhinoscleroma

Rhinoscleroma is a chronic inflammatory condition of the nose and nasopharynx caused by the bacterium *Klebsiella rhinoscleromatis*. The disease is rare but is found worldwide. Patients typically present with a slow growing mass resulting in increasing nasal obstruction over months and usually producing a tumor-like nodule that protrudes from the nostrils (Figs. 2.56, 2.57, 2.58 and 2.59).

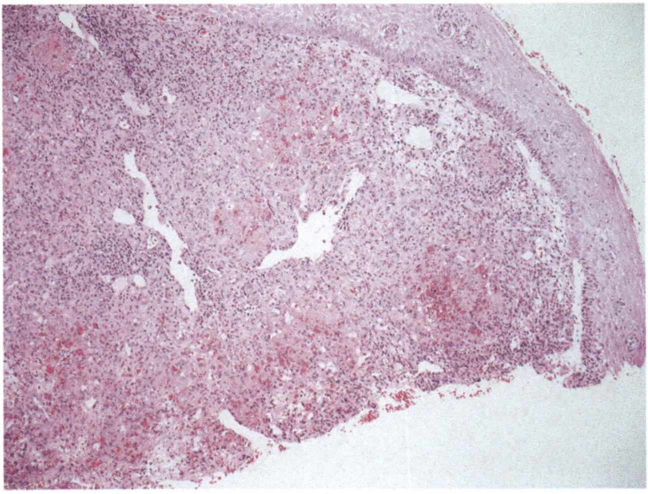

Fig. 2.52 Bacillary angiomatosis presenting in the vaginal wall. The histologic appearance is marked by the proliferation of small, irregularly shaped blood vessels, lined by variably atypical endothelial cells. This is often accompanied by a patchy neutrophilic infiltrate. Abundant extravasated or intravascular red blood cells may be present. The appearance may mimic Kaposis's sarcoma. H&E, 100× magnification

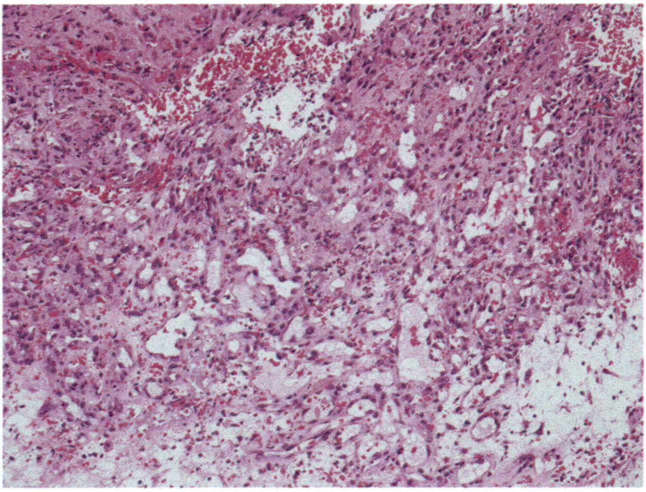

Fig. 2.53 A higher magnification image demonstrating irregularly shaped blood vessels with extravasated erythrocytes and patchy neutrophilic inflammation. H&E, 200× magnification

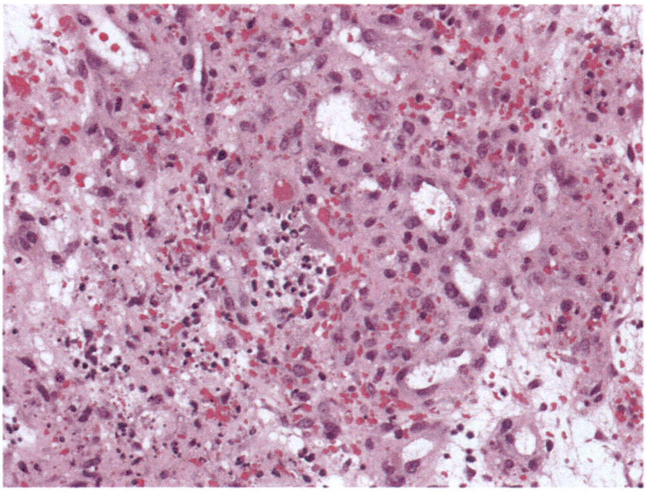

Fig. 2.54 Lesions of bacillary angiomatosis often demonstrate clusters of amorphous, eosinophilic, or amphophilic granular material as seen in the center of the image. H&E, 400× magnification

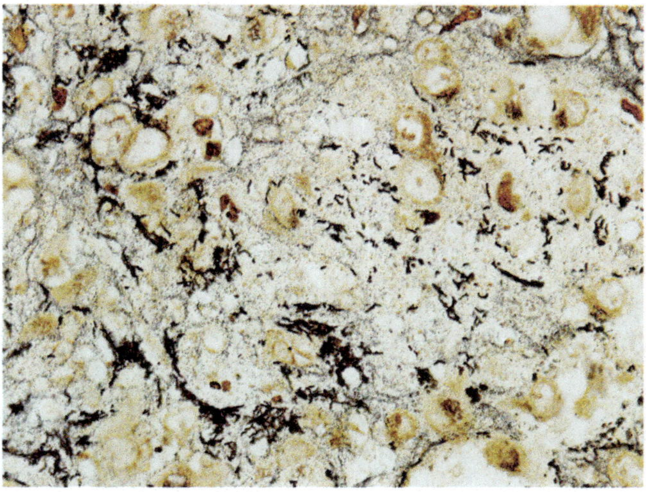

Fig. 2.55 Warthin-Starry stain demonstrating numerous darkly staining bacilli within the stroma of a cutaneous lesion of bacillary angiomatosis. 1000× magnification

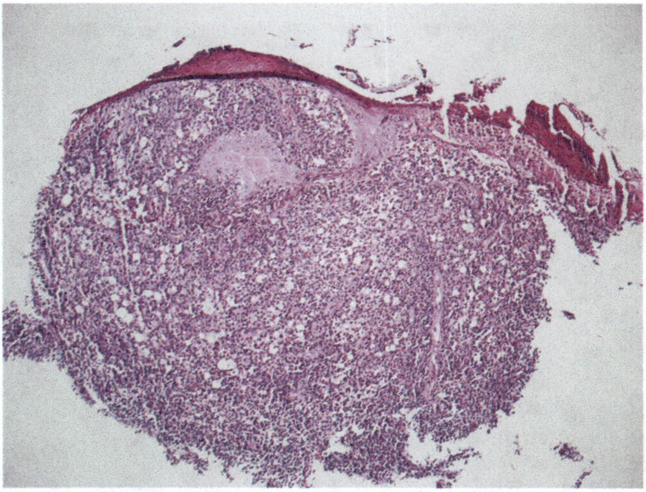

Fig. 2.56 These images were taken from a biopsy of a nasal mass in a patient with rhinoscleroma. Superficial crusting is seen as well as a dense, diffuse, subcutaneous infiltrate of mixed inflammatory cells and prominent clear-appearing histiocytes (Mikulicz cells). H&E, 100× magnification

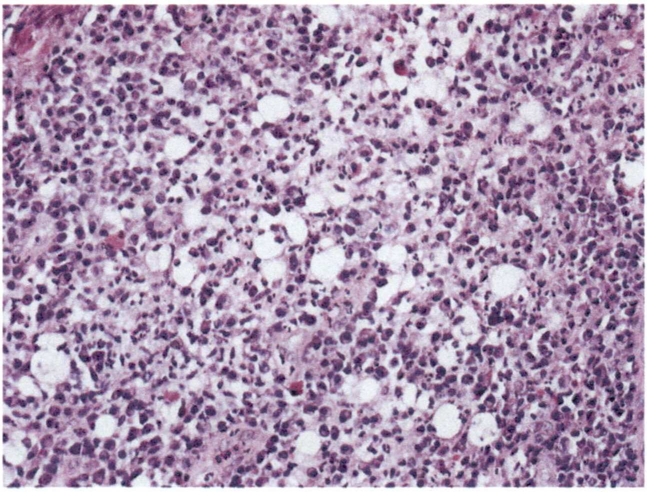

Fig. 2.57 A higher magnification image demonstrates that the inflammatory infiltrate consists predominantly of plasma cells, with the remainder made up of large clear histiocytes, lymphocytes, and neutrophils. H&E, 400× magnification

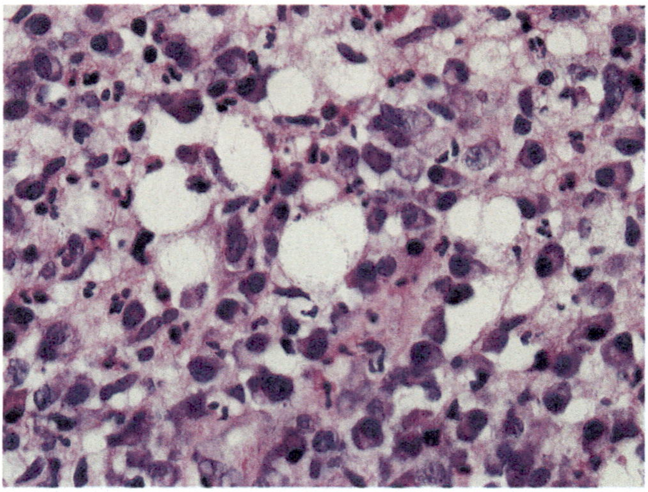

Fig. 2.58 Examination of the Mikulicz cells at higher magnification reveals that they contain numerous rod-shaped bacteria, consistent with the causative agent of this disease, *Klebsiella rhinoscleromatis*. While illustrated well by H&E in this example, other stains, including Giemsa, Warthin-Starry, and PAS, may also be used to highlight this bacteria. H&E, 1000× magnification

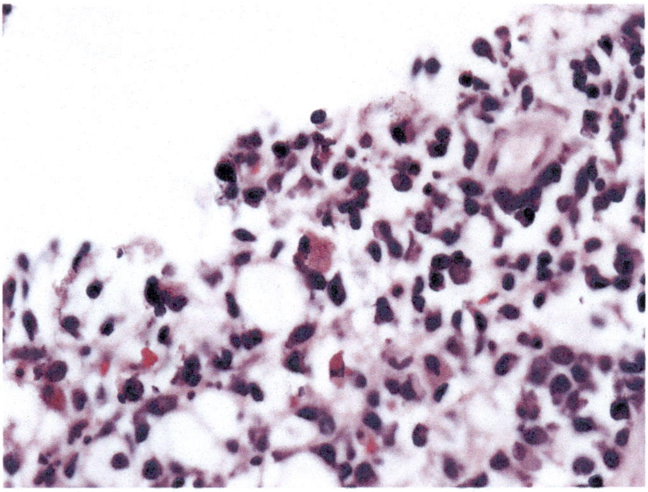

Fig. 2.59 Cases of rhinoscleroma may also exhibit scattered Russell bodies which are eosinophilic inclusions contained within plasma cells caused by excessive production of immunoglobulin. H&E, 1000× magnification

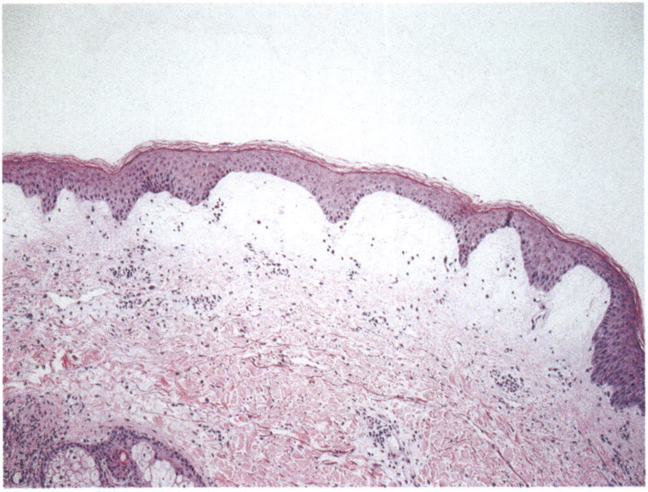

Fig. 2.60 This entity is caused primarily by infections with group A streptococci. Lesions characteristically demonstrate extensive subepidermal edema, with underlying acute inflammation. Vascular ectasia is also usually seen. The epidermal surface is typically uninvolved. H&E, 100× magnification

2.6.3 Erysipelas (Figs. 2.60 and 2.61)

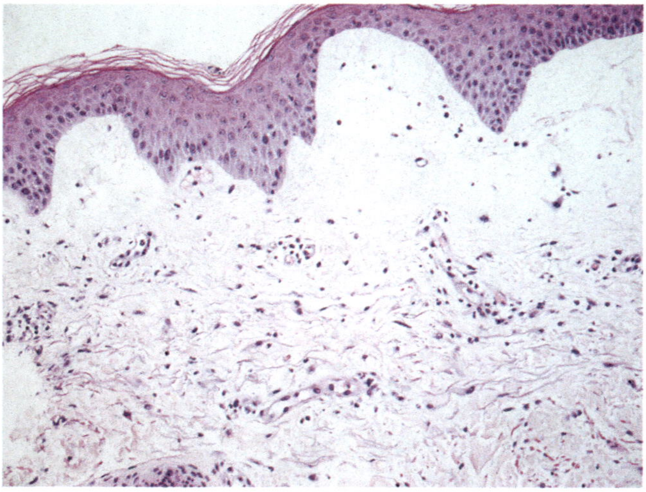

Fig. 2.61 Higher magnification. Note minimal inflammation in the epidermis, subepidermally located edema, and a patchy neutrophilic infiltrate. H&E, 200× magnification

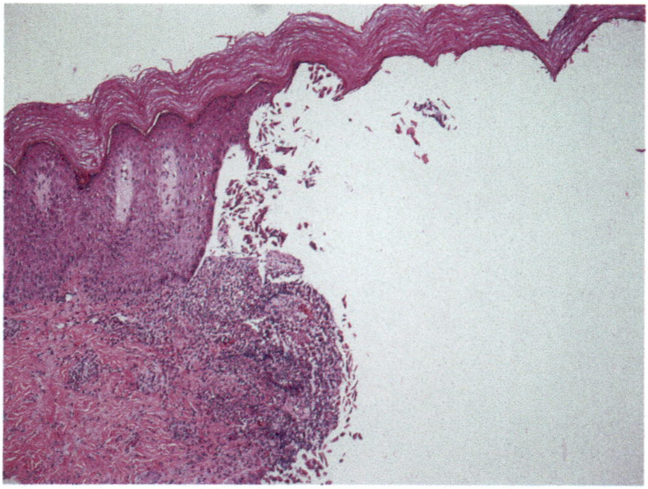

Fig. 2.62 An unroofed bulla in a case of bullous impetigo. Typically, subcorneal bullae are formed with underlying degenerated keratinocytes and few neutrophils. Acantholysis may be present. This entity typically occurs in newborns and young children and is caused by infection with *Staphylococcus aureus* secreting exfoliative toxins A and B. H&E, 200× magnification

2.6.4 Blistering Skin Disorders Caused by Bacterial Infections (Figs. 2.62, 2.63, 2.64 and 2.65)

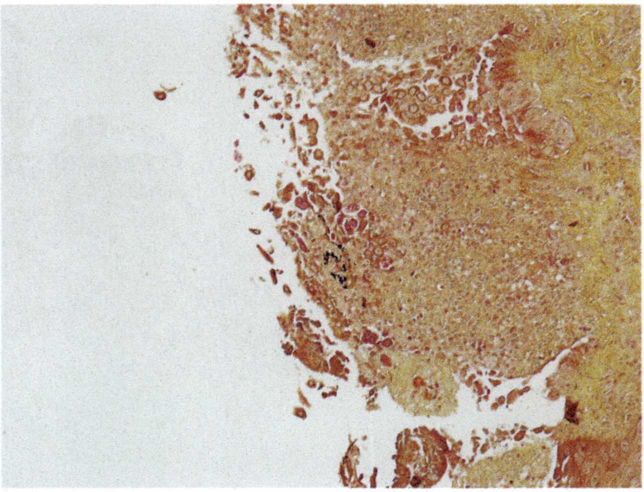

Fig. 2.63 Clusters of Gram-positive organisms may be visualized within the underlying degenerated keratinocytes. Brown and Hopps, 200× magnification

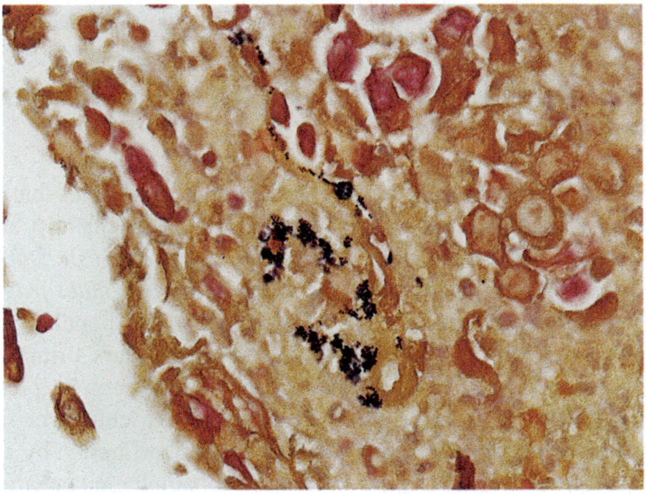

Fig. 2.64 On higher magnification, the bacteria are suggestive of Gram-positive cocci in clusters, consistent with *S. aureus*. Brown and Hopps, 1000× magnification

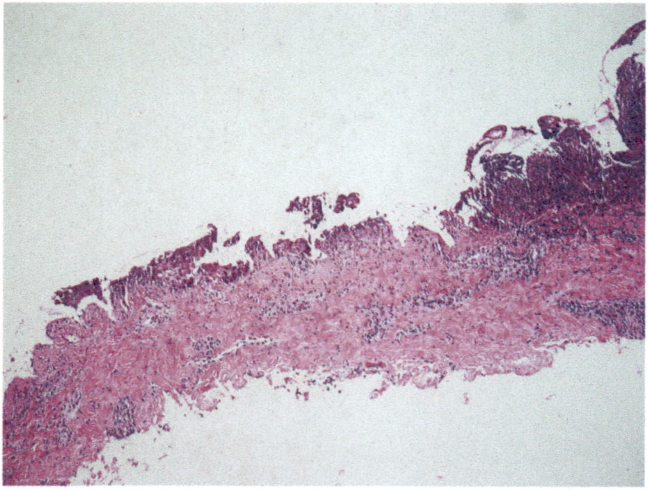

Fig. 2.65 Staphylococcal scalded skin syndrome (SSSS). In contrast to bullous impetigo, SSSS represents widespread and painful blistering of the skin. Like bullous impetigo, this entity is caused by the secretion of exfoliative toxins A and B by *Staphyloccous aureus* that target desmoglein 1. Some literature suggests that toxin B may be more definitively linked to the development of SSSS versus localized bullous impetigo. H&E, 100× magnification

2.6.5 Necrotizing Fasciitis and Clostridial Myonecrosis (Gas Gangrene)

Necrotizing fasciitis denotes infections of the subcutaneous tissues that may spread through fascial planes at a rapid rate. Although most frequently attributed to infection with group A streptococci (*Streptococcus pyogenes), Staphylococcus aureus, Vibrio vulnificus, Aeromonas hydrophila, and Bacteroides fragilis*, among others, are also known causes of necrotizing fasciitis. The popular name "flesh-eating bacteria" is a misnomer as tissue destruction occurs primarily through secretion of toxins. As such, the causative bacteria may not be present within sampled tissue and may not be readily identified through culture or tissue Gram stain. Gas gangrene (clostridial myonecrosis), caused primarily by *Clostridium perfringens* and other clostridial bacteria has a histopathologic appearance similar to that of necrotizing fasciitis; however, prominent and well-circumscribed gas bubbles are seen within skeletal muscle and surrounding soft tissues (Figs. 2.66, 2.67, 2.68, 2.69, 2.70, 2.71, 2.72 and 2.73).

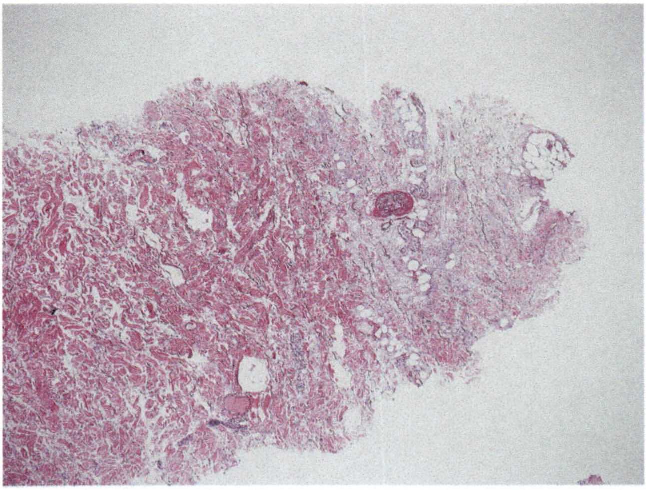

Fig. 2.66 Skin punch biopsy in a case of necrotizing fasciitis demonstrating necrosis of deep subcutaneous tissues. No apparent histopathologic change was noted in the epidermis and superficial dermal layers. H&E, 40× magnification

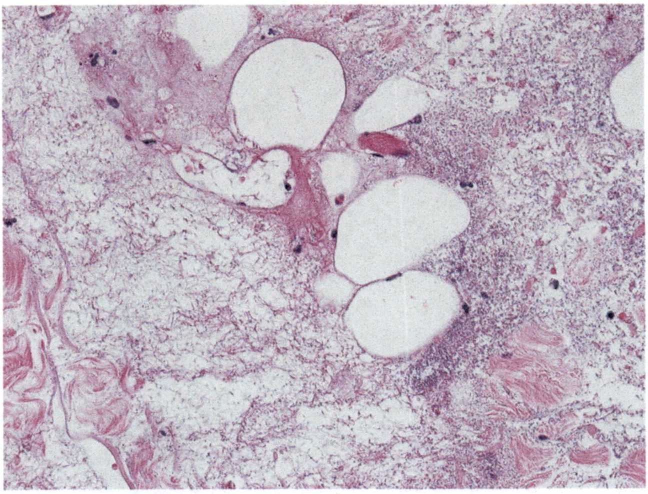

Fig. 2.67 Higher magnification demonstrating extensive destruction of subcutaneus tissue accompanied by relatively minor inflammation. H&E, 400× magnification

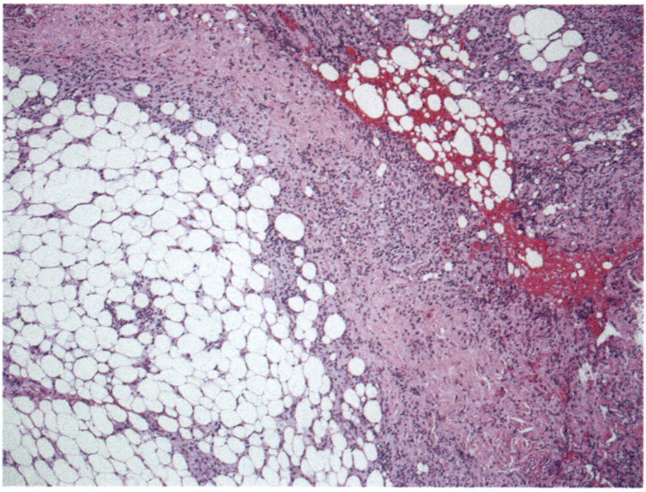

Fig. 2.68 Acute inflammation and necrosis within fibroconnective tissue and surrounding adipose tissue characteristic of necrotizing fasciitis. H&E, 100× magnification

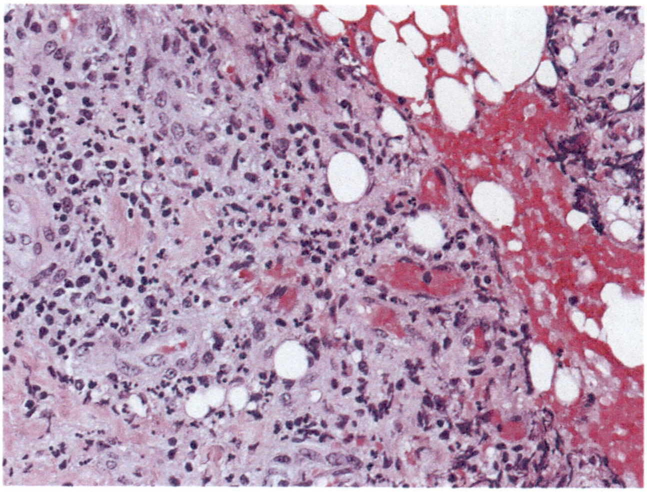

Fig. 2.69 Higher magnification demonstrating acute inflammation within fibroconnective tissue and surrounding adipose tissue. H&E, 400× magnification

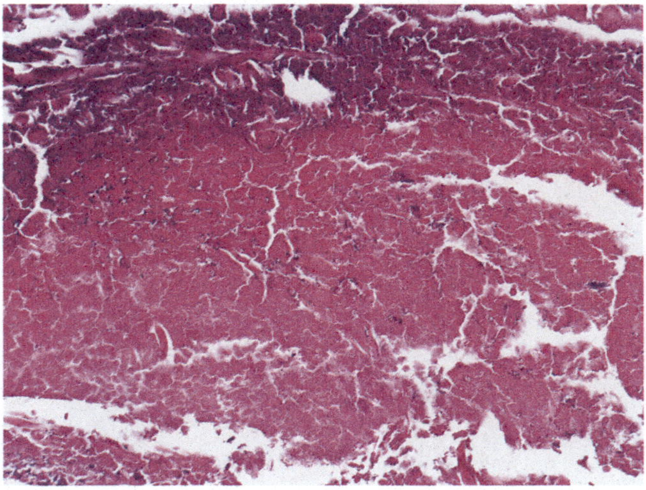

Fig. 2.70 Areas of complete necrosis may be seen, particularly in regions that have been affected by the disease process the longest. The hallmark inflammatory infiltrate may not be present. H&E, 400× magnification

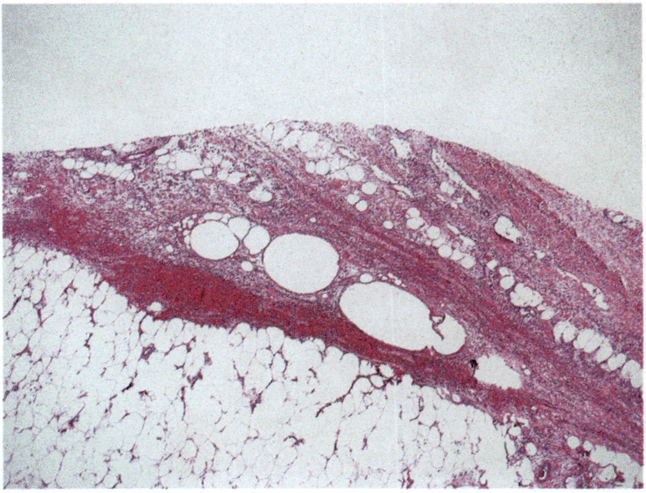

Fig. 2.71 Prominent gas bubble formation, hemorrhage, and acute inflammation in a case of clostridial myonecrosis of the arm. H&E, 40× magnification

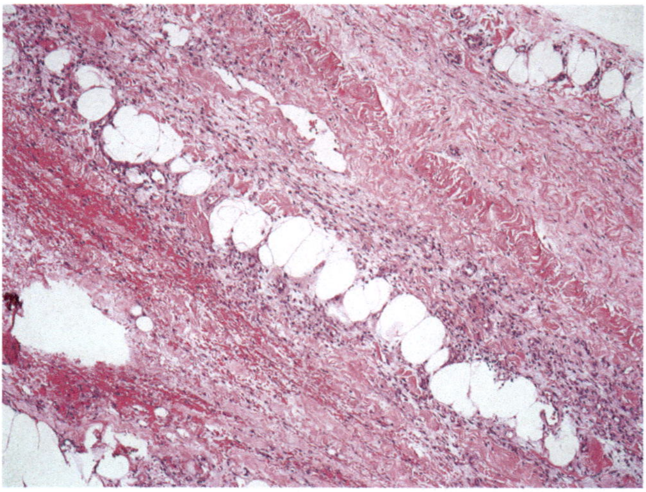

Fig. 2.72 Gas bubble formation in connective tissue associated with clostridial myonecrosis. The gas bubbles usually connect in a linear pattern, vary in size, and do not demonstrate the peripheral nuclei present in adipocytes. H&E, 100× magnification

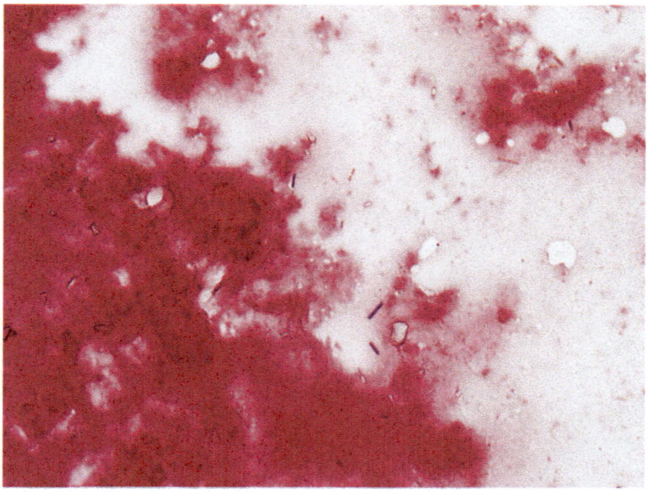

Fig. 2.73 Fine-needle aspirate of a lesion suspected of clostridial myonecrosis. Gram staining demonstrates variably Gram-positive large rods consistent with *Clostridum* species. Cultures later grew *Clostridium perfringens*. Gram stain, 1000× magnification

2.7 Syphilis

Syphilis, caused by *Treponema pallidum,* is known as the "great mimicker" in that it has myriad clinical presentations as well as multiple histopathologic appearances. The clinical history is very important for proper diagnosis and clinical staging. Common presentations are shown here (Figs. 2.74, 2.75, 2.76, 2.77, 2.78, 2.79, 2.80, 2.81 and 2.82).

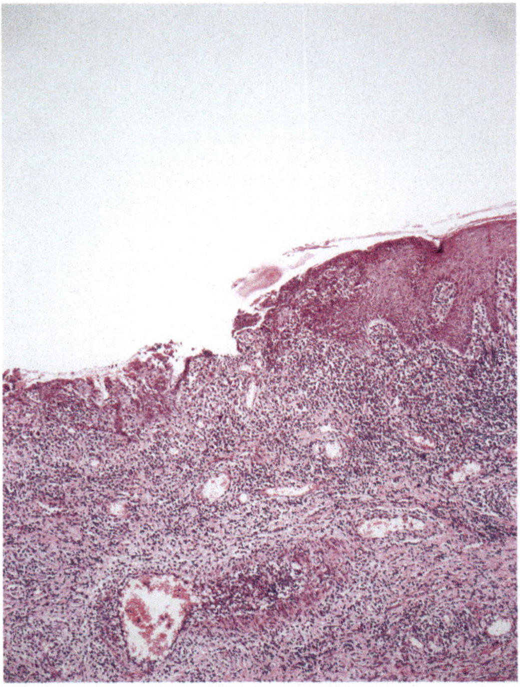

Fig. 2.74 A syphilis chancre, which is the hallmark lesion of primary syphilis. These lesions present as non-painful ulcerations (helping to distinguish them from chancroid caused by *Haemophilus ducreyi*). Underlying the acute inflammation within the ulcer bed is a dense lymphocytic and plasma cell infiltrate. H&E, 100× magnification

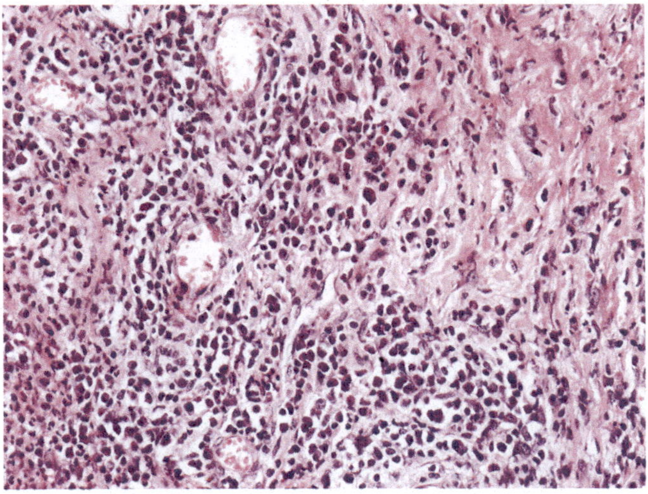

Fig. 2.75 Higher magnification of the area directly under the ulceration. Note a dense infiltrate of lymphocytes and plasma cells. This infiltrate will extend under the epidermis to nonulcerated areas. H&E, 400× magnification

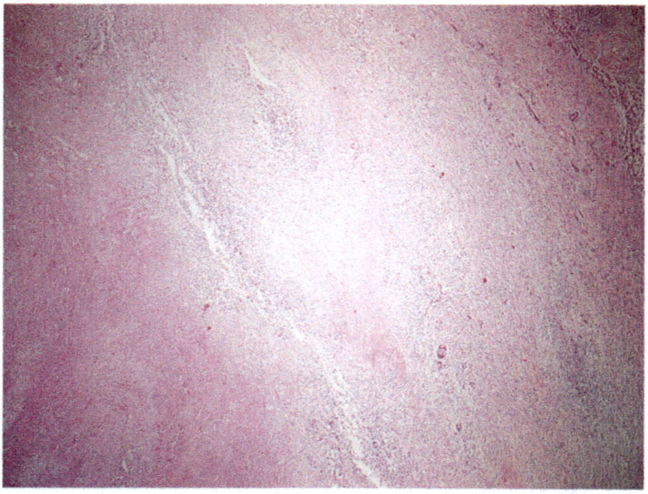

Fig. 2.76 Gumma formation in the liver. This form of the disease is seen in tertiary syphilis, most commonly manifesting in the liver, heart, and brain, although nearly any organ may be affected. Gummas microscopically appear as granulomatous inflammation with a variety of different appearances, depending on the stage. Eventually they undergo fibrous degeneration, which appears as a round scar or nodule. Here, areas of necrosis with surrounding fibrosis and giant cell formation are seen. Residual liver tissue is present to the *right side* of the image. H&E, 40× magnification

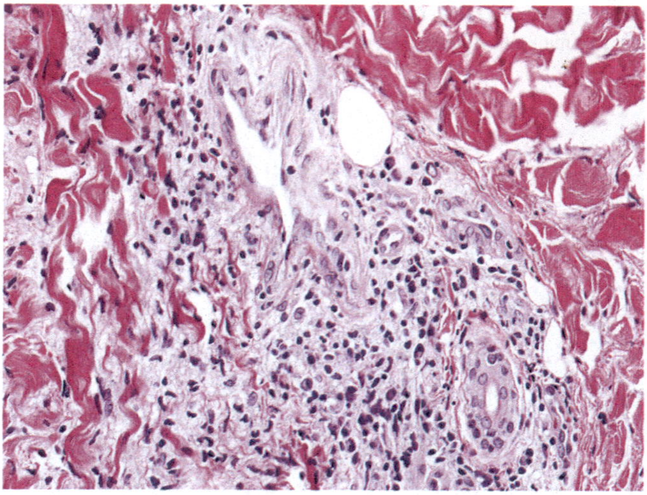

Fig. 2.77 Deep subcutaneous tissue from a skin punch biopsy obtained from a patient with secondary syphilis. Note the predominantly plasma cell perivascular infiltrate, a hallmark of *T. pallidum* infection. H&E, 400× magnification

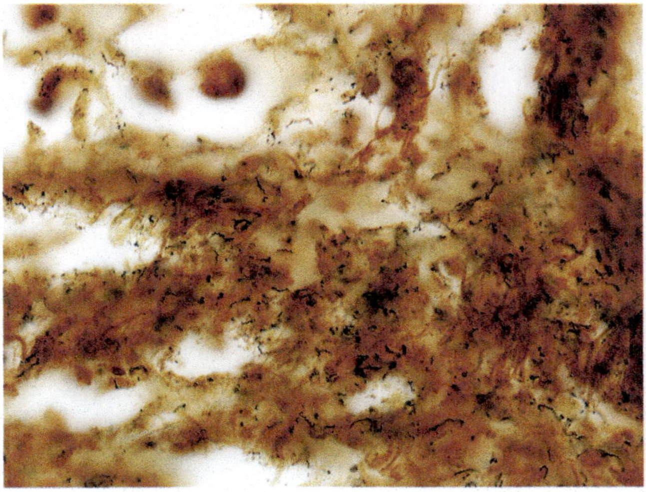

Fig. 2.78 High magnification of a skin punch biopsy demonstrating spiral-shaped organisms consistent with *T. pallidum*. Warthin-Starry stain, 1000× magnification

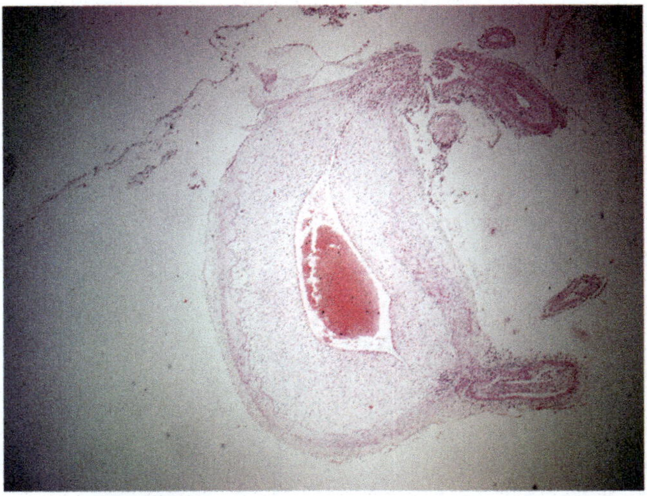

Fig. 2.79 Syphilitic arteritis. This late stage manifestation demonstrates marked intimal proliferation, with degeneration of the tunica media. These changes are most commonly seen in the aortic arch, ascending aorta, and pulmonary artery, although they can manifest throughout the circulatory system. Seen here is syphilitic arteritis of the posterior cerebral artery. H&E, 40× magnification

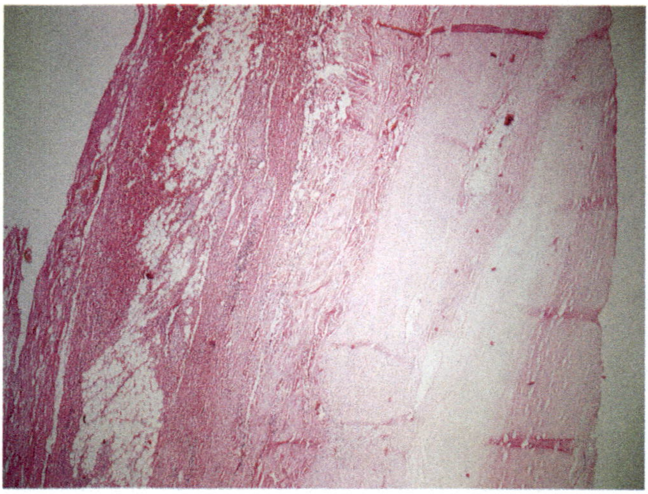

Fig. 2.80 Section through the aorta demonstrating marked thickening of the aortic wall in a case of syphilitic aortitis. The vessels feeding the aorta – the vasa vasorum – become markedly thickened, leading to ischemia of the outer aortic wall. This in turn leads to fibrous scarring of the media and loss of elastin fibers, which may progress to aneurysm formation. H&E, 40× magnification

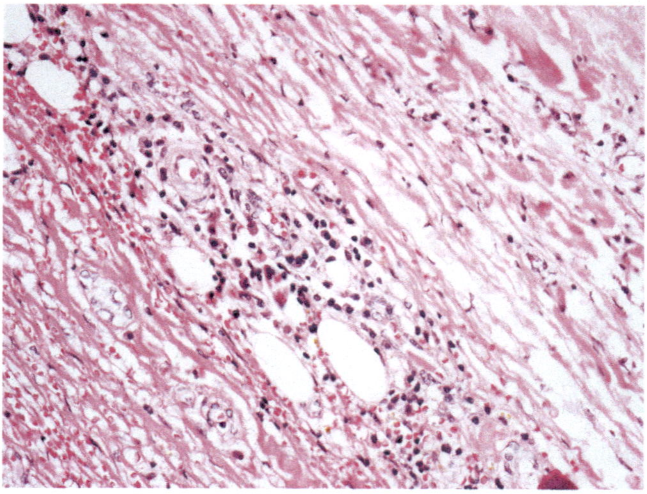

Fig. 2.81 At higher magnification, patchy infiltrates of lymphocytes and plasma cells are seen. This may be most prominent within the adventitia. H&E, 400× magnification

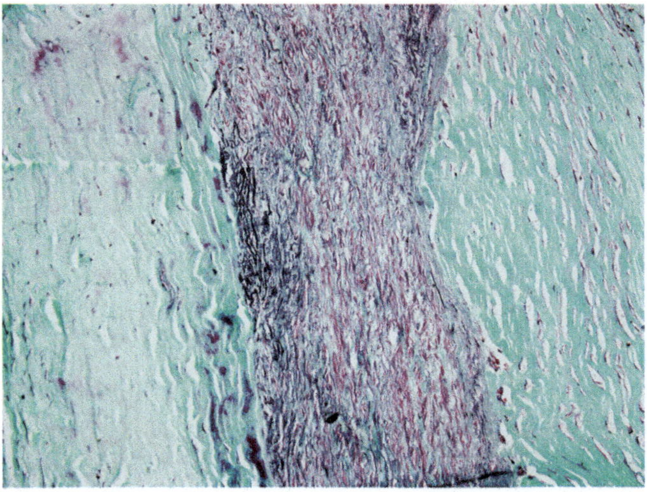

Fig. 2.82 Elastin stain demonstrating patchy loss of what is normally a delicate meshwork of elastin fibers. The loss of elastin fibers and concurrent ischemia and fibrosis of the adventitia and media can lead to aneurysm formation as well as a variety of other clinical complications. H&E, 200× magnification

2.8 Bacterial Lymphadenitis

Lymphadenitis has many bacterial causes. While most cases can be tied to local infections with the commonly encountered human pathogens *Staphylococcus* and *Streptococcus* species, infections with *Bartonella henselae* (cat scratch disease), *Chlamydia trachomatis* (lymphogranuloma venerum) and *Franciscella tularensis* (tularemia) frequently enter the differential diagnosis. Since these diseases all have distinct causes but similar appearances, access to proper patient history is paramount in formulating a differential diagnosis. Cat scratch disease, caused by infection with *Bartonella henselae,* typically manifests as painful regional lymphadenopathy that begins near an area of a cat scratch or cat bite, particularly from a kitten. The organism is difficult to grow in the laboratory and therefore a history of such exposures is helpful. Serologic testing may also provide a useful aid. Lymphogranuloma venerum is caused by the obligate intracellular bacteria *Chlamydia trachomatis* (serovars L1, L2, and L3). The organism is not easily identifiable on routine stains, and being an obligate intracellular organism it requires special procedures to culture that may not be available at a local laboratory service. In addition, cultures are only positive 30–40% of the time. The location of the lesions, generally in the inguinal area, and a history of possible exposure to *C. trachomatis* are helpful in the diagnosis. Tularemia is caused by *Francisella tularensis*. Transmission is associated with a wide variety of generally wilderness-associated vectors. Tick bites, deer fly bites, exposure to lagomorphs (rabbits and hares), and rodents as well as other mammals that hunt them (including felines) have all been

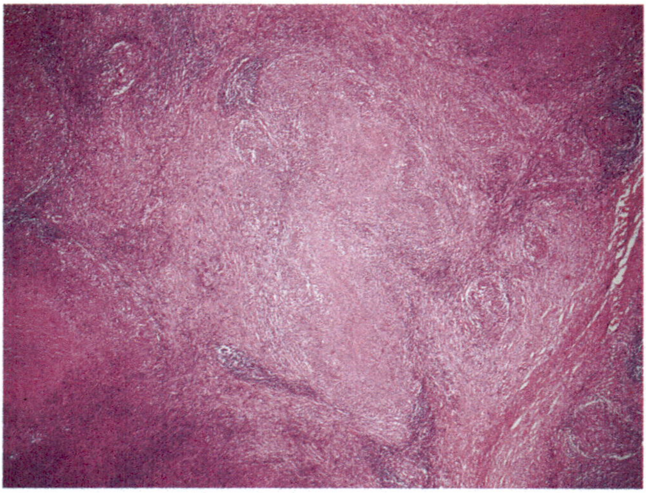

Fig. 2.83 Axillary lymph node from a case of cat scratch disease. Lymph nodes characteristically show necrotizing granulomas surrounded by palisading histiocytes. H&E, 40× magnification

linked to the transmission of tularemia. The most common form seen is ulceroglandular, which is explored here, but it is important to note that the disease may also have pneumonic, typhoidal, oculoglandular, and oropharyngeal forms. A glandular form exists as well that is similar to the ulceroglandular form but does not manifest overlying skin ulceration. Although sporadic cases are seen naturally, at various times in history *Francisella tularensis* has been used or experimented with as an agent of biological warfare. It is thought to be particularly useful for this purpose because the infection dose is very low; as few as ten organisms are required to establish infection via the aerosol route. Therefore if this organism is suspected by means of clinical history and/or histopathology, the microbiology laboratory must be notified so that proper precautions may be taken (Figs. 2.83, 2.84, 2.85, 2.86, 2.87, 2.88, 2.89, 2.90 and 2.91).

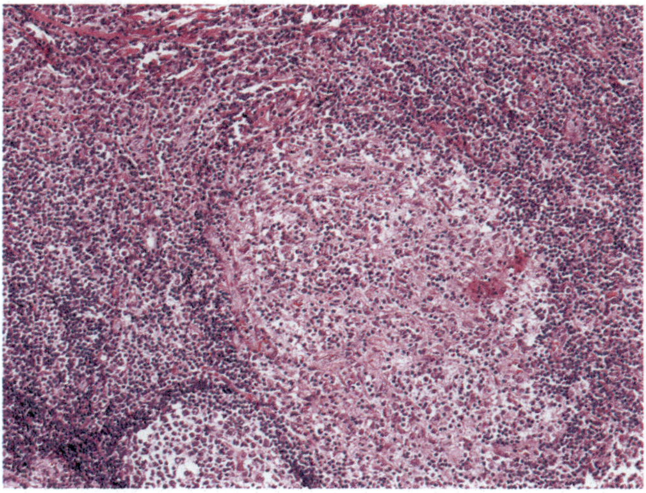

Fig. 2.84 Early lesions may demonstrate some neutrophilic infiltrate with surrounding histiocytes and follicular hyperplasia. H&E, 200× magnification

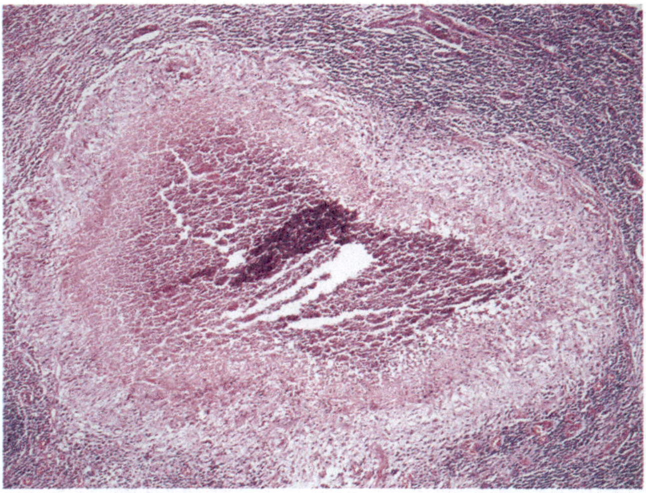

Fig. 2.85 Classically, "stellate" shaped abscesses are present within lymph nodes. Neutrophils are present within and around the necrotic areas surrounded by palisading histiocytes. H&E, 100× magnification

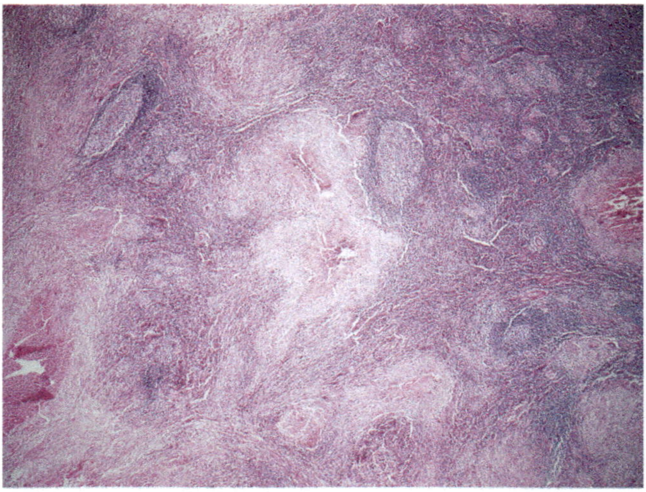

Fig. 2.86 Lymphogranuloma venerum. "Stellate" abscesses similar to those in cat scratch disease can be seen in the lymph nodes. Although they occur most frequently in the inguinal lymph nodes, regional lymph nodes in any area of sexual contact may demonstrate these changes. H&E, 40× magnification

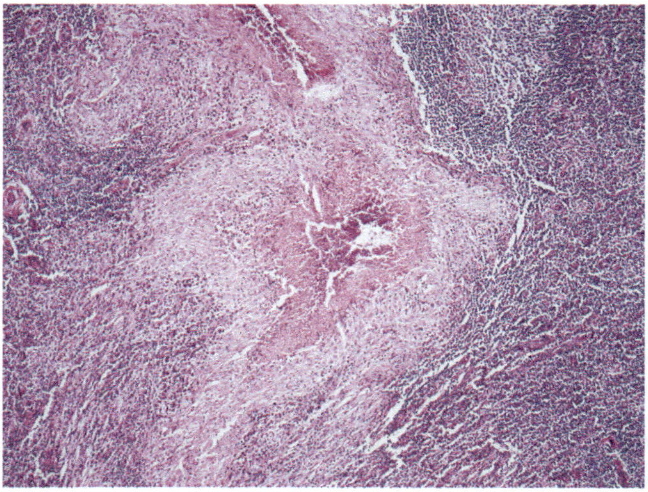

Fig. 2.87 Higher magnification demonstrating stellate abscesses with necrotic centers and surrounding neutrophilic infiltrate in an inguinal lymph node consistent with lymphogranuloma venerum. As lesions progress they continue to enlarge, effacing the lymph node architecture and losing their stellate outlines. H&E, 100× magnification

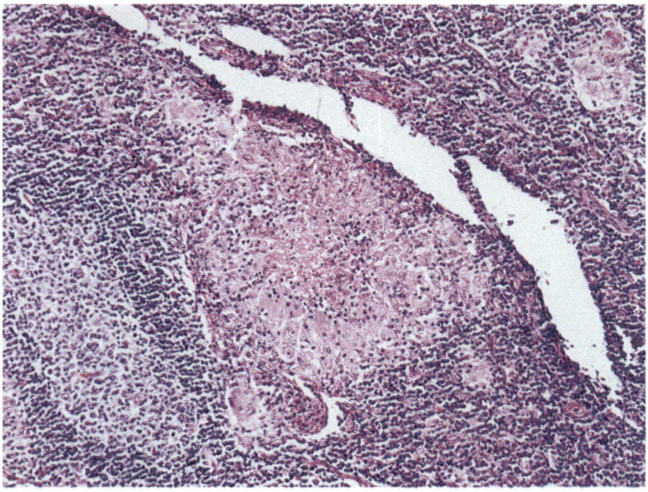

Fig. 2.88 Early development of a microabscess associated with lymphogranuloma venerum. Note the necrotic center with neutrophilic infiltrate and surrounding histiocytes. H&E, 200× magnification

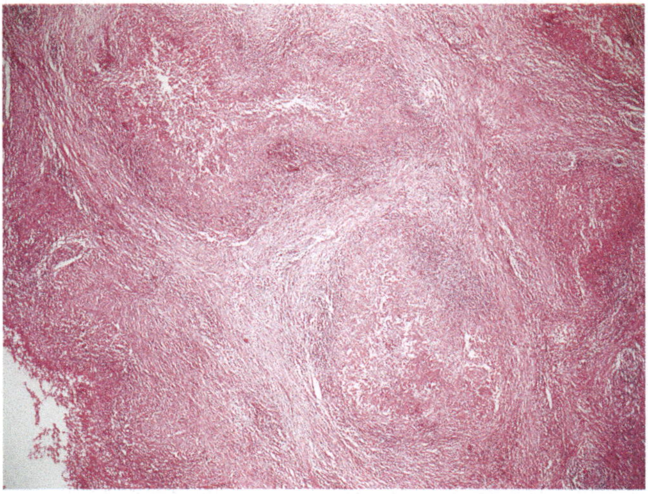

Fig. 2.89 Lymph node in ulceroglandular tularemia. Nodes demonstrate a progression of appearances beginning with mild reactive changes shortly after infection; this progresses to centralized necrosis with surrounding granulomatous inflammation. Stellate abscesses similar to those in cat scratch disease may also be seen and may complicate the differential diagnosis because this disease may also be transmitted by felines. Several necrotic foci with surrounding granulomatous inflammation are seen. H&E, 40× magnification

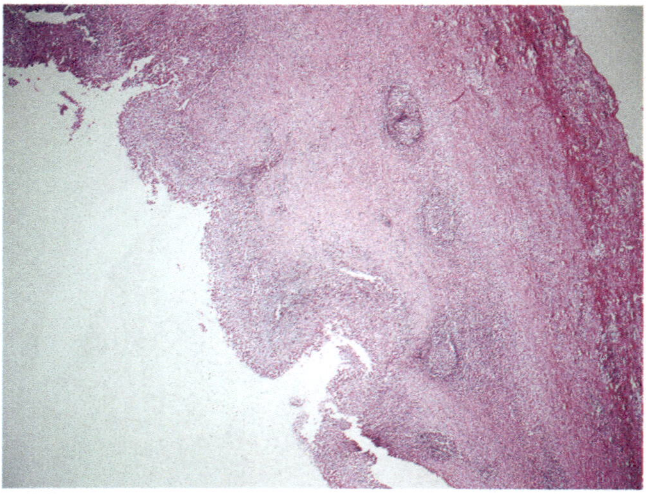

Fig. 2.90 Later stage glandular infection may show large areas of central necrosis. Note the loss of the central portion of the lymph node with residual lymphoid tissue remaining at the edges. H&E, 40× magnification

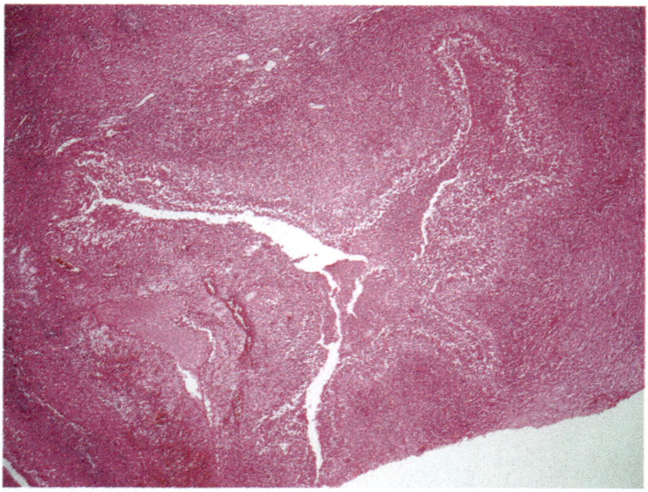

Fig. 2.91 Stellate-shaped abscesses similar to those classically seen in cat scratch disease may be identified. H&E, 40× magnification

2.9 Waterhouse-Friderichsen Syndrome

Waterhouse-Friderichsen syndrome is a fulminant bacterial infection characterized by severe sepsis leading to hemorrhagic adrenalitis and a cascade of effects, including adrenal insufficiency, systemic shock, disseminated intravascular coagulation, and multiple organ failure. While *Neisseria meningitidis* is the most frequently associated organism, other bacteria including *Pseudomonas, Streptococcus,* and *Staphylococcus* species have also been implicated. Characteristic findings of hemorrhagic adrenalitis are seen here (Figs. 2.92 and 2.93).

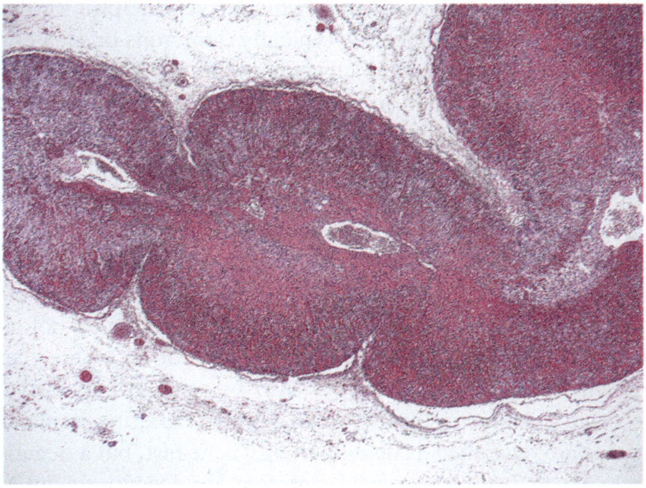

Fig. 2.92 Waterhouse-Friderichsen syndrome. Typical acute inflammation with prominent hemorrhage and necrosis throughout both the medulla and cortex of the adrenal gland. H&E, 40× magnification

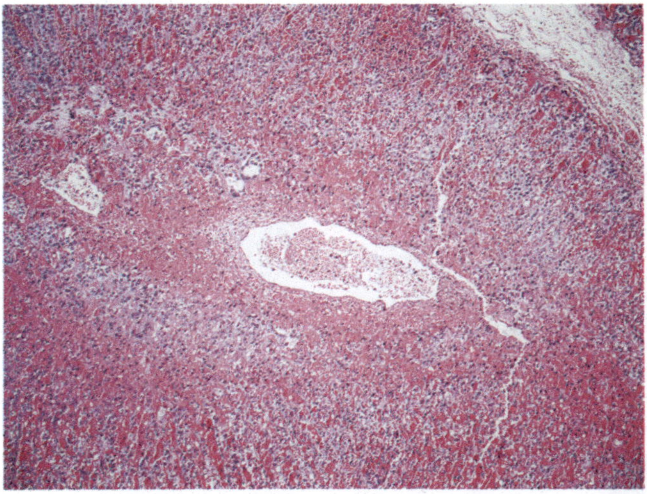

Fig. 2.93 Higher magnification demonstrating extensive hemorrhage throughout the adrenal gland, *centered* particularly around the adrenal vasculature. Acute inflammation is also present. These changes typically affect the entire gland, which is not usually seen in adrenal infarct or trauma. H&E, 100× magnification

2.10 Actinomycosis

Actinomycosis is a relatively rare infection caused by anaerobic, Gram-positive, filamentous, branching bacteria. Being a member of the Actinomycetes, these bacteria often demonstrate branching hyphal-like growth. In general, bacterial pathogens are less than 1 micron in width, which is very helpful for distinguishing them from filamentous fungi, which are typically 3 microns or greater in width. In general, actinomycotic infections are subacute to chronic and may be present in a variety of locations, often related to where the body is colonized. Cervicofacial, abdominal, and pelvic infections are most common, but thoracic infections are not unheard of. Histopathologically, Gram-positive to Gram variable, filamentous, branching bacteria are seen. The appearance of these bacteria is very similar to that of *Nocardia* species, another member of the actinomycetes. Grossly, *Actinomyces* is well known for the production of "sulfur granules," so named because of their yellow appearance. Microscopically, they appear as lamellated, generally basophilic mats, often demonstrating mixed bacterial morphologies. Sulfur granules are frequently encountered in tonsillar resections, where they generally exist as commensal organisms; they may also be seen in pelvic cytology or in surgically resected specimens from women with intrauterine implanted devices. *Nocardia* species are described as being partially acid-fast, but a negative acid-fast stain does not confirm that *Actinomyces* is present nor does it rule out *Nocardia*, as more infrequently encountered pathogens such as *Streptomyces* may be present, and *Nocardia* species do not always stain acid-fast (Figs. 2.94, 2.95, 2.96, 2.97, 2.98 and 2.99).

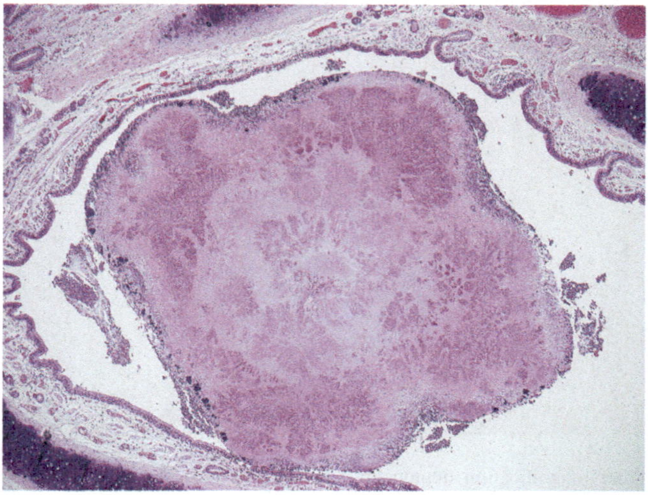

Fig. 2.94 A typical actinomycotic sulfur granule. Note the layered fungal-like growth. H&E, 40× magnification

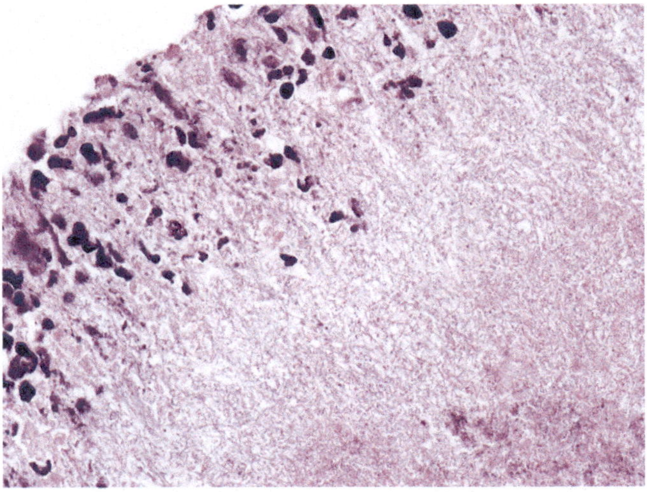

Fig. 2.95 Higher magnification image demonstrating an intricate meshwork of filamentous branching bacteria consistent with an actinomycotic granule. H&E, 1000× magnification

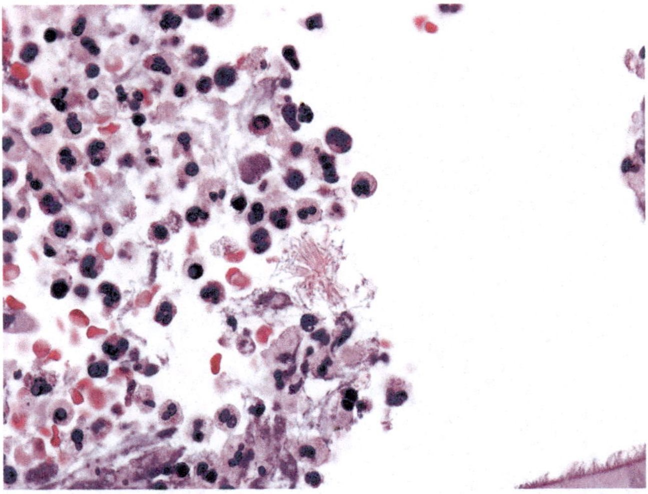

Fig. 2.96 Eosinophilic "asteroid bodies" may be seen in actinomycotic infections. These formations are caused by the Splendore-Hoeppli phenomenon, which creates eosinophilic "star-burst" crystalline formations consisting primarily of immunoglobulin around bacteria, fungi, and some parasites

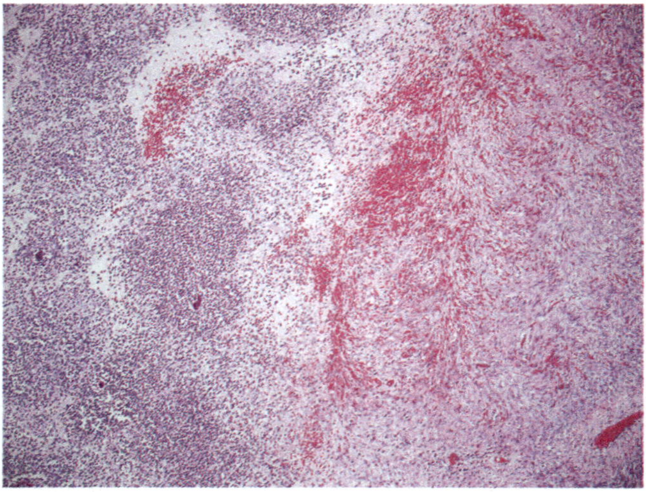

Fig. 2.97 Ovarian infection attributable to *Actinomyces* species. Note a dense, predominantly acute inflammatory infiltrate to the *left* of the image with hemorrhage in the remaining ovarian tissue to the *right*. Bacterial colonies typical of actinomycotic infection are visible. H&E, 100× magnification

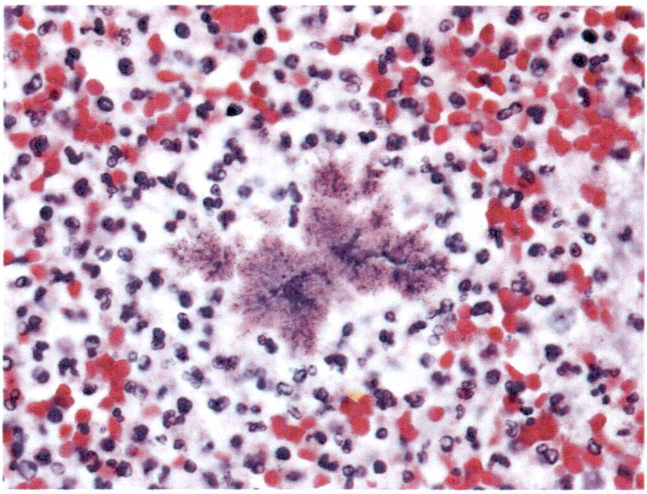

Fig. 2.98 Higher magnification of an ovarian infection caused by *Actinomyces* species. Note the typical sulfur granule appearance and beaded staining. The surrounding inflammation is largely neutrophilic. H&E, 1000× magnification

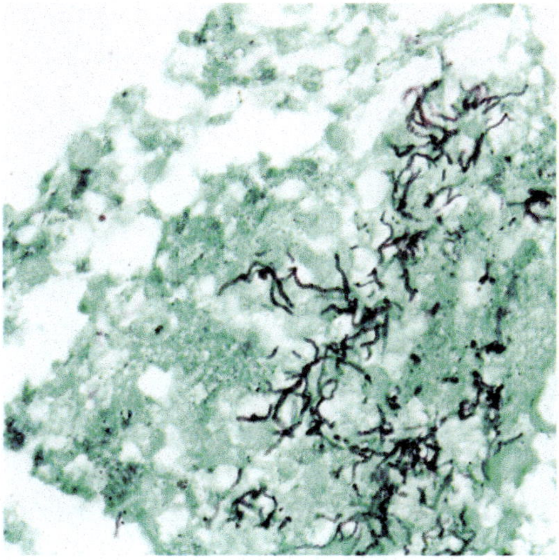

Fig. 2.99 Gomori methenamine silver stain of a brain abscess caused by *Actinomyces* species. These filamentous branching bacteria may mimic the appearance of filamentous fungi, demonstrating the appearance of "septations" and acute or wide angle branching. While silver stains such as this are typically used for the identification of fungal organisms, it is important to note that Gram-positive bacteria in particular may stain "positive." Measurement is important in these cases because bacteria are typically 1 micrometer or less in width. Gomori methenamine silver stain, 1000× magnification

2.11 Nocardial Infections

Like *Actinomyces* species, *Nocardia* species are Gram-positive, filamentous branching bacteria. While *Actinomyces* prefer growth in anaerobic conditions, *Nocardia* are aerobic. Most species are partially acid-fast; as such, it is recommended that a modified Kinyoun or a Fite stain be used to assess this characteristic. As previously noted, *Nocardia* may not always stain acid-fast even using these methods, so caution must be used if trying to differentiate *Nocardia* from other filamentous branching bacteria such as *Actinomyces*, based on a negative stain. These bacteria can be involved in infections at any site but are particularly noted to cause infections of the lung, since the primary route of initial infection is usually by inhalation. These cases may appear as a single nodule or abscess but may demonstrate multiple lung nodules on radiologic examination, similar to the appearance of miliary tuberculosis. Nocardial infections also frequently behave in a metastatic fashion; the classic scenario is dissemination from the lung to the central nervous system, leading to multiple brain abscesses (Figs. 2.99, 2.100, 2.101, 2.102, 2.103, 2.104 and 2.105).

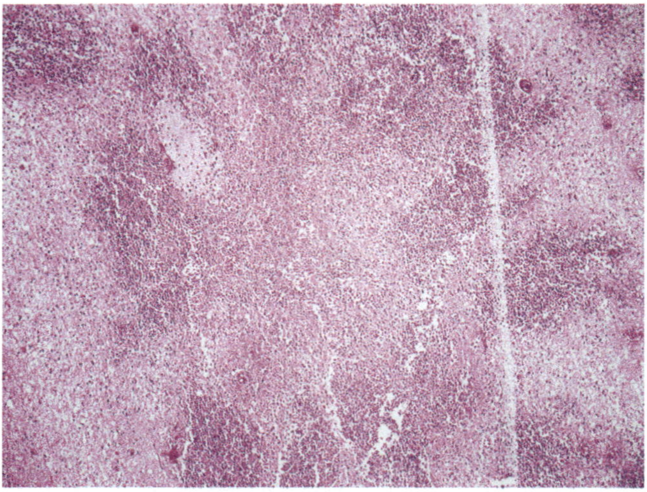

Fig. 2.100 Nocardial brain abscess. While *Nocardia* species are filamentous branching bacteria like *Actinomyces* species, they do not usually form granules. Note that a predominantly acute inflammatory response is seen with no readily apparent identifiable bacteria. H&E, 100× magnification

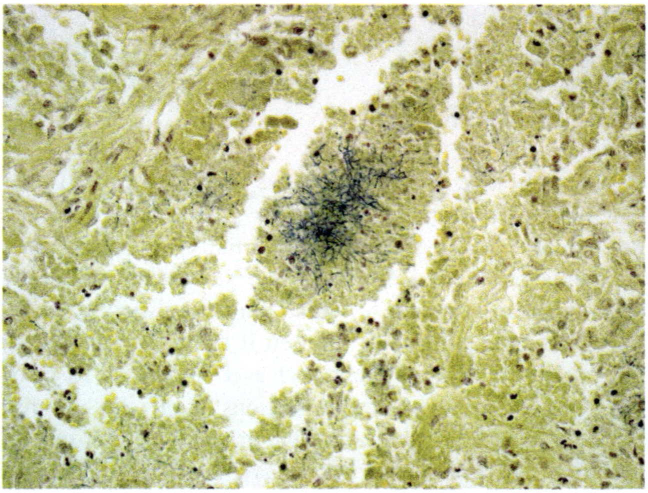

Fig. 2.101 Nocardial lung abscess. Note the similarity to other filamentous branching bacteria, such as *Actinomyces* species. Brown and Brenn, 400× magnification

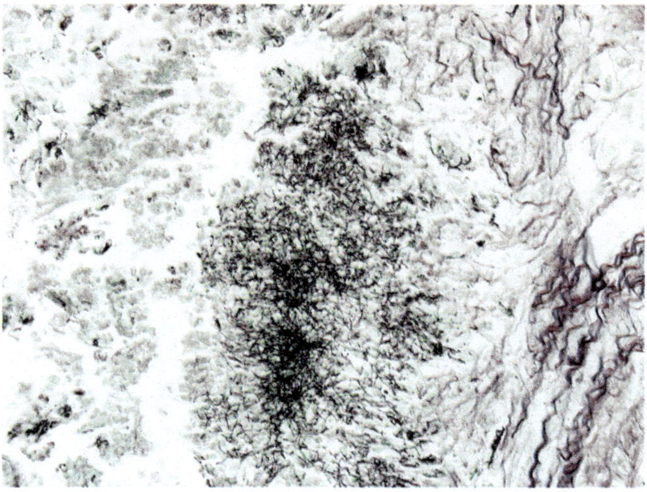

Fig. 2.102 Nocardial lung abscess. Note that these bacteria stain positive with Gomori methenamine silver and other silver-based stains. Although they may appear very similar to fungal hyphae, the size of the bacteria distinguishes them from most fungal organisms; they are around 1 micrometer or less in width. Gomori methenamine silver stain, 400× magnification

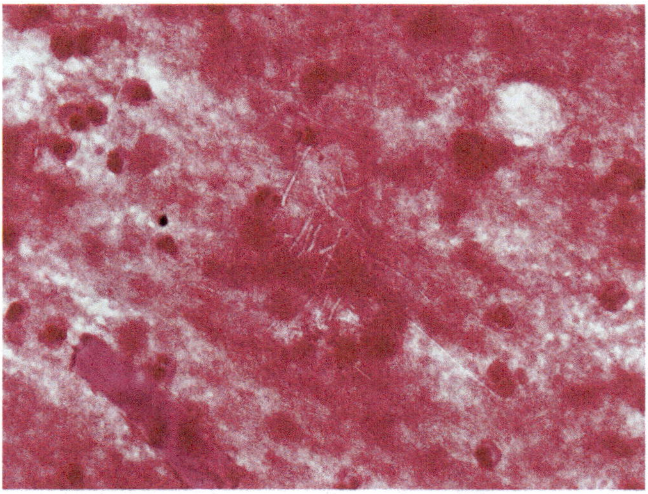

Fig. 2.103 "Negative image" created by *Nocardia* that did not retain the crystal violet stain. This feature can be seen frequently in drug treated cases of nocardiosis and may lead to missed identifications of the organism. Bronchoalveolar lavage, Gram stain, 1000× magnification

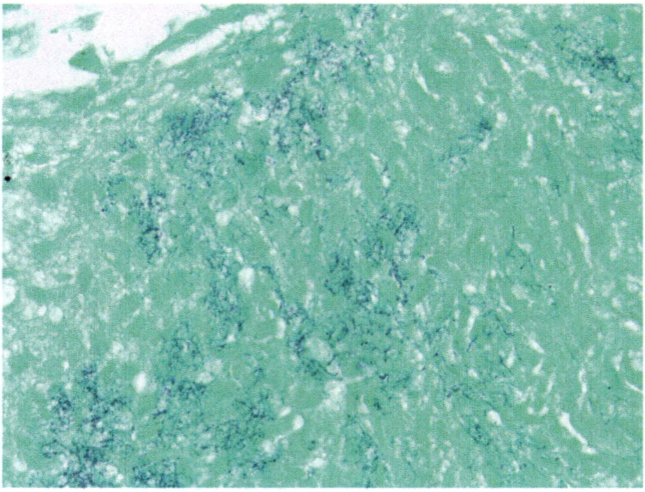

Fig. 2.104 In cases in which *Nocardia* stains poorly, a silver stain such as Gomori methenamine silver may highlight the organisms. This case was negative by Gram stain alone. Transbronchial biopsy, Gomori methenamine silver stain, 1000× magnification

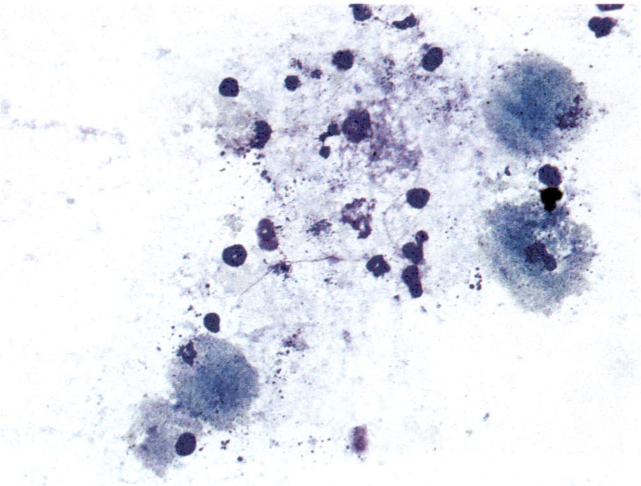

Fig. 2.105 *Nocardia* typically stains "partially acid fast." Note that often the Ziehl-Neelsen stain is too harsh to demonstrate the acid-fast properties of *Nocardia*. For this reason, modified Kinyoun or Fite stains are recommended. Even with these methods, *Nocardia* may still fail to stain pink or may only stain weakly, such as in this example. Bronchoalveolar lavage, modified Kinyoun method, 1000× magnification

2.12 Mycobacterial Infections Including Leprosy

Mycobacteria are often broadly classified as the most important pathogen of the species, *Mycobacterium tuberculosis* or as nontuberculous mycobacteria (NTMs). The NTMs can be further classified as rapid growers, such as *M. abscessus* and *M. fortuitum*, which typically grow in 7 days or less, and other groups (photochromagens, scotochromagens, nonchromogens) based on pigment production of cultured bacteria. While it is important to note that there are other acid-fast bacteria, so called because they retain carbol-fuschin after decolorization with acid-alcohol, mycobacteria are likely the most important for their pathogenic potential. With the exception of *M. leprae*, these bacteria typically stain well with classic Ziehl-Neelsen or Kinyoun stains. Fite stain combines peanut- or a vegetable-based oil with xylene, minimizing exposure of the mycolic acids to organic solvents. This method is particularly useful for the staining of *M. leprae*, which will usually stain acid-fast negative using harsher methods. Of note, *M. leprae* cannot be grown using traditional laboratory methods; therefore identification using microscopy may be the only initial indication that *M. leprae* is present (Figs. 2.105, 2.106, 2.107, 2.108, 2.109, 2.110, 2.111, 2.112, 2.113, 2.114, 2.115, 2.116, 2.117, 2.118, 2.119 and 2.120).

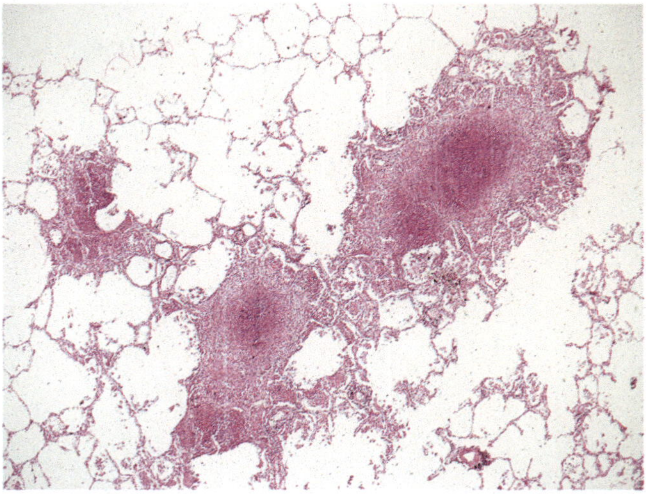

Fig. 2.106 Miliary tuberculosis of the lung. This entity is so named because it produces disseminated small opacities on radiographic examinations. The appearance is reminiscent of scattered millet seed. On histopathology, discrete, scattered granulomas are identified. While these findings may be seen in other infections, notably in pulmonary nocardial infections and infections with the dimorphic fungus *Histoplasma capsulatum*, they are classically associated with infection with *Mycobacterium tuberculosis*. H&E, 40× magnification

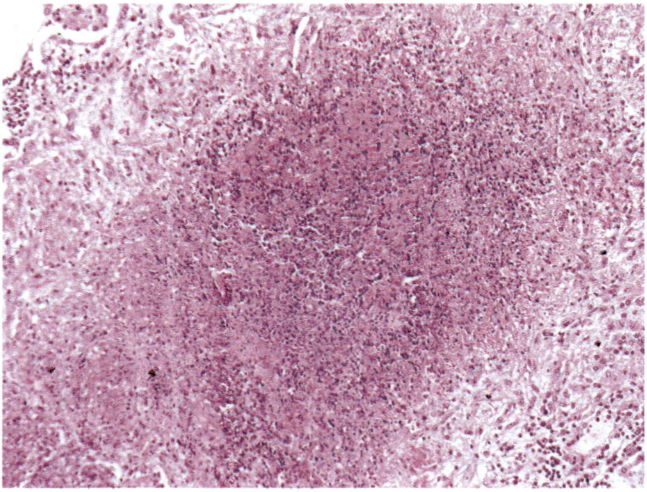

Fig. 2.107 Necrotizing granuloma in lung tissue caused by infection with *M. tuberculosis*. Grossly, these appear as caseating granulomas, that is, that they appear caseous or cheese-like. While they are classically attributed to *M. tuberculosis* infection, similar lesions may also be credited to a variety of other agents, including *H. capsulatum* and nocardial infections. H&E, 200× magnification

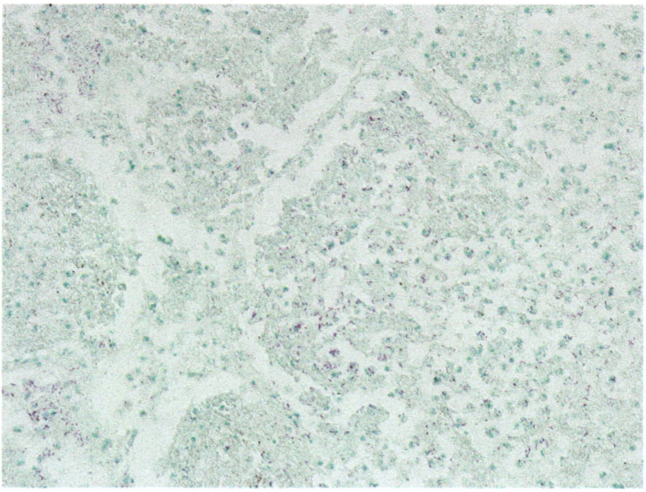

Fig. 2.108 Ziehl-Neelsen stain of lung tissue infected with *M. tuberculosis*. In heavy infections, the acid-fast bacilli are relatively easy to spot on lower magnifications. However, it is important to note that some mycobacterial infections will demonstrate very few organisms, and may require the use of oil-assisted magnification to identify. 400× magnification

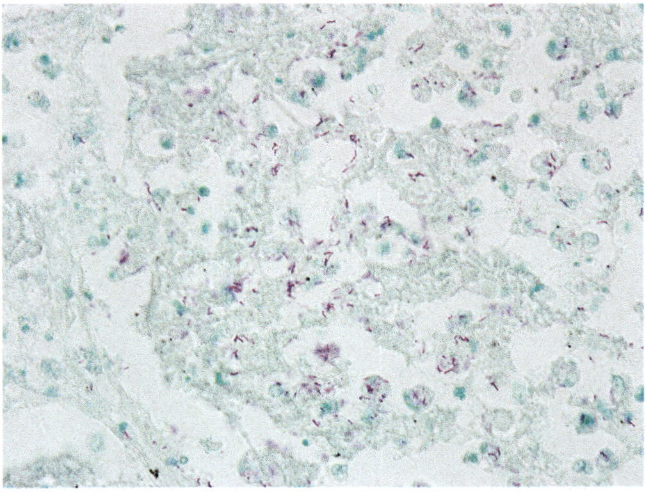

Fig. 2.109 Higher magnification image of the case illustrated in Fig. 2.96 demonstrating the typical morphology of *M. tuberculosis*. Ziehl-Neelsen stain, 1000× magnification

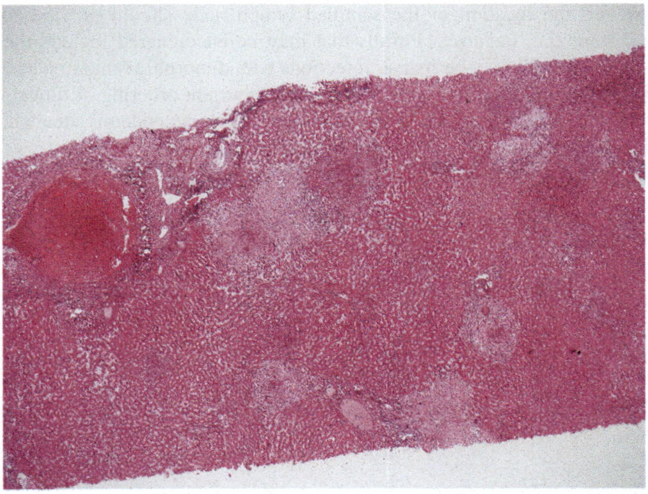

Fig. 2.110 Miliary tuberculosis of the liver. It is important to note that mycobacteria, in particular *M. tuberculosis*, may affect every organ system. Seen here is a miliary pattern of infection in the liver. H&E, 40× magnification

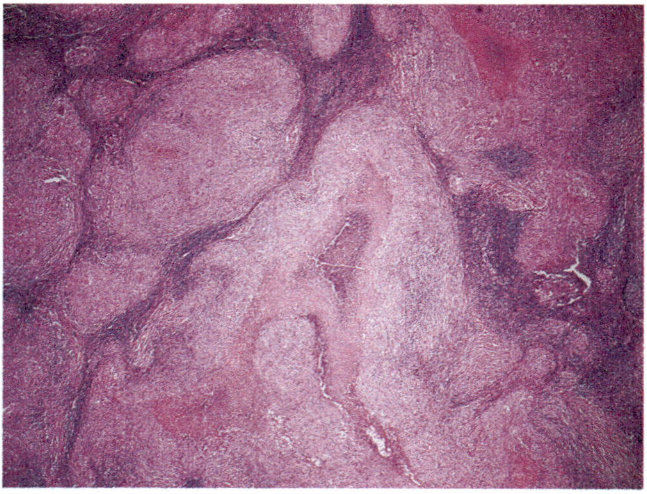

Fig. 2.111 Invasion of local lymph nodes, particularly in the case of pulmonary tuberculosis, is common. Shown here is a mediastinal lymph node affected by *M. tuberculosis* in a patient with a primary lung infection. Note that necrotizing granulomas are commonly seen and may appear similar to stellate lymph node abscesses in other disease entities such as infection with *Bartonella henselae*. However, the location of the sampled lymph node should provide some guidance regarding the differential diagnosis. Pitfalls that may be encountered include the fact that the presence of acid-fast bacilli may be sparse. Infections with dimorphic fungi in particular may also produce a similar appearance and should prompt the concurrent ordering of fungal stains such as Gomori methenamine silver, particularly if the patient is from an endemic area where dimorphic fungal infections are encountered. H&E, 40× magnification

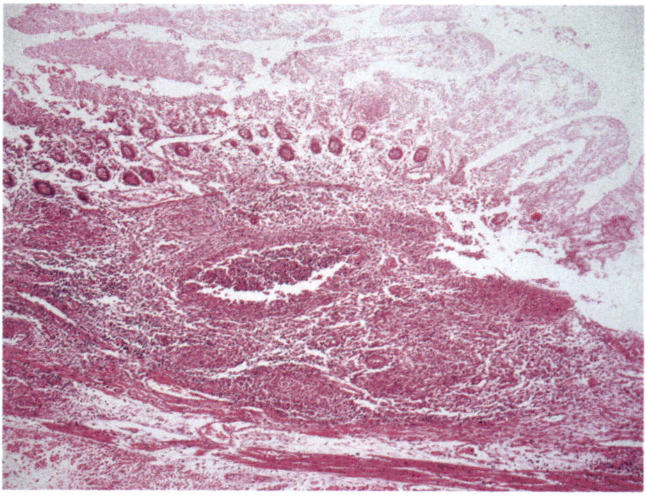

Fig. 2.112 As previously mentioned, mycobacterial infections may affect any organ system. Shown here is an infection of the ileum with *M. tuberculosis* causing full-thickness coagulative necrosis. H&E, 100× magnification

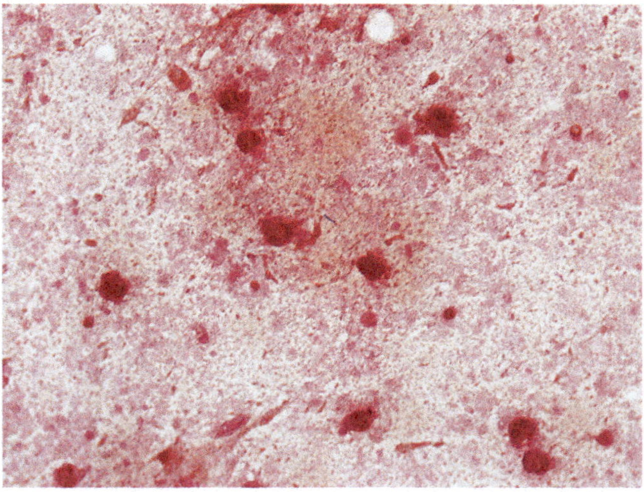

Fig. 2.113 A single mycobacterium seen on Gram stain of a bronchoalveolar lavage specimen. Mycobacteria, particularly those that are rapid growers, are sometimes able to be detected using traditional Gram staining methods. As seen here, a beaded retention of the crystal violet stain (appearing *purple*) is characteristic. In this case, *M. abscessus* was identified by culture. See Fig. 2.114, which demonstrates the same case using a modified acid-fast stain in which the organism is much more readily seen. 1000× magnification

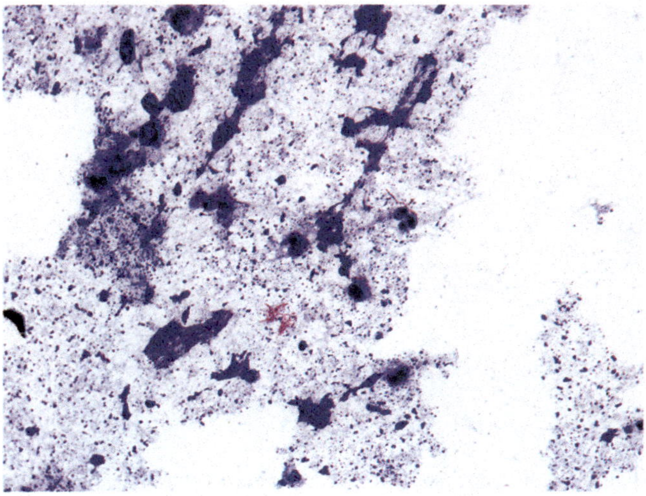

Fig. 2.114 Modified Kinyoun method demonstrating much more consistent staining of *M. abscessus* from the previous case. 1000× magnification

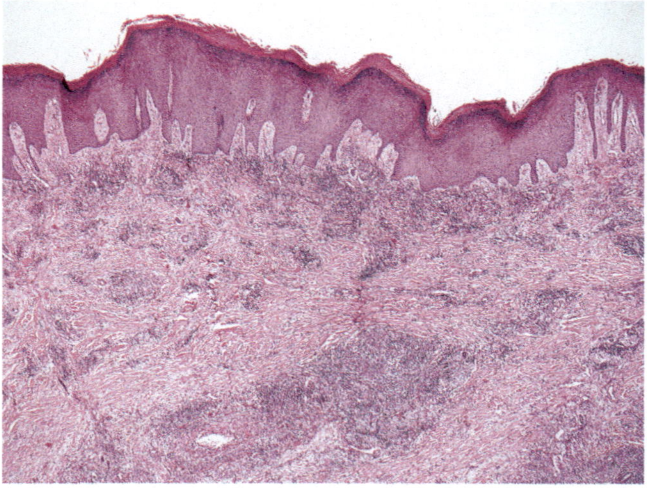

Fig. 2.115 *Mycobacterium leprae*. Leprosy is classified primarily as lepromatous leprosy or tuberculoid leprosy. It is important to note that an indeterminate form with features of both is also recognized. Lepromatous leprosy, illustrated here in a finger lesion, is characterized by loose aggregates of macrophages, often associated with a sparse inflammatory infiltrate consisting of lymphocytes and plasma cells. H&E, 40× magnification

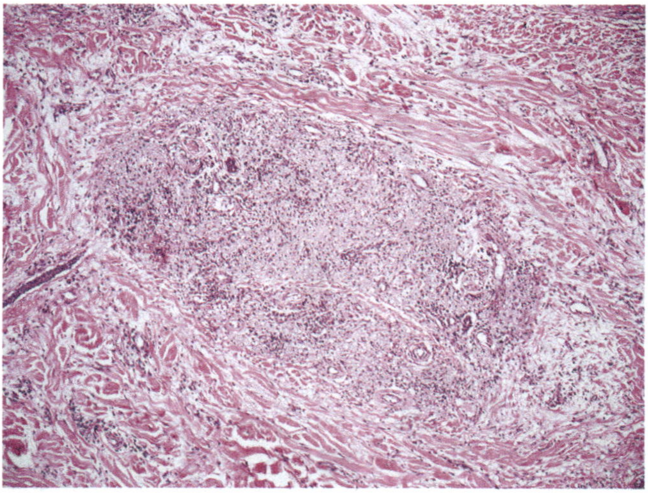

Fig. 2.116 High magnification image of tissue obtained from a finger demonstrating loose aggregates of macrophages typical of lepromatous leprosy. The macrophages often have a foamy-appearing cytoplasm, which reflects that they are filled with bacilli. As such, they are usually easily identifiable in this state using a Fite stain. Other methods, including modified Kinyoun stains, will destroy the delicate mycolic acid structures, and the bacteria will appear acid-fast negative or may not be identified at all. H&E, 100× magnification

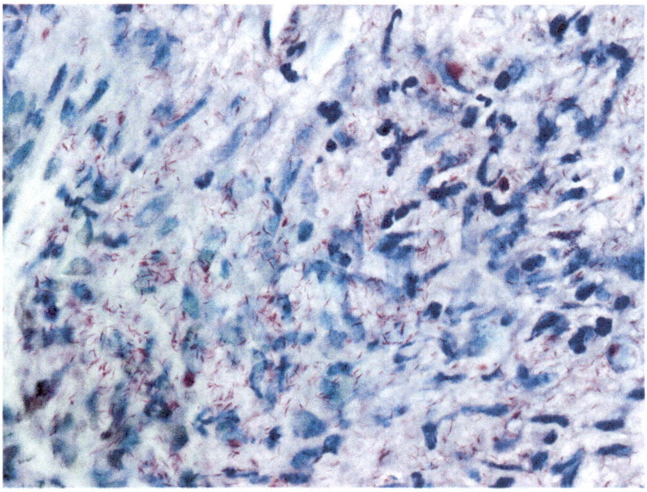

Fig. 2.117 A Fite stain of a finger biopsy within lepromatous leprosy demonstrating many thin and delicately staining acid-fast bacilli. 1000× magnification

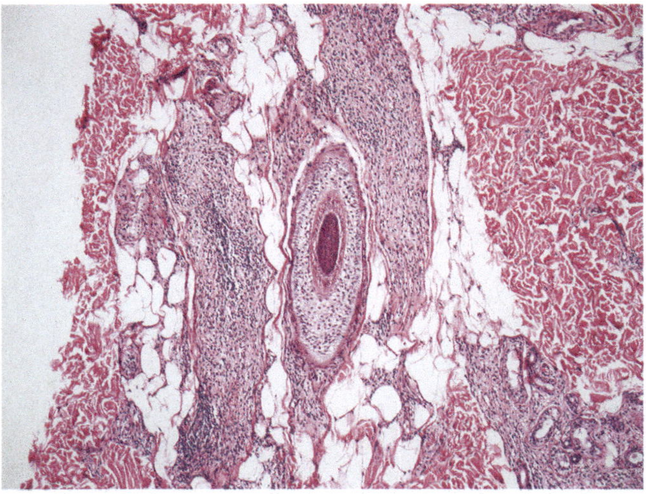

Fig. 2.118 Turberculoid leprosy demonstrating well-formed sarcoidal granulomas featuring macrophages in tight clusters. A few scattered lymphocytes may be present. The infiltrate characteristically surrounds hair and adnexal structures (shown here) as well as peripheral nerves. Organisms are typically scant and may not be identified, even with Fite staining. H&E, 100× magnification

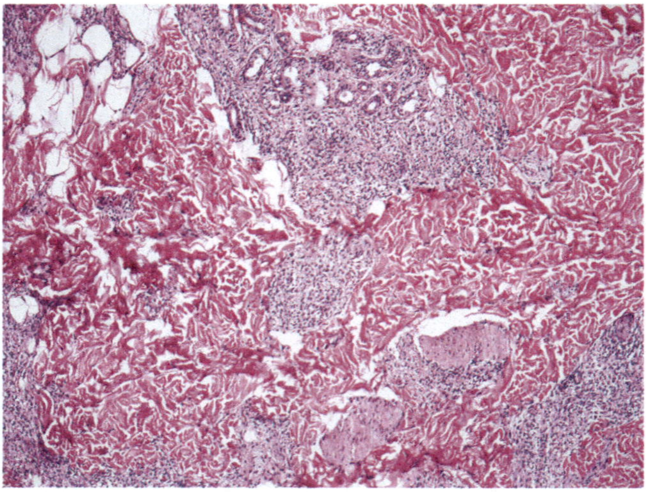

Fig. 2.119 Tuberculoid leprosy demonstrating well-formed granulomas that surround peripheral nerves and adnexal structures. H&E, 100× magnification

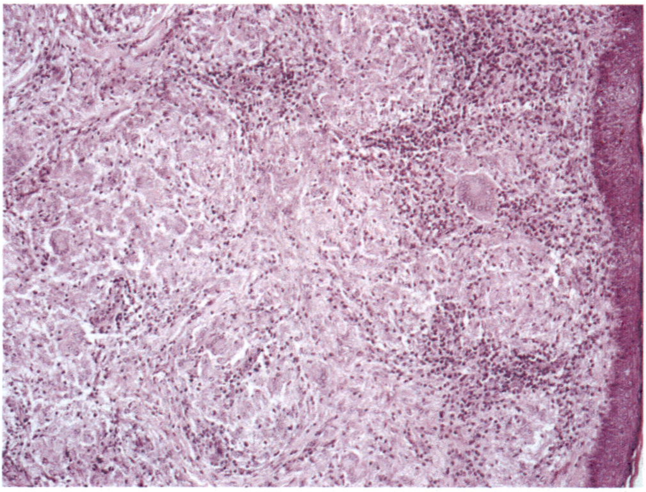

Fig. 2.120 Multinucleated Langhans cells can also be frequently found associated with granulomas in cases of tuberculoid leprosy. H&E, 200× magnification

Suggested Reading

Allen SD. Pig-bel and other necrotizing disorders of the gut involving *Clostridium perfringens*. In: Connor DH, editor. Pathology of infectious diseases, vol I. New York: Appleton and Lange; 1997. p. 717–24.

Anaya DA, Dellinger EP. Necrotizing soft-tissue infection: diagnosis and management. Clin Infect Dis. 2007;44:705.

Brook I, Frazier EH. Clinical and microbiological features of necrotizing fasciitis. J Clin Microbiol. 1995;33:2382.

Cooke RA. Leprosy. In: Infectious diseases, atlas, cases, text. Sydney/New York: McGraw-Hill; 2008a. p. 65–104.

Cooke RA. Tuberculosis. In: Infections diseases, atlas, cases, text. Sydney/New York: McGraw-Hill; 2008b. p. 39–64.

Cotell SL, Noskin GA. Bacillary angiomatosis. Clinical and histologic features, diagnosis, and treatment. Arch Intern Med. 1994;154:524.

Dennis DT, Inglesby TV, Henderson DA, Bartlett JG, Ascher MS, Eitzen E, et al. Tularemia as a biological weapon: medical and public health management. JAMA. 2001;285:2763.

Efstratiou A, Engler KH, Mazurova IK, Glushkevich T, Vuopio-Varkila J, Popovic T. Current approaches to the laboratory diagnosis of diphtheria. J Infect Dis. 2000;181(Suppl 1):S138.

Engelkens HJ, ten Kate FJ, Vuzevski VD, van der Sluis JJ, Stolz E. Primary and secondary syphilis: a histopathological study. Int J STD AIDS. 1991;2:280–4.

Farver C. Bacterial pneumonia. In: Procop GW, Pritt BS, editors. Pathology of infectious diseases. Philadelphia: WB Saunders; 2015. p. 247–64.

Golden MR, Marra CM, Holmes KK. Update on syphilis: resurgence of an old problem. JAMA. 2003;290:1510.

Hagley M, Carne CA, Gorgees N. A case of cat scratch disease masquerading as lymphogranuloma venereum. Int J STD AIDS. 1999;10:334.

Könönen E, Wade WG. Actinomyces and related organisms in human infections. Clin Microbiol Rev. 2015;28:419.

Larson MA, Fey PD, Hinrichs SH, Iwen PC. Francisella tularensis bacteria associated with feline tularemia in the United States. Emerg Infect Dis. 2014;20:2068–71.

Lucas SB. Histopathology of leprosy and tuberculosis – an overview. Br Med Bull. 1988;44:584–99.

Mabeza GF, Macfarlane J. Pulmonary actinomycosis. Eur Respir J. 2003;21:545.

Massone C, Belachew WA, Schettini A. Histopathology of the lepromatous skin biopsy. Clin Dermatol. 2015;33:38–45.

Monteil RA, Michiels JF, Hofman P, Saint-Paul MC, Hitzig C, Perrin C, et al. Histological and ultrastructural study of one case of oral bacillary angiomatosis in HIV disease and review of the literature. Eur J Cancer B Oral Oncol. 1994;30B:65.

Pathela P, Blank S, Schillinger JA. Lymphogranuloma venereum: old pathogen, new story. Curr Infect Dis Rep. 2007;9:143.

Raoult D, La Scola B, Lecocq P, Lepidi H, Fournier PE. Culture and immunological detection of *Tropheryma whippelii* from the duodenum of a patient with Whipple disease. JAMA. 2001;285:1039.

Rodig SJ, Dorfman DM. Splendore-Hoeppli phenomenon. Arch Pathol Lab Med. 2001;125:1515–6.

Scollard DM, Adams LB, Gillis TP, Krahenbuhl JL, Truman RW, Williams DL. The continuing challenges of leprosy. Clin Microbiol Rev. 2006;19:338.

Spach DH, Koehler JE. Bartonella-associated infections. Infect Dis Clin N Am. 1998;12:137.

Wilson JW. Nocardiosis: updates and clinical overview. Mayo Clin Proc. 2012;87:403–7.

3 Viral Infections

Ryan F. Relich

Despite major advances in basic and applied research and the availability of several vaccines, viral diseases still account for a large proportion of the human infectious disease burden. Many viruses cause self-limiting and relatively mild infections, but several, including human immunodeficiency virus and influenza virus, are responsible for millions of deaths every year throughout the world. Several factors contribute to the enormous impact that viruses have on human health. For example, there are very few therapeutic options available for the treatment of viral infections, and many of those that are available possess a limited spectrum of activity or are designed for the treatment of diseases caused by specific viruses (e.g., oseltamivir is intended for the treatment of influenza only). In addition, the rapid evolution of viruses has led to the emergence of drug-resistant strains against which no currently available therapeutics are effective. Coupled with these and other issues are the appearance of never before seen viruses and the emergence of known but previously underappreciated viruses. Since the beginning of the twenty-first century, numerous "new" viruses, including the coronaviruses responsible for severe acute respiratory syndrome (SARS) and Middle East respiratory syndrome (MERS), the 2009 pandemic influenza A virus, and Lujo hemorrhagic fever virus, have made their debut and have proved to be formidable threats to human health. Recently, the appearance of Ebola (*Zaire ebolavirus*) virus in West Africa, a region that has not previously seen an outbreak of this virus, was marked by an epidemic that afflicted nearly 30,000 individuals and killed more than 11,000 of those who were infected. Most recently, the far-reaching and rapid spread of Zika virus, a mosquito-borne virus that was discovered in the 1940s in Uganda, in the Western Hemisphere has invoked considerable public and scientific attention and has given rise to perhaps the largest concerted effort by scientists to rapidly develop a vaccine to halt the

R.F. Relich (✉)
Department of Pathology and Laboratory Medicine, Indiana University School of Medicine, Indianapolis, IN, USA
e-mail: rrelich@iupui.edu

B.H. Schmitt (ed.), *Atlas of Infectious Disease Pathology*,
Atlas of Anatomic Pathology, DOI 10.1007/978-3-319-54702-2_3

transmission of a virus. Each of these points underscores the importance of further research into improved surveillance, diagnosis, treatment, and prevention of viral diseases.

The diagnosis of viral infections has traditionally relied upon the observation of clinical signs and symptoms alone or in conjunction with analysis of clinical specimens. Historical laboratory methods, including direct analysis of clinical specimens by transmission electron microscopy, immunofluorescence, and inoculation of cultured cells for recovery of infectious viruses have largely been supplanted by rapid immunoserologic and molecular methods that provide definitive answers in as little as a few hours or less. Despite their waning presence in clinical laboratories, these historical methods remain important for the detection and characterization of rare or new viruses and for basic virology research, among other things. The microscopic examination of fixed and paraffin-embedded tissue and fixed cell concentrates also plays an important role in the diagnosis of many viral infections. The recognition of virus infection–associated tissue architectural and cytologic changes (cytopathic effects) and the judicious use of immunohistochemical methods afford anatomic pathologists the ability to provide clinically meaningful information to healthcare providers regarding the type and extent of a viral infection. Chief among the requirements for optimal visualization of virus-induced histopathology and cytopathology is the procurement of high-quality clinical specimens, such as tissue biopsy specimens and body fluids. Sections of tissue destined for histopathologic examination should immediately be placed into an appropriate fixative (e.g., 10% buffered formalin) and allowed to thoroughly fix prior to processing, staining, and examination. Specimens for other viral diagnostic studies, including viral cultures, may not be possible using formalin-fixed specimens; therefore separate sections of tissue should be submitted in transport media appropriate for the desired test(s). The same general considerations should be given when bodily fluids or exfoliated cell preparations are harvested for cytopathologic analysis.

In this chapter, representative photomicrographs of histopathologic and cytopathologic features of several viral infections are presented with brief descriptions of the viruses that cause them. Viral infections with readily detectable and distinguishing features that are likely to be encountered by anatomic pathologists in routine private and academic settings are presented along with a few examples of uncommonly encountered viral diseases.

3.1 Viral Classification and Genomics

Viruses are most commonly grouped by the type of nucleic acid, either DNA or RNA, that comprises their genomes and by the means by which their genomes are transcribed into messenger RNA. So far, seven distinct viral genome types are known and, to date, all characterized viruses possess one of these seven types. DNA genomes can exist either as double-stranded (dsDNA), gapped-double-stranded (g-dsDNA), or as single-stranded molecules (ssDNA). RNA genomes can also be double-stranded (dsRNA) or single-stranded (ssRNA). ssRNA genomes are further divided into three distinct types, including negative-sense ssRNA (−ssRNA), positive-sense ssRNA (+ssRNA), and positive-sense ssRNA that is reverse transcribed into a DNA intermediate (+ssRNA-RT). This generalized system for categorization of viruses is the backbone of the most widely used grouping system for viruses, the Baltimore classification system.

Viruses are also formally categorized according to conventional Linnaean taxonomic classification into orders, families, subfamilies, genera, and species. As of this writing and according to the latest virus taxonomy release of the International Committee on Taxonomy of Viruses, there are seven accepted orders, 122 families (of which 84 are not assigned to an order), 35 subfamilies, and many genera and species. Most of these viruses are not human pathogens, however. Examples of human viruses categorized according to genome type and formal taxonomic naming are listed in Table 3.1. For the most up-to-date information regarding viral systematics, please refer to the viral taxonomy listing of the International Committee on Taxonomy of Viruses (https://talk.ictvonline.org/taxonomy/).

3.2 Human Adenoviruses

In immunocompetent hosts, human adenoviruses (HAdVs) are common causes of usually self-limited respiratory tract and extrapulmonary infections, including coryza, conjunctivitis, and gastroenteritis; however, severe respiratory tract infections have been reported in otherwise healthy adults. Infections of immunosuppressed patients can lead to severe and sometimes fatal infections such as pneumonia, neurologic diseases, and diseases of the gastrointestinal and urinary tracts. Currently, there are 57 HAdV types spanning seven species (*Human mastadenovirus A-G*) that belong to the genus *Mastadenovirus*. Like all members of the family *Adenoviridae*, HAdV possess monopartite, linear dsDNA genomes that are covalently linked to a terminal protein (TP) at the 5′-ends of both DNA strands. HAdV genomes measure approximately 36 kilobase pairs (kbp) in length and encode roughly 40 proteins. Once susceptible and permissive host cells are infected, viral replication and particle assembly occurs within the host cell nucleus (Figs. 3.1 and 3.2).

3.3 Human Herpesviruses

The family *Herpesviridae* is currently organized into three subfamilies, including *Alphaherpesvirinae*, *Betaherpesvirinae*, and *Gammaherpesvirinae*, and a single unassigned genus. Scattered among these subfamilies are nine human herpesviruses (*see* Table 3.2). Although it is not considered a human herpesvirus, *Macacine alphaherpesvirus 1* (herpes virus B or "B" virus) is a zoonotic agent that is associated with severe and often fatal central nervous system infections in human hosts that acquire the virus through bites from infected macacine nonhuman primates (e.g., rhesus macaques). Virions are enveloped and contain an amorphous

Table 3.1 Human viruses according to genome type, ranked according to formal taxonomic hierarchy

Common name	Genome	Order	Family	Sub-family	Genus	Species
Herpes simplex virus-1	dsDNA	*Herpesvirales*	*Herpesviridae*	*Alphaherpesvirinae*	*Simplexvirus*	*Human alphaherpesvirus 1*
Human adenovirus	dsDNA	Unassigned	*Adenoviridae*	Unassigned	*Mastadenovirus*	*Human mastadenovirus A–G*
Hepatitis B virus	g-dsDNA	Unassigned	*Hepadnaviridae*	Unassigned	*Orthohepadnavirus*	*Hepatitis B virus*
Human parvovirus B19	ssDNA	Unassigned	*Parvoviridae*	Unassigned	*Erythroparvovirus*	*Primate erythroparvovirus 1*
Torque teno virus	ssDNA	Unassigned	*Anelloviridae*	Unassigned	*Alphatorquevirus*	*Torque teno virus 1*
Colorado tick fever virus	dsRNA	Unassigned	*Reoviridae*	*Spinareovirinae*	*Coltivirus*	*Colorado tick fever virus*
Rotavirus	dsRNA	Unassigned	*Reoviridae*	*Sedoreovirinae*	*Rotavirus*	*Rotavirus A–I*
Ebola virus	−ssRNA	*Mononegavirales*	*Filoviridae*	Unassigned	*Ebolavirus*	*Zaire ebolavirus*
Influenza A virus	−ssRNA	Unassigned	*Orthomyxoviridae*	Unassigned	*Influenzavirus A*	*Influenza A virus*
Hepatitis C virus	+ssRNA	Unassigned	*Flaviviridae*	Unassigned	*Hepacivirus*	*Hepacivirus C*
Zika virus	+ssRNA	Unassigned	*Flaviviridae*	Unassigned	*Flavivirus*	*Zika virus*
Human immunodeficiency virus-1	+ssRNA-RT	Unassigned	*Retroviridae*	*Orthoretrovirinae*	*Lentivirus*	*Human immunodeficiency virus 1*
Human T-lymphotropic virus-1	+ssRNA-RT	Unassigned	*Retroviridae*	*Orthoretrovirinae*	*Deltaretrovirus*	*Primate T-lymphotropic virus 1*

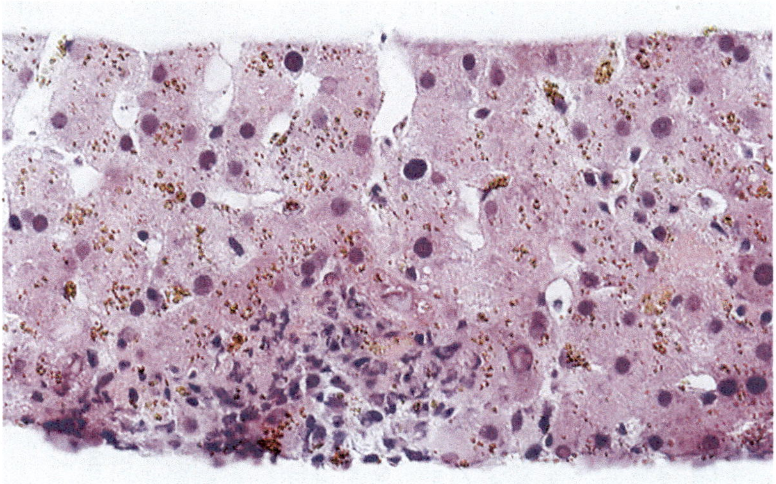

Fig. 3.1 Replication of adenoviruses results in cytopathic effects that are largely restricted to the nucleus, which is the site of adenoviral replication. Early in the viral infectious cycle, discrete eosinophilic inclusions composed of nascent particles are visible at relatively low magnifications. Continued assembly of new particles leads to expansion of these inclusions, which, over time, tend to stain more basophilic. In the terminal stages of progeny virus production, the nuclear membrane degenerates, imparting a blurred or smudged appearance to the nucleus. In the above image of an hematoxylin and eosin (H&E)-stained liver core biopsy section, both early- and late-stage cytopathic effects are visible throughout the field. Bile crystals are also seen dispersed throughout the tissue, underscoring the importance of careful interpretation of observations, since pigment granules (e.g., bile, lipofuscin, anthracotic pigment) can sometimes be confused with nuclear and cytoplasmic viral inclusions. Original magnification, 400×

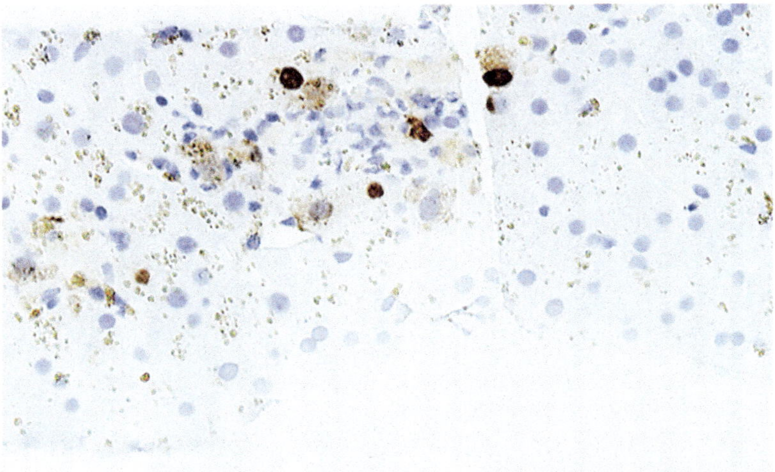

Fig. 3.2 Immunohistochemical staining permits confirmation of human adenovirus infection in tissue sections. In this example, a murine-derived pan-adenoviral antibody was used for detection of adenoviral antigens within a liver core biopsy section. Intense nuclear staining and less intense cytoplasmic staining are observable. Bile crystals are also seen dispersed throughout the tissue, which highlights the importance of careful interpretation of immunohistochemistry stains, especially in tissues in which endogenous pigment granules (e.g., bile, lipofuscin, anthracotic pigment) are commonly found, as some pigments may be confused with positive immunohistochemical staining. Original magnification, 400×

Table 3.2 Human herpesviruses according to common name, formal taxonomic hierarchy, and common disease associations

Common name	Subfamily	Genus	Species	Associated disease(s)
Herpes simplex virus-1	*Alphaherpesvirinae*	*Simplexvirus*	*Human alphaherpesvirus 1*	Orolabial lesions (common), genital lesions (less common), conjunctivitis, CNS diseases, disseminated infections, etc.
Herpes simplex virus-2	*Alphaherpesvirinae*	*Simplexvirus*	*Human alphaherpesvirus 2*	Genital lesions (common), orolabial lesions (less common), conjunctivitis, CNS diseases, disseminated infections, etc.
Varicella-zoster virus	*Alphaherpesvirinae*	*Varicellovirus*	*Human alphaherpesvirus 3*	Chickenpox (varicella), shingles (zoster), CNS diseases, disseminated infections, etc.
Epstein-Barr virus	*Gammaherpesvirinae*	*Lymphocryptovirus*	*Human gammaherpesvirus 4*	Infectious mononucleosis (IM), Burkitt lymphoma, Hodgkin lymphoma, etc.
Human cytomegalovirus	*Betaherpesvirinae*	*Cytomegalovirus*	*Human betaherpesvirus 5*	IM/glandular fever-like syndrome, various infections of the immunosuppressed, etc.
Human herpesvirus-6A	*Betaherpesvirinae*	*Roseolovirus*	*Human betaherpesvirus 6A*	Roseola, IM-like syndrome, encephalitis, mesial temporal lobe epilepsy, various infections of the immunosuppressed, etc.
Human herpesvirus-6B	*Betaherpesvirinae*	*Roseolovirus*	*Human betaherpesvirus 6B*	Roseola, IM-like syndrome, encephalitis, mesial temporal lobe epilepsy, various infections of the immunosuppressed, etc.
Human herpesvirus-7	*Betaherpesvirinae*	*Roseolovirus*	*Human betaherpesvirus 7*	Roseola, febrile seizures, pityriasis rosea (possibly), various infections of the immunosuppressed, etc.
Kaposi sarcoma-associated herpesvirus (HHV-8)	*Gammaherpesvirinae*	*Rhadinovirus*	*Human gammaherpesvirus 8*	Febrile illness with rash, Kaposi sarcoma

tegument within the space between the viral membrane and the nucleocapsid. Herpesvirus genomes contain linear, monopartite dsDNA that ranges in length from approximately 120–140 kbp. As with many other DNA viruses, herpesvirus replication occurs within the nucleus, and infection with many of these viruses results in obvious cytopathic effects. Many herpesviruses, including HSV and CMV, can be detected by immunohistochemistry (Figs. 3.3, 3.4, 3.5, 3.6, 3.7, 3.8, 3.9, 3.10, 3.11, and 3.12).

3.4 Human Papillomaviruses

The family *Papillomaviridae* is comprised of 49 genera and numerous species of nonenveloped, dsDNA viruses containing genomes of approximately 8 kbp in length that produce particles that measure approximately 60 nm in size. Interestingly, papillomaviral genomes are complexed with cellular histones, a feature also seen in polyomaviruses. Human papillomaviruses (HPV) are the causative agents of warts, genital cancers, anal dysplasia, focal epithelial hyperplasia, oropharyngeal cancer, and a host of other dermatologic and mucous membrane-associated diseases. Of the 170 types of HPV currently recognized, only a small subset is associated with head, neck, anal, and genital cancers (e.g., HPV 16, 18, 31, 45).

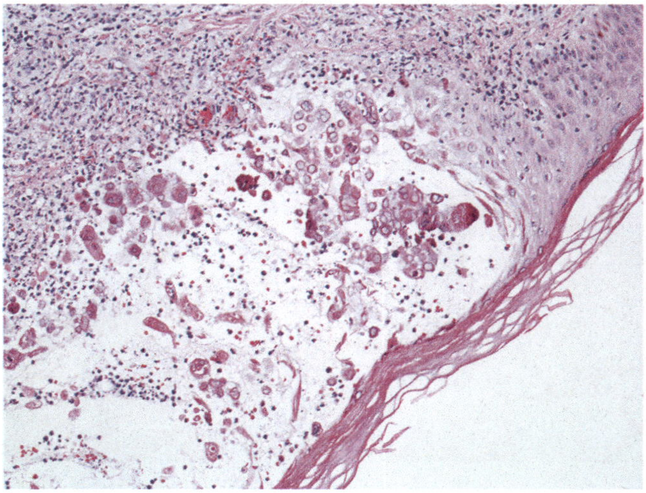

Fig. 3.3 Herpes simplex viruses-1 and -2 (HSV-1 and -2) are the causative agents of orolabial and genital herpes, but among other maladies they can also cause conjunctivitis, central nervous system diseases, and disseminated infections in the very young and immunosuppressed. Although HSV-1 and HSV-2 are often attributed to orolabial and genital herpes, respectively, detection of HSV-1 in genital lesion specimens and HSV-2 in orolabial lesion specimens is not uncommon. Typical cytopathic effects seen in HSV-infected cells include nuclear enlargement, margination of chromatin, nuclear molding, and multinucleation resulting from fusion of adjacent infected cells. The above photomicrograph of an H&E-stained skin biopsy section reveals the presence of numerous HSV-infected cells, especially around the periphery of the lesion, and an acute inflammatory infiltrate admixed with necrotic debris. Original magnification, 200×

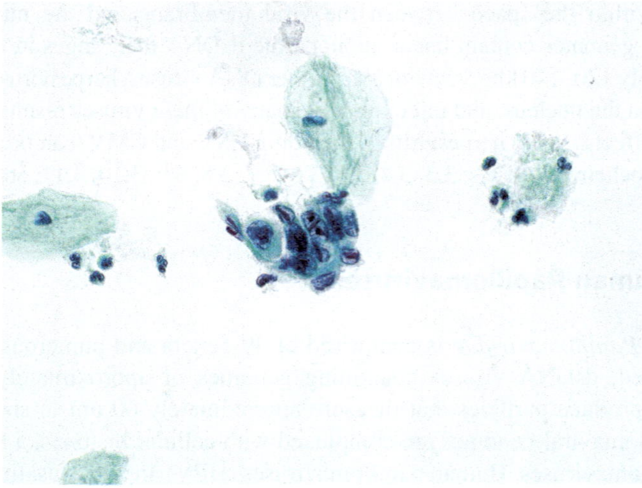

Fig. 3.4 Numerous HSV-infected epithelial cells displaying characteristic cytopathic effects are seen in this Papanicolaou-stained cervical brush specimen. Prominent, dense intranuclear viral inclusion bodies surrounded by marginated chromatin are seen in many of the infected cells. In addition, multinucleation and nuclear molding are apparent. Immunohistochemistry staining using HSV-1- and HSV-2-specific primary antibodies can distinguish infection with these two viruses if warranted. Original magnification, 600×

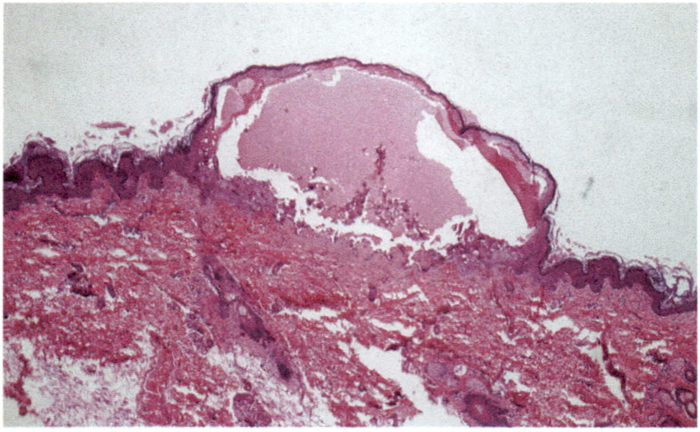

Fig. 3.5 Low-magnification view of a skin biopsy section from a patient with varicella (chickenpox) showing an intraepidermal vesicle containing edema, necrotic debris, acantholytic squamous cells, and neutrophils. Original magnification, 40×

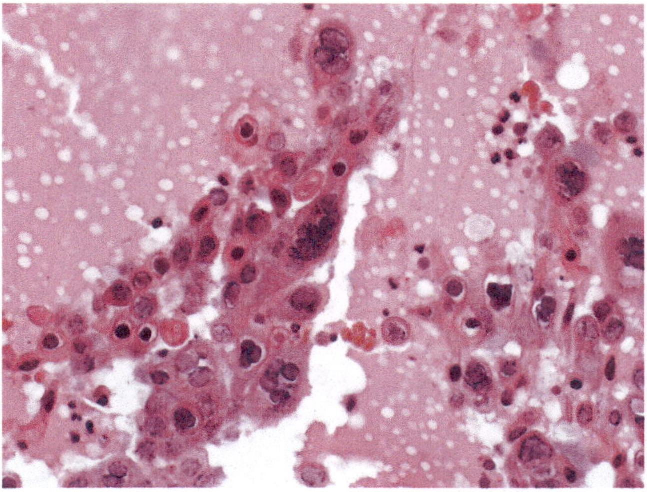

Fig. 3.6 Higher-power view of the skin biopsy shown in Fig. 3.5 reveals the presence of numerous varicella zoster-infected cells displaying cytopathic effects within edema fluid. Salient morphologic features also include fusion of neighboring infected cells to produce multinucleate giant cells, nuclear enlargement with margination of chromatin, and molding of adjacent nuclei. Infections with HSV and varicella-zoster virus induce identical cytopathic effects, but immunohistochemistry permits differentiation of HSV and varicella-zoster infections. Original magnification, 400×

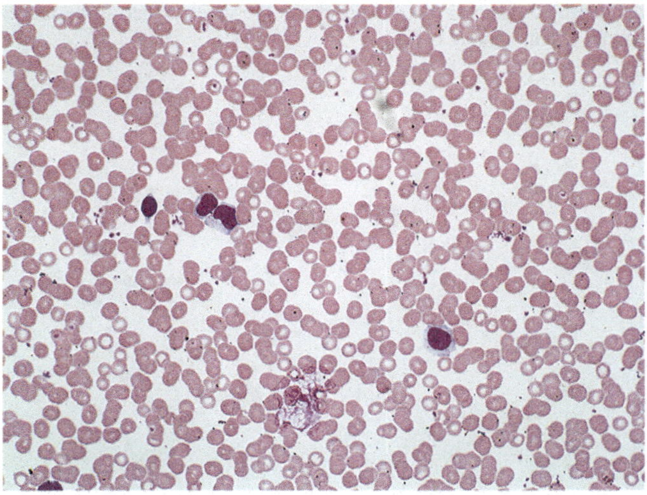

Fig. 3.7 Epstein-Barr virus (EBV) is the principal causative agent of infectious mononucleosis (IM), a disease that primarily affects adolescents and young adults (e.g., college students). EBV is also associated with a number of malignant neoplastic diseases (e.g., Burkitt lymphoma, nasopharyngeal carcinoma) and post-transplant lymphoproliferative disorder, the latter occurring in both hematopoietic stem cell and solid organ transplant recipients. Typical symptoms of IM include fever, pharyngitis, cervical and axillary lymphadenitis, extreme fatigue, and hepatosplenomegaly, among others. Because lesions are generally not produced in primary Epstein-Barr virus infection, histopathology is generally of little value when diagnosing infectious mononucleosis. Instead, immunoserologic testing is the mainstay for IM diagnosis. In most cases of IM, examination of peripheral blood smears reveals the presence of atypical lymphocytes such as those seen in this Wright-Giemsa-stained preparation. Original magnification, 500×

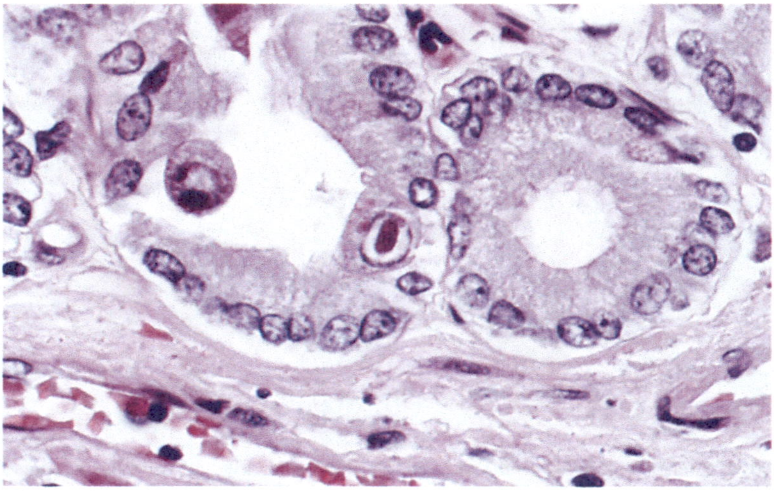

Fig. 3.8 Primary exposure of immunocompetent hosts to human cytomegalovirus (CMV) can result in either a subclinical infection or one with mild, IM-like symptoms. Reactivation of latent infections during states of immunosuppression can lead to focal or disseminated infections that range in severity from mild to fatal. Cytopathic features of CMV infection include cytomegaly and the presence of nuclear and/or cytoplasmic inclusions. The photomicrograph above shows a characteristic "owl's eye" inclusion within the nucleus of a CMV-infected colonic epithelial cell. This inclusion consists of a central solitary viral inclusion surrounded by a zone of pallor, which is surrounded by chromatin that is apposed to the inner leaflet of the nuclear membrane. H&E stain; original magnification, 600×

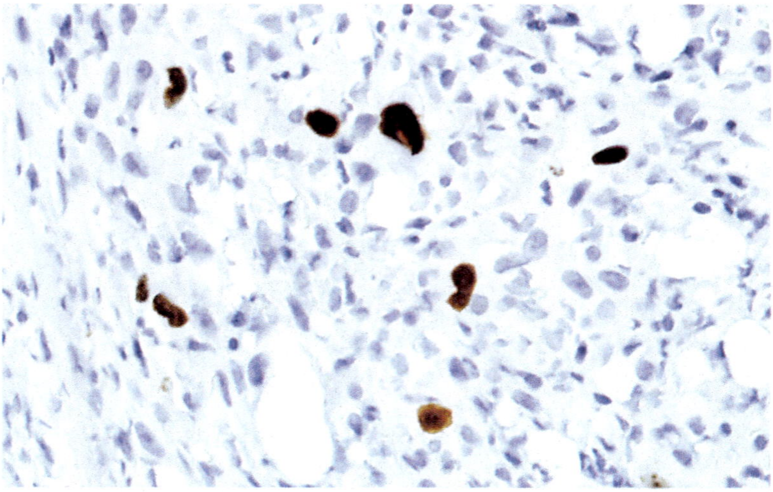

Fig. 3.9 Immunohistochemical staining permits confirmation of CMV infection in tissue sections. In this example, an anti-CMV immediate early antigen monoclonal antibody was used for detection of CMV infected cells. Brown staining highlights the presence of CMV immediate early antigens within the nuclei of colonic stromal cells. Original magnification, 600×

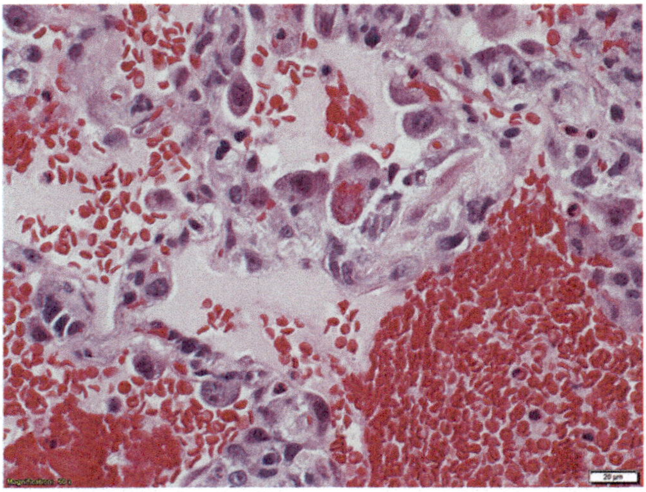

Fig. 3.10 Cytoplasmic CMV inclusions (*center*) often stain deeply eosinophilic when stained with H&E and appear as one or many smooth granules within the cytoplasmic compartment of infected cells. Original magnification, 600×

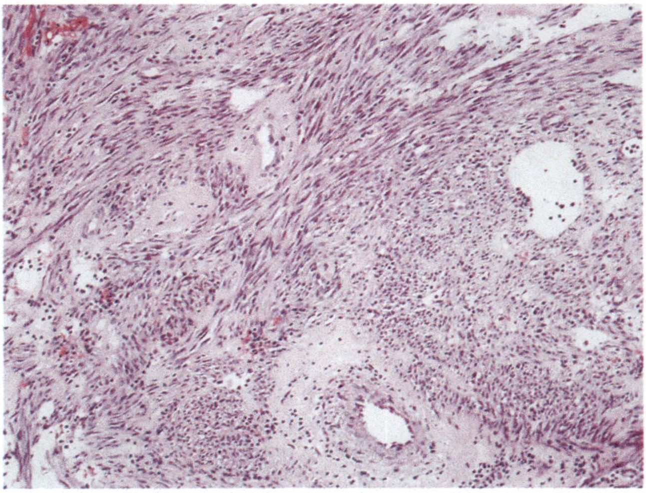

Fig. 3.11 The histopathologic features of Kaposi sarcoma (KS) are rather distinctive, and KS lesions are generally described based upon the stage (e.g., plaque stage, nodular stage) of tumor maturity. There are also several histopathologic variants of KS, including anaplastic, ecchymotic, intravascular, keloidal, and pyogenic-granuloma-like, among others. Lesions appear as dermal nodules comprised of proliferating endothelial cells that create slit-like vascular spaces and spindle cells forming fascicles, sometimes likened to schools of fish. The image above of an H&E-stained skin biopsy section from a KS patient shows a dermal tumor composed of slightly atypical spindle cells in sheets and fascicles with focal slit-like vascular lumen formation. Original magnification, 200×

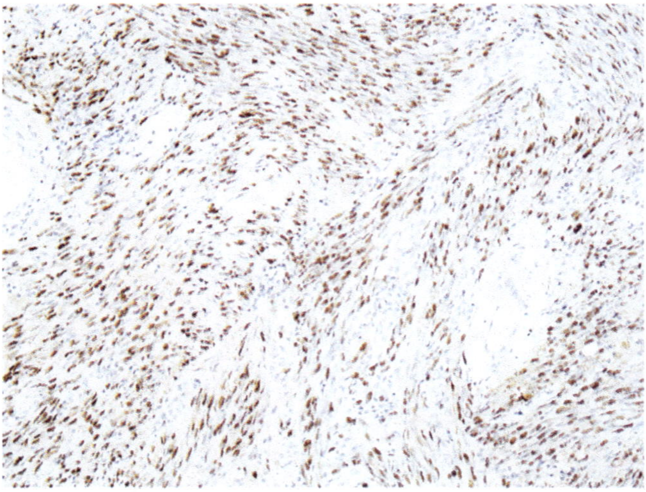

Fig. 3.12 Immunohistochemical staining permits confirmation of HHV-8 infection in tissue sections. In this example, immunohistochemical staining using an HHV-8 latent nuclear antigen 1 antibody reveals prominent nuclear staining and less intense cytoplasmic staining in infected spindle cells. Original magnification, 200×

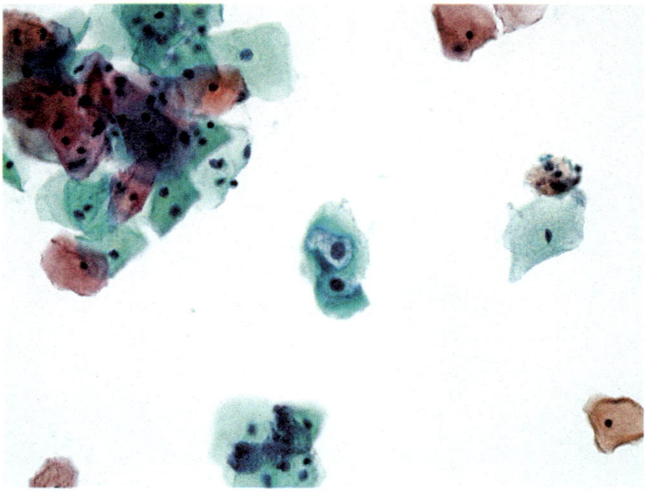

Fig. 3.13 Exfoliated HPV-infected epithelial cells (*center*) often demonstrate nuclear enlargement, nuclear hyperchromasia, irregular nuclear membrane contouring, and the presence of a perinuclear halo. These cells are called koilocytes, and their presence within cytopathologic and histopathologic preparations should prompt typing of the strain to ascertain the risk for cancer development to the infected patient. Papanicolaou stain; original magnification, 400×

Replication of HPV is restricted to stratified epithelial basal cells; therefore, efforts to detect HPV should focus largely on molecular and histopathologic methods using exfoliative cytologic preparations and tissue biopsies (Figs. 3.13, 3.14 and 3.15).

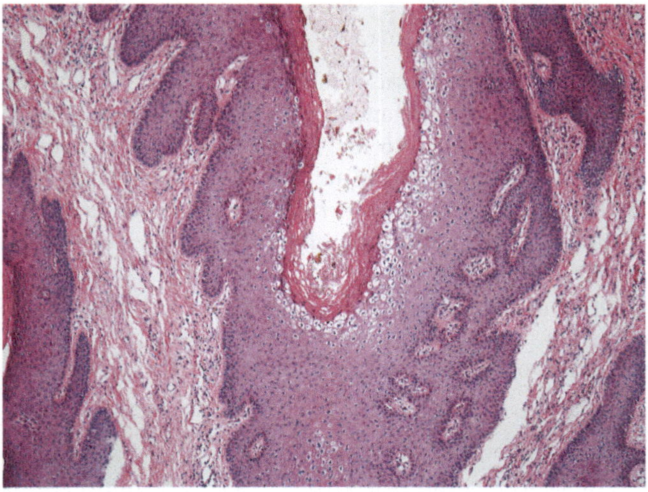

Fig. 3.14 Diffuse epidermal hyperplasia and numerous fibrovascular stalks are notable in H&E-stained sections of warts. In addition, numerous koilocytes are seen within the corneum spinosum. Original magnification, 100×

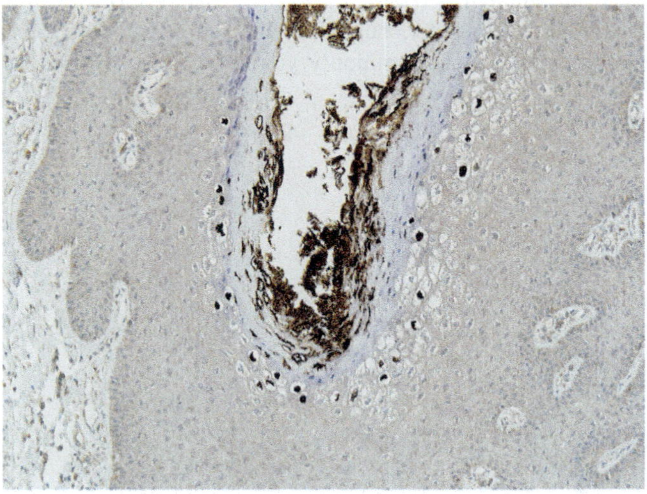

Fig. 3.15 Immunohistochemical staining permits confirmation of human papilloma virus (HPV) infection in tissue sections. In this photomicrograph, HPV antigens are detectable within the stratum corneum and within the nuclei of koilocytes present in the stratum spinosum. Original magnification, 200×

3.5 Human Parvoviruses

Parvoviruses are nonenveloped viruses that possess short (4–6 kbp) linear ssDNA genomes. Parvoviral particles are among the smallest known, with average sizes ranging from approximately 18–26 nm. To date, only two parvoviruses, human parvovirus B19 and human bocavirus, are known to cause human disease. Human parvovirus B19 (*Primate erythroparvovirus 1*) is the causative agent of erythema infectiosum (fifth disease), a common childhood illness, and human bocavirus (*Primate bocaparvovirus1* and *2*) has been suggested to cause gastroenteritis and lower respiratory tract infections. Parvoviruses, like many other DNA viruses, replicate within the cell nucleus and cause morphologic alterations, including nuclear swelling, chromatin margination, and inclusion production (Figs. 3.16 and 3.17).

3.6 Human Polyomaviruses

To date, there have been at least 13 species of human polyomavirus, including BK polyomavirus (*Human polyomavirus1*), JC polyomavirus (*Human polyomavirus 2*), and Merkel cell polyomavirus (*Human polyomavirus 5*) shown to infect humans. Most species are not pathogenic, but those that are cause very mild diseases in immunocompetent hosts, most commonly young children. Severe polyomavirus-

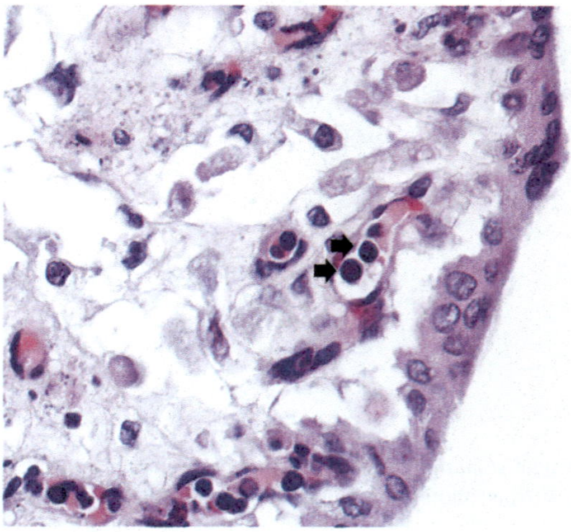

Fig. 3.16 Human parvovirus B19 (B19) is capable of attaching to and penetrating host cells expressing P antigen, which include erythroid precursor cells, endothelial cells, megakaryocytes, and others. Productive infection seems to be limited to the erythroid precursors BFU-E (erythroid burst-forming unit) and CFU-E (erythroid colony-forming unit) within the bone marrow and sites of extramedullary hematopoiesis. Like with many other DNA viruses, viral replication and particle assembly occur within the nucleus, leading to peripheral aggregation of chromatin and formation of variably-sized eosinophilic viral inclusions (*arrows*). Original magnification, 1000×

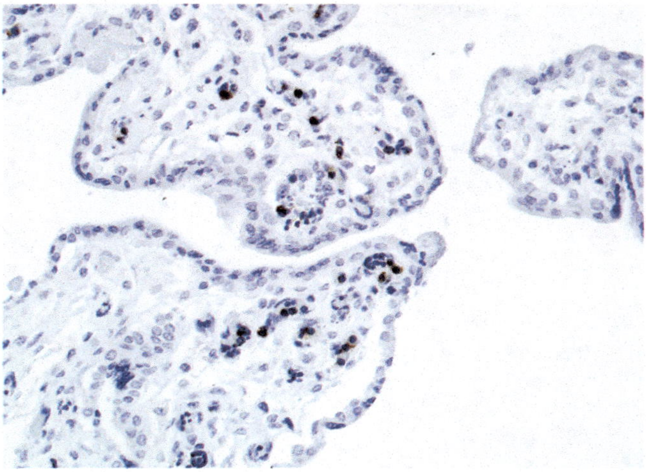

Fig. 3.17 Immunohistochemical staining permits confirmation of B19 infection in tissue sections. In this example, intense brown staining within the nuclei and lighter cytoplasmic staining highlight B19-infected cells. Original magnification, 200×

associated infections are most common in immunosuppressed hosts, including kidney and hematopoietic stem cell transplant recipients, and the spectrum of diseases in these individuals includes progressive multifocal leukoencephalopathy, nephropathy, hemorrhagic cystitis, and Merkel-cell carcinoma. Polyomavirus particles are roughly 50 nm in size, are nonenveloped, and contain a dsDNA genome that measures approximately 5 kbp in length. Like with papillomaviruses, the genomes of polyomaviruses are complexed with histones derived from host cells. Replication of polyomaviral genomes and assembly of new particles occurs within the cell nucleus (Figs. 3.18, 3.19 and 3.20).

3.7 Paramyxoviruses

Several viruses that are classified in the family *Paramyxoviridae* are human pathogens and cause diseases that range in severity from relatively mild respiratory tract infections to severe, life-threatening respiratory and central nervous system infections. Viruses belonging to this family that cause human disease are listed in Table 3.3. Like other members of the order *Mononegavirales*, paramyxoviruses have nonsegmented–ssRNA genomes that measure approximately 15 kbp in length and form complexes with viral structural proteins to produce helical nucleocapsids. Nascent particles bud from the cytoplasmic membrane, during which they are enveloped; resulting particles are roughly spherical or filamentous. Paramyxoviruses are transmitted between humans via aerosolized infectious respiratory secretions, through fomites, and some, the henipaviruses, are transmissible from infected animals such as bats, pigs, and horses (Figs. 3.21 and 3.22).

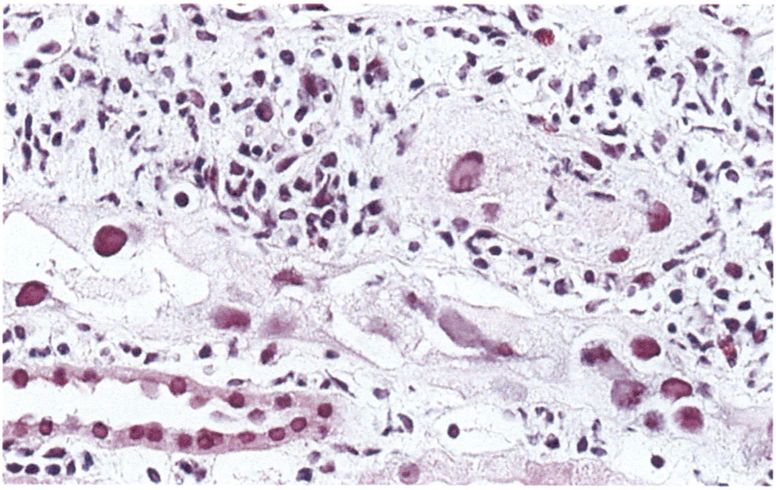

Fig. 3.18 BK polyomavirus infection of renal transplant recipients can result in ureteral stenosis and virus-induced nephropathy, which can lead to graft loss. Hemorrhagic cystitis, another manifestation of urogenital BK polyomavirus infection, is more common in hematopoietic stem cell transplant recipients, especially within the first few months following transplantation. Intranuclear viral replication leads to displacement of the cellular chromatin, imparting darker peripheral staining of the nucleus. As viral replication progresses, the accumulation of progeny particles leads to swelling of the nucleus and eventual degeneration of the nuclear membrane. Both early- and late-stage cytopathic effects are apparent in the renal tubular epithelium and surrounding cells in the above photomicrograph of an H&E-stained kidney biopsy section from a renal transplant patient with tubulointerstitial nephritis. Original magnification, 400×

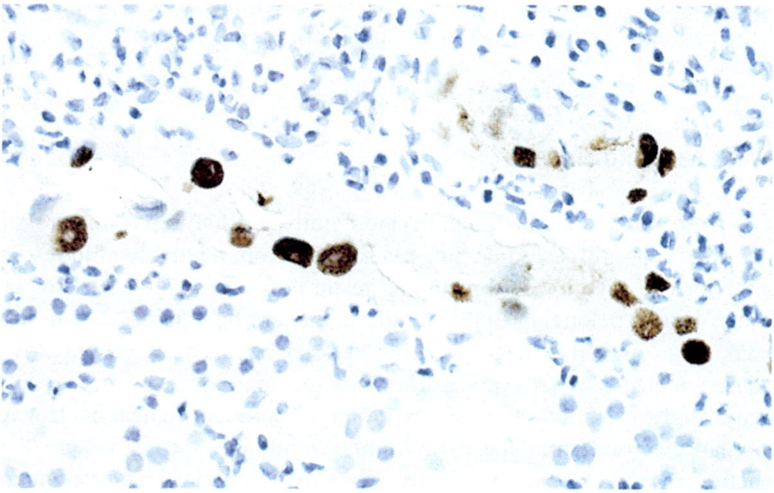

Fig. 3.19 Immunohistochemical staining permits confirmation of BK polyomavirus infection in tissue sections. In this example, BK polyomavirus antigens are detected within the nucleus of infected renal tubular epithelial cells. Original magnification, 400×

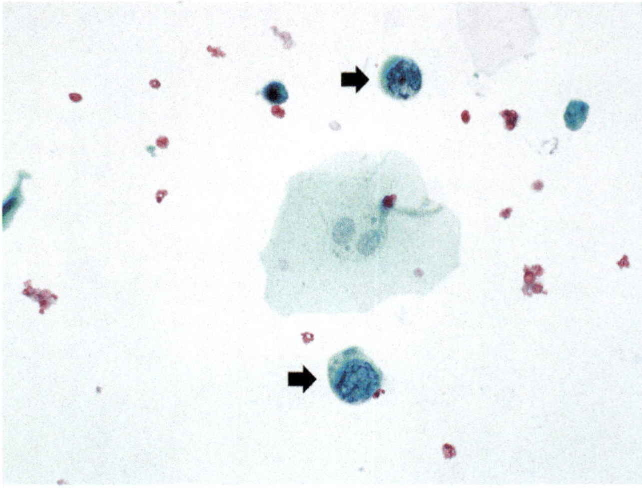

Fig. 3.20 A Papanicolaou-stained urine sediment containing exfoliated BK polyomavirus-infected urothelial cells (*decoy cells; arrows*) from a patient with hemorrhagic cystitis. Decoy cells were given their name because of their resemblance to malignant urothelial cells. They characteristically have a large nucleus that may contain one or more basophilic inclusions surrounded by chromatin, which sometimes gives the nucleus a ground-glass appearance. Original magnification, 600×

Table 3.3 Examples of human-pathogenic paramyxoviruses listed according to common name, formal taxonomic hierarchy, and disease associations

Common name	Genus	Species	Associated disease(s)
Respiratory syncytial virus	*Orthopneumovirus*	*Human orthopneumovirus*	Mild-to-severe bronchiolitis and pneumonia, coryza
Human parainfluenza virus	*Respirovirus* *Rubulavirus*	*Human respirovirus 1* *Human respirovirus 3* *Human rubulavirus 2* *Human rubulavirus 4*	Mild-to-severe upper and lower respiratory tract infections (e.g., croup), meningitis (rare)
Mumps virus	*Rubulavirus*	*Mumps rubulavirus*	Mumps, meningoencephalitis (rare)
Measles virus	*Morbillivirus*	*Measles morbillivirus*	Measles, subacute sclerosing panencephalitis
Hendra virus	*Henipavirus*	*Hendra henipavirus*	respiratory infections, meningitis, encephalitis
Nipah virus	*Henipavirus*	*Nipah henipavirus*	respiratory infections, meningitis, encephalitis

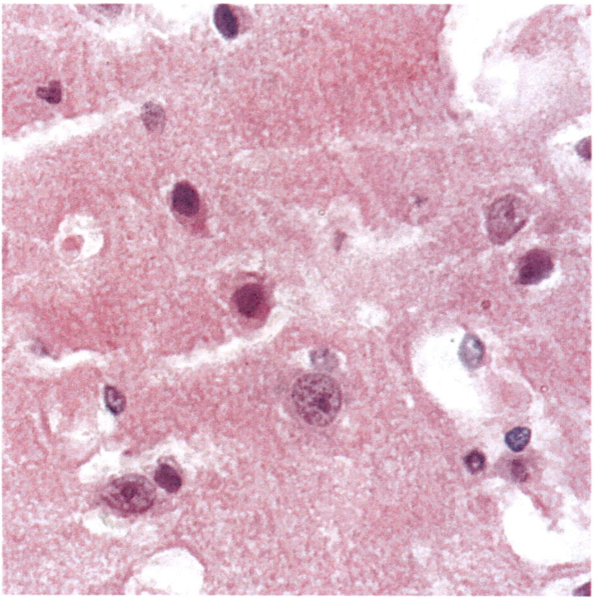

Fig. 3.21 Although relatively uncommon in the developed world, measles remains a significant cause of human morbidity and mortality throughout the developing world, where vaccination against the virus is uncommon or inaccessible. The majority of measles virus infections occur during childhood and are characterized by fever, nonproductive cough, conjunctivitis, coryza, and a maculopapular rash. The disease is generally self-limiting, but serious or fatal sequelae, including pneumonia and subacute sclerosing panencephalitis (SSPE), can occur. In this photomicrograph of an H&E-stained section of brain tissue from a patient who died from measles inclusion-body encephalitis several years after initial measles virus infection, multiple measles virus-infected neurons are present. In this example, the cytoplasm of infected neurons is shrunken and deeply eosinophilic and a few eosinophilic inclusions are evident. In measles-infected lymphoid tissue, large multinucleate cells (Warthin-Finkeldey cells) are usually seen. Original magnification, 1000×

3.8 Poxviruses

Some poxviruses (e.g., molluscum contagiosum virus) are common human pathogens; however, natural variola virus transmission has been eradicated from the planet, and the last human cases of smallpox were witnessed in the later part of the 1970s. Poxviruses possess some of the largest genomes of any virus known to infect humans. On average, the linear dsDNA genomes of these viruses measure approximately 170–250 kbp in length and encode numerous proteins. Unlike many other DNA viruses, replication of poxvirus genomes and particle assembly occurs within the cytoplasmic compartment of host cells, a feature that is made possible by viral proteins encoded within poxviral genomes. Consequently, light microscopic examination of stained tissue sections often permits visualization of intracytoplasmic inclusions of poxviruses such as Guarnieri bodies and molluscum bodies seen in variola virus- and molluscum contagiosum virus-infected cells, respectively (Figs. 3.23, 3.24, 3.25 and 3.26).

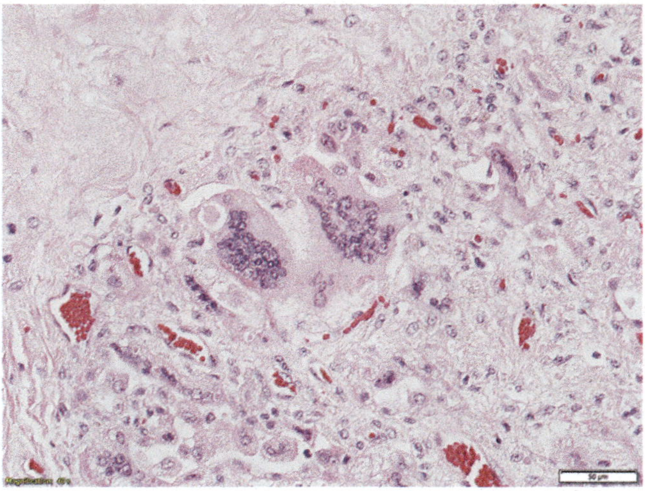

Fig. 3.22 Many infections caused by paramyxoviruses result in the formation of syncytia (*above*). Infected cells express viral fusion proteins on the cell surface that, at physiologic pH, mediate fusion of the cytoplasmic membranes of adjacent cells. Cell-cell fusion permits the spread of virions from infected cells to naïve cells, which affords virions some level of protection from host defenses. The photomicrograph above shows numerous syncytia in an H&E-stained section of lung tissue from an infant that died from severe parainfluenza virus infection. Original magnification, 400×

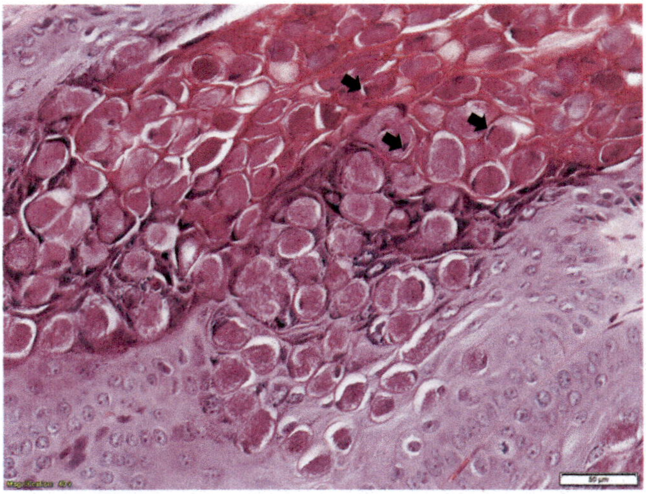

Fig. 3.23 Molluscum contagiosum virus is the agent of a mild and often benign skin disease called molluscum contagiosum. This virus is cosmopolitan in distribution and is transmitted from person-to-person by direct contact and via fomites, such as contaminated towels, razors, and toys. Viral replication is restricted to the epidermis, where it causes enlargement of infected cells, which produce very large and intensely eosinophilic cytoplasmic inclusions (molluscum bodies) that displace organelles. The nucleus of infected cells is often seen pressed against the cytoplasmic membrane, as seen in the H&E-stained skin biopsy section above (*arrows*). Original magnification, 400×

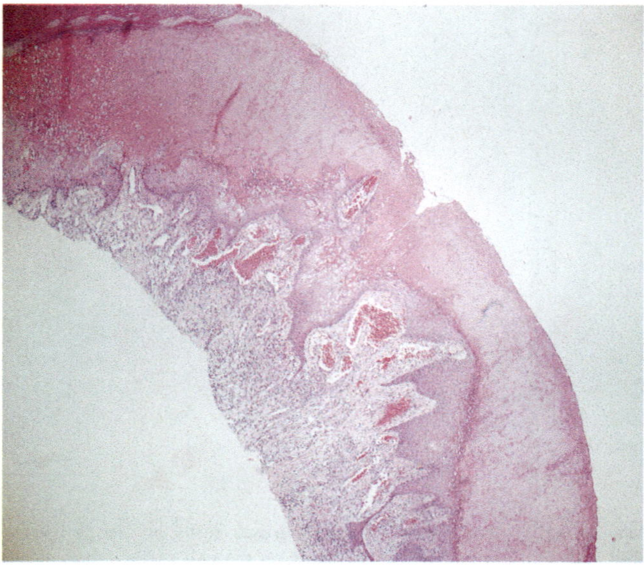

Fig. 3.24 The Orf virus is a zoonotic agent that primarily affects goats and sheep, but other mammals, including humans, can become infected. Transmission of orf virus occurs by direct contact with infected animals, and human infections lead to the formation of one or more papules at sites of infection, which can include the fingers, hands, and arms among other sites. Orf virus infection of humans is generally benign and self-limiting. Salient histopathologic features include spongiosis, ballooning degeneration, and superficial necrosis of the epidermis. High-power examination reveals small, eosinophilic cytoplasmic viral inclusions in some cells. H&E stain; original magnification, 40×

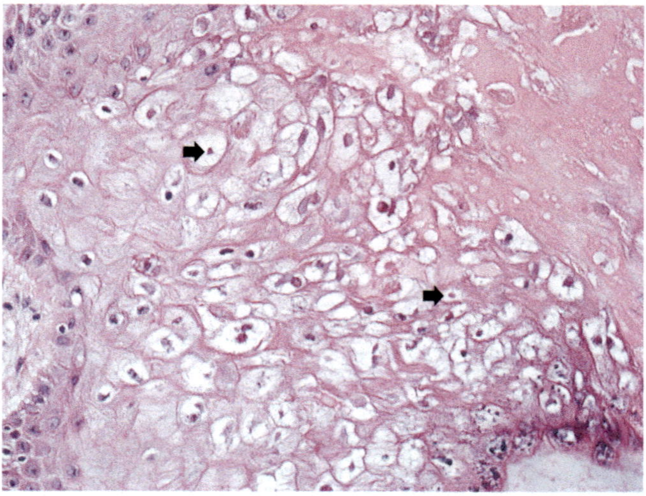

Fig. 3.25 Ballooning degeneration and viral inclusions (*arrows*) are seen in a high-power photomicrograph of the specimen from Fig. 3.24. Original magnification, 400×

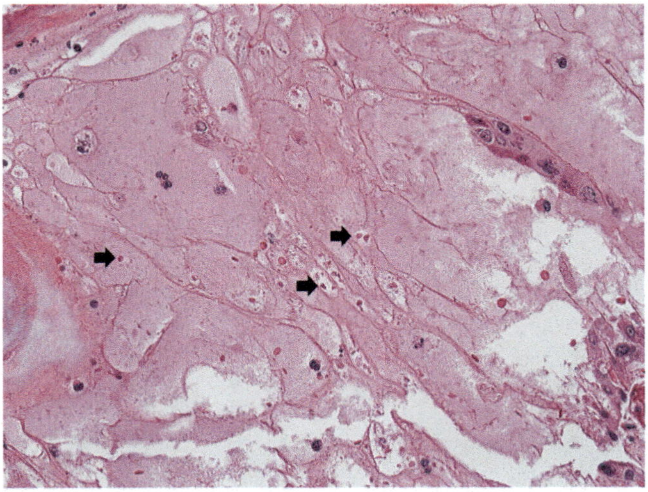

Fig. 3.26 The dermatologic manifestations of smallpox include both raised (vesicular) and flat lesions; the latter predominate in cases of hemorrhagic smallpox. Variola virus has a relatively broad host cell tropism and infects cells of the respiratory tract, endothelial and epithelial cells, hepatocytes, and numerous others. In this example from an archival case dating back to the 1920s, examination of an H&E-stained skin biopsy section reveals epidermal necrosis with ballooning reticular degeneration, resulting in vesicle formation. Rare intracytoplasmic eosinophilic inclusions (Guarnieri bodies) are visible under high-power magnification (*arrows*). Original magnification, 400×. (Slide of H&E-stained tissue provided by Dr. Bobbi Pritt, Division of Clinical Microbiology, Mayo Clinic, Rochester, MN)

3.9 Hemorrhagic Fever Viruses and Miscellaneous Human-Pathogenic Viruses

The following figures represent a broad diversity of viruses that can cause hemorrhagic fever or other severe infectious diseases that are rarely encountered in most developed nations. Included among this group are the filoviruses (e.g., Ebola virus), flaviviruses (e.g., yellow fever virus), hantaviruses (e.g., Sin Nombre virus), and rabies virus (Figs. 3.27, 3.28, 3.29 and 3.30).

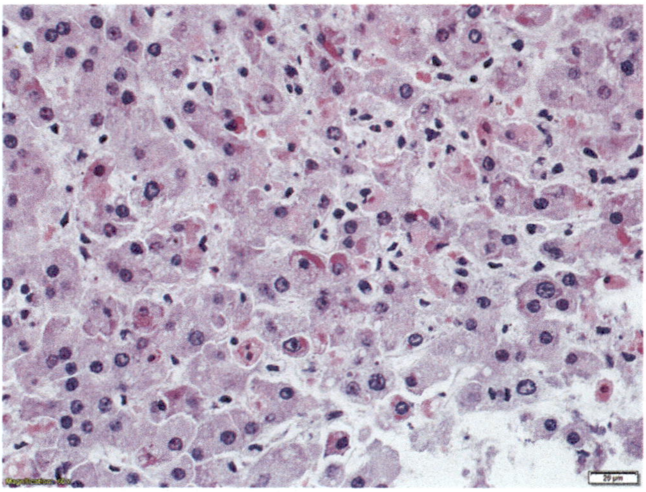

Fig. 3.27 Filoviruses, including ebolaviruses and marburgviruses, cause severe and often life-threatening infectious diseases in humans and other animals. Hallmarks of filoviral infections include the abrupt onset of fever, weakness, and severe head and body aches followed by the development of a rash, severe gastrointestinal symptoms, red eyes, and in a variable proportion of infected individuals, eventual development of hemorrhagic manifestations, including bleeding of the gums, the gastrointestinal tract, and from needle puncture sites. The incubation period for filoviral disease ranges from a few days to a few weeks following exposure, and infected individuals are contagious once symptoms appear. Ebola virions have been recovered from various body fluids, including blood, feces, urine, breast milk, and semen, among others. Filoviruses have a broad cell tropism; susceptible and permissive cells include monocytes, macrophages, dendritic cells, hepatocytes, endothelial cells, adrenal cortex cells, and others. The image above is a high-power view of an H&E-stained liver core biopsy section from a patient infected with *Zaire ebolavirus* (Ebola virus). In this example, there exists the conspicuous absence of a robust acute inflammatory response and the presence of apoptotic lymphocytes. Numerous Ebola virus-infected hepatocytes are present, and many contain eosinophilic, rope-like, football-shaped, or pleomorphic cytoplasmic inclusions. Original magnification, 600×. (Slide of H&E-stained tissue section provided by Dr. Sherif Zaki, Infectious Diseases Pathology Branch, U.S. Centers for Disease Control and Prevention, Atlanta, GA)

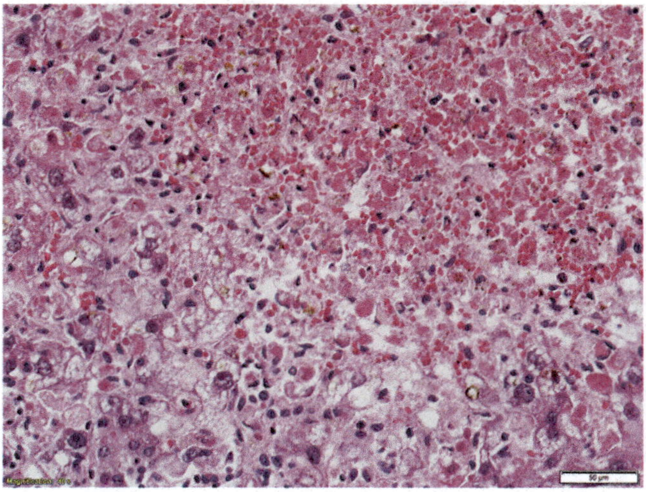

Fig. 3.28 The family *Flaviviridae* includes numerous viruses associated with hemorrhagic fever, including yellow fever virus, dengue viruses, Alkhurma hemorrhagic fever virus, Omsk hemorrhagic fever virus, and Kyasanur forest disease virus. These viruses are zoonotic agents that are largely transmitted by contact with infected animals or through the bites of infected mosquitoes or ticks. The specific means of transmission, symptoms, treatment, and prevention measures for the various viruses within this family are beyond the scope of this text, but refer to the section "Suggested Reading" for additional details. The photomicrograph above is an H&E-stained liver biopsy section from a patient with yellow fever and shows diffuse hepatocyte necrosis, parenchymal hemorrhage, and numerous Councilman bodies (apoptotic hepatocytes). Original magnification, 400×. (Slide of H&E-stained tissue section provided by Dr. Sherif Zaki, Infectious Diseases Pathology Branch, U.S. Centers for Disease Control and Prevention, Atlanta, GA)

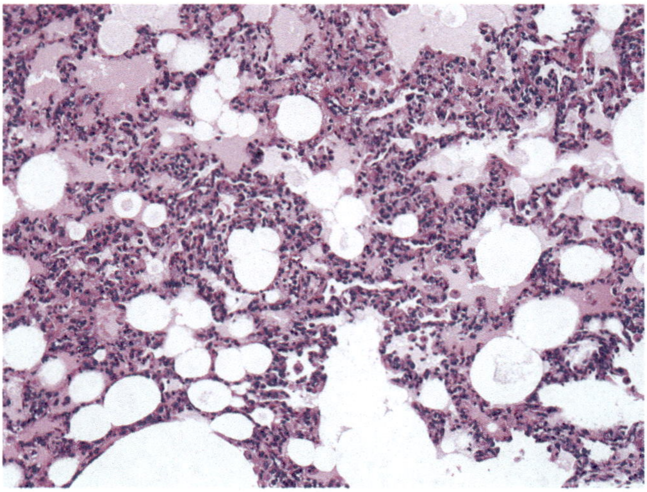

Fig. 3.29 Numerous hantaviruses are known to cause cardiopulmonary disease and hemorrhagic fever with renal syndrome. In nature, these viruses are carried by rodents such as deer mice, and human infections occur by inhalation of virion-laden aerosols generated by disturbance of rodent excreta. Replication of hantaviruses associated with cardiopulmonary disease occurs within pulmonary vascular endothelial cells, pulmonary macrophages, follicular dendritic cells, and within the vascular endothelium of myocardial capillaries. Cytoplasmic inclusions can be seen within pulmonary vascular endothelial cells, but immunohistochemical staining provides a more specific and reliable means for viral detection. The massive pulmonary edema seen in hantavirus cardiopulmonary syndrome patients is associated with virus-induced impairment of the pulmonary vascular endothelium. Hantavirus particles are enveloped, measure approximately 80–120 nm in size, and contain a tripartite genome composed of linear –ssRNA molecules. The photomicrograph above is that of an H&E-stained lung section from a nonhuman primate that was experimentally infected with Sin Nombre virus, the hantavirus associated with the 1993 Four Corners region hantavirus cardiopulmonary syndrome outbreak. Nonhuman primate models provide valuable insight into the pathogenesis and pathology of hantavirus infections, and they also recapitulate the disease processes seen in humans with relatively high fidelity. This photomicrograph shows the intra-alveolar edema and fibrin deposition, hyaline membrane formation, and interstitial pneumonitis. Original magnification, 200×. (Slide of H&E-stained tissue section provided by Dr. Dana Scott, Chief of Pathology, National Institutes of Health Rocky Mountain Laboratories, Hamilton, MT)

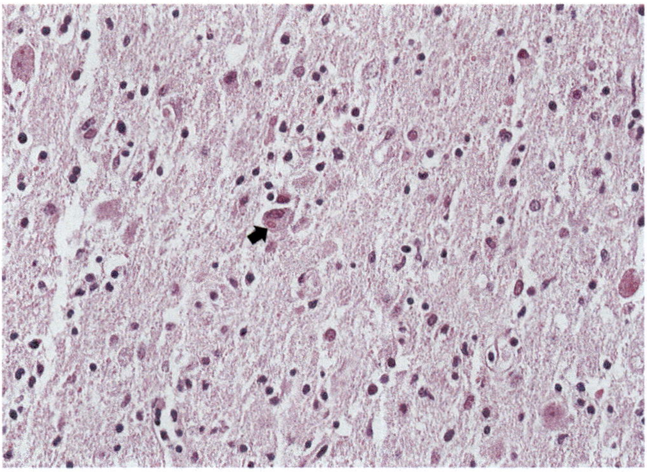

Fig. 3.30 Despite the availability of highly effective postexposure prophylaxis, rabies virus remains a significant cause of human mortality in regions of the world where animal and human vaccines are not readily accessible. Rabies virus is a zoonotic virus that is most frequently transmitted to humans by the bites of infected canids, although a small percentage of human infections result from the bites of other infected carnivores and bats, while an even smaller percentage of infections are transmitted by other means, including through allogeneic tissue transplants received from infected donors. Following inoculation, rabies virus can access the central nervous system via infection of peripheral nerves, which serve as conduits through which rabies virus travels to the brain. Myocytes and presumably other cell types at the site of rabies virus inoculation can also host rabies virus infection, but detection of the virus in these cells is difficult. With the exception of limited tissue necrosis, neuronal loss, and the appearance of characteristic cytoplasmic inclusion bodies (Negri bodies) within infected neurons, rabies virus induces little pathologic change to infected tissues. Rabies virus is a member of the order *Mononegavirales*, family *Rhabdoviridae,* and possesses a –ssRNA within a helical nucleocapsid that forms a bullet-shaped particle that is enveloped during budding through the cytoplasmic membrane. The image above is from an H&E-stained cerebellar section from an adolescent patient that died from rabies. Numerous rabies virus-infected neurons are present within the Purkinje layer, and the arrow points to a Negri body. Original magnification, 400×

Acknowledgments The author wishes to thank Dr. Sherif Zaki (Infectious Diseases Pathology Branch, U.S. Centers for Disease Control and Prevention), Dr. Bobbi Pritt (Division of Clinical Microbiology, Mayo Clinic), and Dr. Dana Scott (National Institutes of Health Rocky Mountain Laboratories) for provision of slides of H&E-stained tissue sections of Ebola and yellow fever virus-infected tissues, variola virus-infected tissue, and hantavirus-infected nonhuman primate tissue, respectively. In addition, Dr. Relich wishes to thank Drs. Bryan Schmitt, Theodore Kieffer, Matthew Kuhar, Simon Warren, Mercia Gondim, and Dibson Gondim (Department of Pathology and Laboratory Medicine, Indiana University School of Medicine, Indianapolis, IN) for their professional consultations and interpretations of many of the images shown.

Suggested Reading

Brackney DE, Armstrong PM. Transmission and evolution of tick-borne viruses. Curr Opin Virol. 2016;21:67–74.

Burke DS. Evolvability of emerging viruses. In: Nelson AM, Horsburgh CR, editors. Pathology of emerging infections 2. Washington, DC: ASM Press; 1998. p. 1–10.

Caruso JL, Childs JM, Howell DN. Surgical pathology and diagnostic cytology of viral infections. In: Jerome KR, editor. Lennette's laboratory diagnosis of viral infections. 4th ed. New York: Informa Healthcare; 2010. p. 151–72.

Dash AP, Bhatia R, Sunyoto T, Mourya DT. Emerging and re-emerging arboviral diseases in Southeast Asia. J Vector Borne Dis. 2013;50(2):77–84.

Feldmann H, Geisbert TW. Ebola hemorrhagic fever. Lancet. 2011;377(9768):849–62.

Goldsmith CS, Whistler T, Rollin PE, Ksiazek TG, Rota PA, Bellini WJ, et al. Elucidation of Nipah virus morphogenesis and replication using ultrastructural and molecular approaches. Virus Res. 2003;92(1):89–98.

Goldsmith CS, Ksiazek TG, Rollin PE, Comer JA, Nicholson WL, Peret TC, et al. Cell culture and electron microscopy for identifying viruses in diseases of unknown cause. Emerg Infect Dis. 2013;19(6):886–91.

Jaffe HW, Frankel SS. Kaposi's sarcoma and human herpesvirus 8. In: Horsburgh CR, Nelson AM, editors. Pathology of emerging infections. Washington, DC: ASM Press; 1997. p. 107–18.

Landry ML, Caliendo AM, Ginocchio CC, Tang Y-W, Valsamakis A. Algorithms for detection and identification of viruses. In: Jorgensen JH, Pfaller MA, Carroll KC, Funke G, Landry ML, Richter SS, et al. Manual of clinical microbiology, Vol. 2, 11th Ed. Washington, DC: ASM Press; 2015. pp. 1432–1436.

Mayer SV, Tesh RB, Vasilakis N. The emergence of arthropod-borne viral diseases: a global prospective on dengue, chikungunya and zika fevers. Acta Trop. 2016;166:155–63.

Miller SE. Electron microscopy of viral infections. In: Jerome KR, editor. Lennette's laboratory. Diagnosis of viral infections. 4th ed. Informa Healthcare: New York; 2010. p. 173–96.

Molina-Ruiz AM, Santonja C, Rütten A, Cerroni L, Kutzner H, Requena L. Immunohistochemistry in the diagnosis of cutaneous viral infections – part I. Cutaneous viral infections by herpesviruses and papillomaviruses. Am J Dermatopathol. 2015a;37 (1):1–14.

Molina-Ruiz AM, Santonja C, Rütten A, Cerroni L, Kutzner H, Requena L. Immunohistochemistry in the diagnosis of cutaneous viral infections – part II. Cutaneous viral infections by parvoviruses, poxviruses, paramyxoviridae, picornaviridae, retroviruses and filoviruses. Am J Dermatopathol. 2015b;37(2):93–106.

Peters CJ, Zaki SR. Hantavirus pulmonary syndrome. In: Horsburgh CR, Nelson AM, editors. Pathology of emerging infections. Washington, DC: ASM Press; 1997. p. 95–106.

Shibl A, Senok A, Memish Z. Infectious diseases in the Arabian Peninsula and Egypt. Clin Microbiol Infect. 2012;18(11):1068–80.

Solomon IH, Milner Jr DA. Histopathology of vaccine-preventable diseases. Histopathology. 2017;70(1):109–22.

Vasilakis N, Weaver SC. Flavivirus transmission focusing on Zika. Curr Opin Virol. 2016;22:30–5.

Zaki SR, Kilmarx PH. Ebola virus hemorrhagic fever. In: Horsburgh CR, Nelson AM, editors. Pathology of emerging infections. Washington, DC: ASM Press; 1997. p. 299–312.

Fungal Infections

4

Bryan H. Schmitt

Many fungal pathogens are ubiquitous in the environment as well as being human commensal organisms. Minor infections such as athlete's foot or other superficial dermatoses are very common but are relative inconveniences that are easily treated with over-the-counter antifungal preparations. Discounting superficial infections, fungal etiologies are an infrequently encountered cause of serious disease. However, with the increasing number of medical innovations that involve immunosuppressive therapy, patients are more frequently faced with life-threatening infections with typically opportunistic fungal pathogens. For the pathologist, fungal infections represent some of the most serious, rapidly progressive, and most difficult to treat infectious conditions. It is therefore paramount to have the ability to correctly categorize and eventually identify fungal pathogens. Some fungal infections, such as rhinocerebral zygomycosis, are particularly aggressive and require swift identification in order for the surgical and infectious disease teams to proceed appropriately.

This chapter will initially discuss specific fungi, beginning with the frequently encountered *Candida* species, and then progress to less encountered species that usually have very specific presentations. The dimorphic fungi as well as the hyaline fungi, including *Aspergillus* species, and the zygomycetes, and to an extent the dematiaceous fungi, have typical presentations but can also affect essentially any organ system. Therefore, the remainder of the chapter will focus on narrowing the causative agent to specific categories of fungal pathogens with further direction being given by fungal culture, special stains, or other ancillary testing.

B.H. Schmitt (✉)
Department of Pathology and Laboratory Medicine, Indiana University School of Medicine, Indianapolis, IN, USA
e-mail: bhschmit@iupui.edu

B.H. Schmitt (ed.), *Atlas of Infectious Disease Pathology*,
Atlas of Anatomic Pathology, DOI 10.1007/978-3-319-54702-2_4

4.1 Infections Caused by *Candida* Species

Candida species are likely the most frequently encountered fungi in the majority of anatomic pathology practices. Being normal flora, most of the time that these fungi are encountered they are representative of the normal microbiota of the patient and can be safely disregarded as such. In rare cases, particularly in immunocompromised patients, especially those who have received an organ transplant and in neonates, *Candida* can become a pathogen. Therefore, it is important to be able to recognize *Candida* species, both as a contaminant and when they are the likely cause of disease. *Candida* may also mimic several well-known fungal pathogens, notably *Histoplasma capsulatum* and *Malassezia* species. This is particularly a problem with *Candida glabrata,* which produces small round to oval yeasts without production of pseudohyphae, the presence of which is typically a strong indicator of *Candida* species. Gram staining, while usually utilized for the identification and classification of bacteria, can also prove useful in the identification of yeast. The majority of the time *Candida* species will retain the crystal violet stain and will appear purple, similar to a Gram-positive reaction. Other small round to oval yeast pathogens, such as *Histoplasma capsulatum,* do not generally retain the crystal violet stain and appear pink, similar to a Gram-negative reaction, or they do not stain at all. As discussed later, *Cryptococcus* species as well as *Sporothrix schenkii* complex can also partially retain the crystal-violet stain, often with a beaded or granular appearance. These genera of fungal pathogens have other distinguishing features that should help differentiate them from infection with *Candida* species (Figs. 4.1, 4.2, 4.3, and 4.4).

4.2 *Malassezia* Infections

Malassezia species are relatively commonly seen in superficial skin infections but are also rare agents of invasive fungal infection. The most commonly implicated species, *Malassezia furfur,* is seen most frequently in dermatologic specimens, in which it causes tinea versicolor as well as inflammatory dermatitis and a variety of other superficial skin infections. The yeast cells are very small, generally 2–3 microns, which may initially cause confusion with *Histoplasma capsulatum,* particularly if they are encountered in respiratory specimens. One distinguishing factor is that budding yeast forms of *Malassezia* species may demonstrate a characteristic "collarette" seen at the base of the bud. This creates the classic "bowling pin" or "Coke bottle" appearance. It is important that most but not all *Malassezia* species require long-chain fatty acids to grow. As such, if cultures are requested, the microbiology laboratory must be notified that a *Malassezia* species is suspected so that a lipid overlay, typically olive oil, can be placed on the culture plates. It is

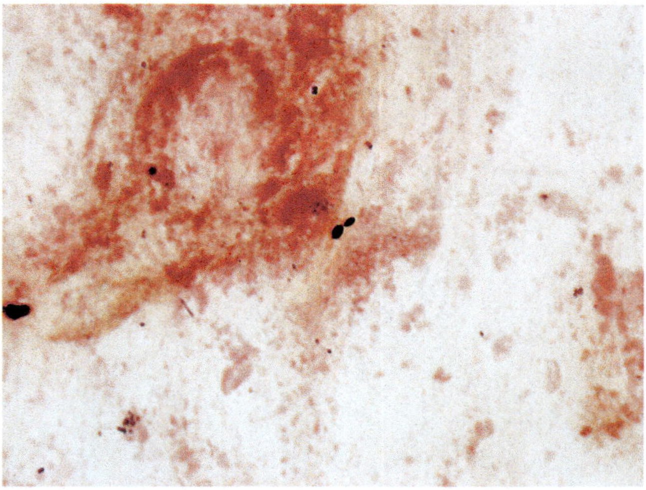

Fig. 4.1 Yeast forms of *Candida albicans* as seen on Gram stain of a sputum specimen. On a properly decolorized Gram stain, most pathogenic fungi, with the notable exceptions of *Candida* and *Cryptococcus* species and *Sporothrix schenkii* complex, do not retain the crystal violet stain and appear pink or nonstaining. This feature can at times be helpful with identification. 1000× magnification

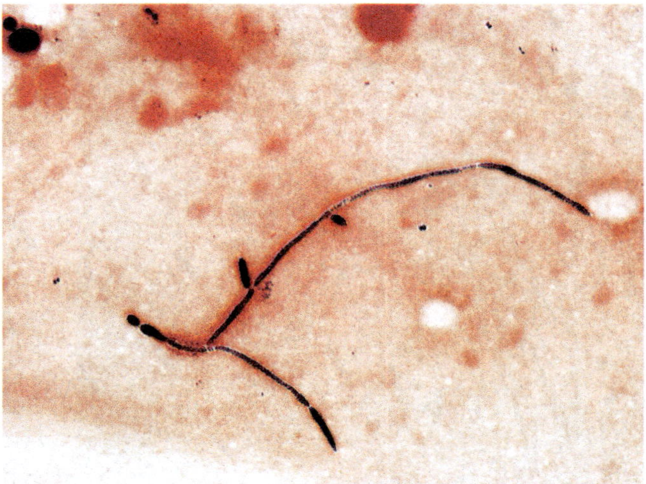

Fig. 4.2 Gram stain of a sputum specimen demonstrating pseudohyphae of *C. albicans,* which usually retain the crystal violet stain. Pseudohyphae generally demonstrate a pinched appearance at the "septations," which are truly boundaries between discrete budding cells with no connecting cytoplasm. 1000× magnification

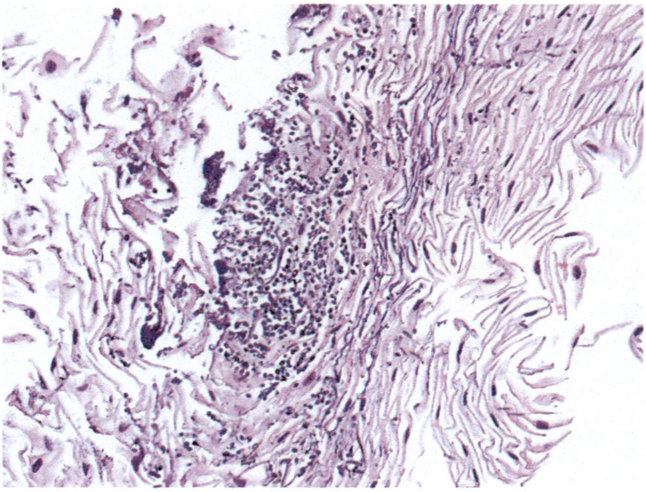

Fig. 4.3 *Candida* species are colonizers of the skin, gastrointestinal tract, and nearly every mucosal surface of the body. As such, it is important to recognize that they may be harmlessly present in surgical pathology specimens. Frank invasion, such as in this case of candidal esophagitis, is evidence that *Candida* is behaving in a pathogenic manner. Hematoxylin and eosin (H&E), 400× magnification

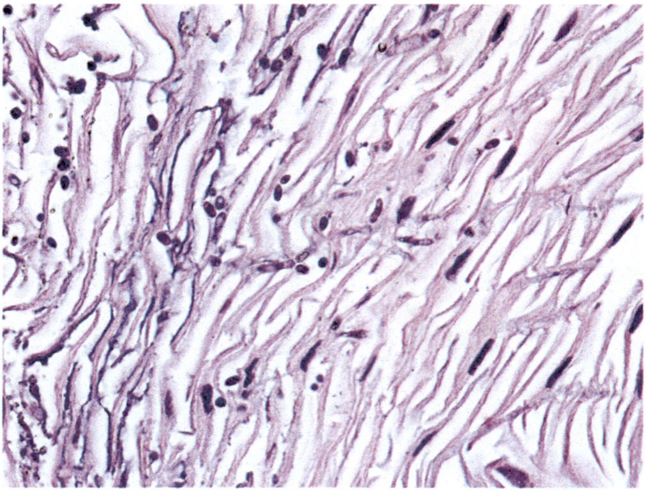

Fig. 4.4 Higher magnification image demonstrating pseudohyphae invading through the keratinized layers of esophageal tissue. H&E, 1000× magnification

important to note that total parenteral nutrition solutions often have a high lipid content, which may rarely create the opportunity for patients to develop systemic infections with *Malassezia* species (Figs. 4.5, 4.6, 4.7, 4.8, 4.9, 4.10, 4.11, and 4.12).

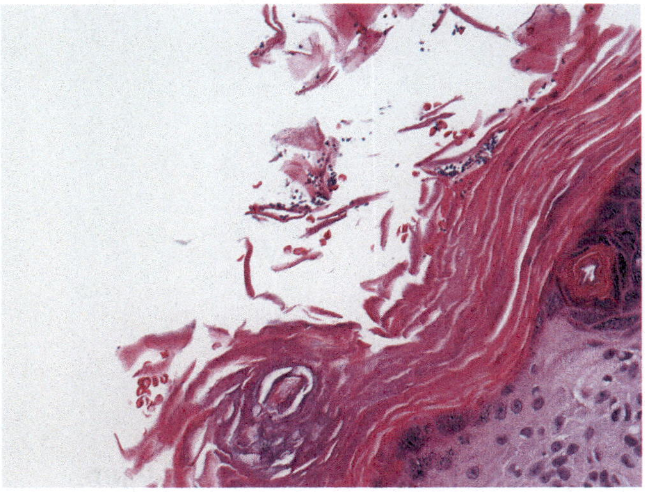

Fig. 4.5 Typical appearance of *Malassezia* species in the skin. Classically, the yeast cells are intermingled with thin hyphae, giving a "spaghetti and meatballs" appearance. The hyphae are better visualized using periodic acid–Schiff or Gomori methenamine silver staining. H&E, 400× magnification

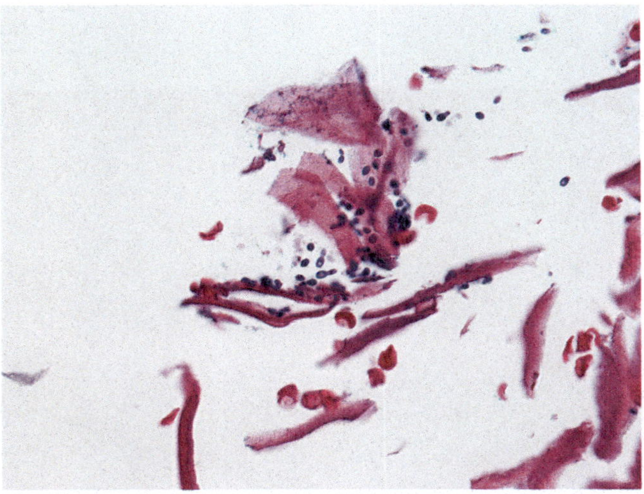

Fig. 4.6 Higher magnification demonstrating the prominent collarette (*center of image*) characteristic of *Malassezia* species. H&E, 1000× magnification

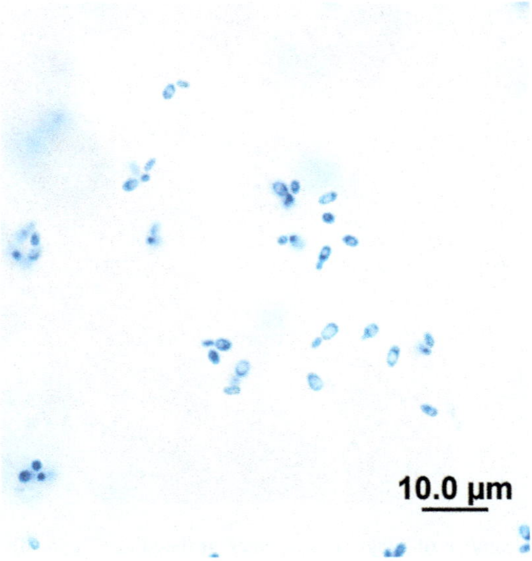

Fig. 4.7 Lactophenol cotton blue preparation of cultured *M. furfur*. Note the small size, generally 2–3 microns, and the prominent collarette, appearing here as a clear space between the bud and mother cells. 1000× magnification

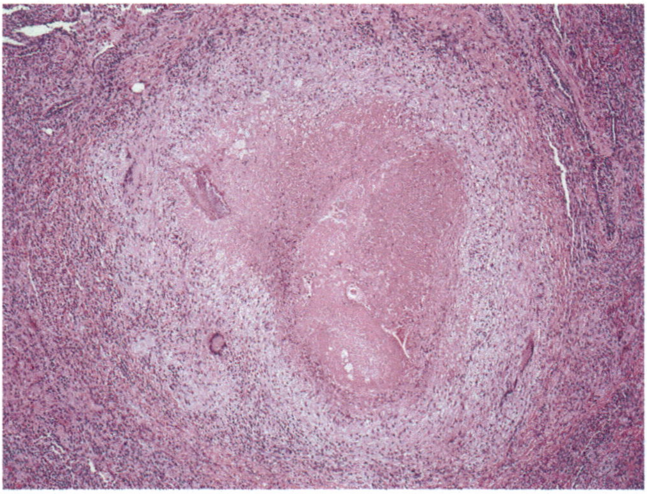

Fig. 4.8 Necrotizing granulomas seen in a lung infection with *M. furfur*. This patient was on total parenteral nutrition owing to short gut syndrome. H&E, 100×

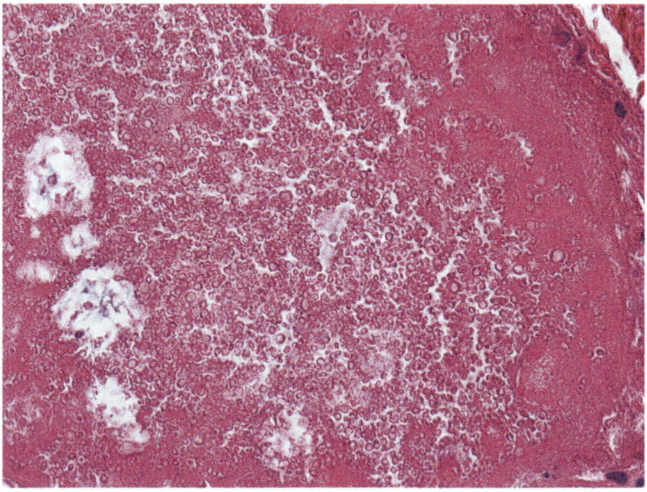

Fig. 4.9 At higher magnification, numerous eosinophilic yeast forms of *M. furfur* can be seen within the necrotic portion of a granuloma. H&E, 1000×

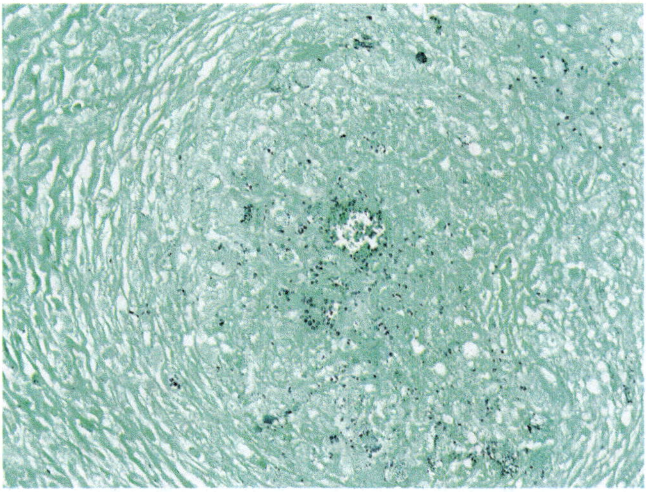

Fig. 4.10 At first glance, these small round to oval yeast cells appear very similar in size and shape to the yeast forms of *Histoplasma capsulatum*. Both are also found predominantly within necrotizing and non-necrotizing granulomas. Gomori methenamine silver stain, 400× magnification

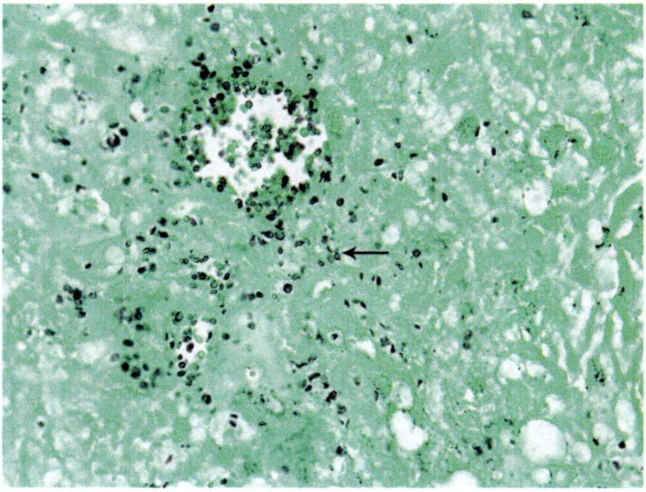

Fig. 4.11 At higher magnification, prominent collarette formation can be seen in some of the yeast cells (*arrow*). If the identification is still uncertain, additional ancillary patient testing, such as histoplasma antigen assays, may be helpful to rule out other pathogens. Gomori methenamine silver stain, 1000× magnification

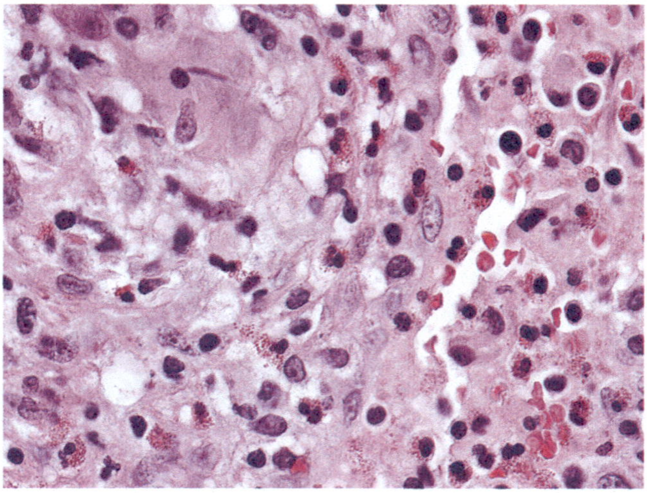

Fig. 4.12 Both superficial and systemic infections with *M. furfur* can elicit a strong eosinophilic response, as seen here in a lung wedge resection from a patient with *M. furfur* infection. H&E, 1000× magnification

4.3 Cryptococcal Infections

Cryptococcal infections are most commonly caused by the species *Cryptococcus neoformans* and *Cryptococcus gatti*, although others, including *C. laurentii* and *C. albidus,* have also been implicated. Pathogenic *Cryptococcus* species nearly always demonstrate a true capsule which, along with considerable size variation (generally from 2 to 15 microns), is a diagnostic feature of the organism. The capsule is usually easily visualized on histopathologic examination, but it is important to note that capsule-deficient cryptococci can occasionally be seen. Cryptococcal infections are most frequently identified in the lungs and within the central nervous system of immunocompromised individuals. However, it is also important to mention that this organism has the capacity to infect virtually every organ system. India ink staining, particularly from cerebrospinal fluid, is the classic rapid method of identification from clinical specimens, however, sensitivity is poor, between 40% and 60%. Cryptococcal antigen detection, which can be performed on a variety of different specimen types including cerebrospinal fluid, pleural fluid, serum, and urine, is the current best available adjunct method for rapid identification of cryptococcal infections (Figs. 4.13, 4.14, 4.15, 4.16, 4.17, 4.18, 4.19, and 4.20).

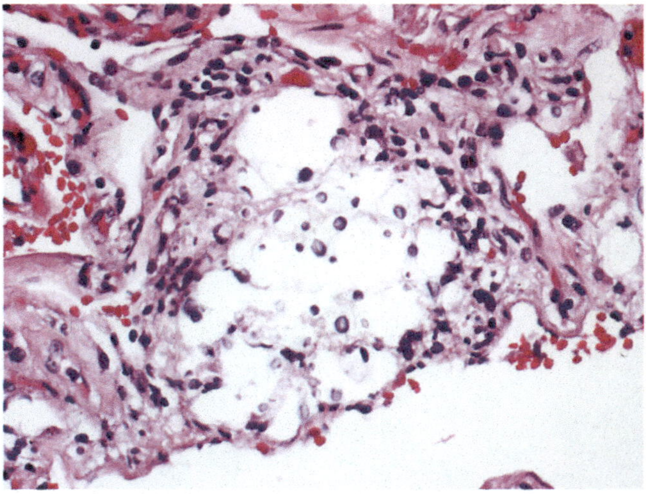

Fig. 4.13 Cryptococcosis of the lung. The basophilic staining cryptococcal yeast demonstrates considerable size variation, which is a hallmark of this organism. Also note the very prominent clearing or halo surrounding the organism, which is representative of the capsule. The absence of such a capsule does not rule out the presence of *Cryptococcus* species, since capsule-deficient cryptococci may also be infrequently encountered. H&E, 600× magnification

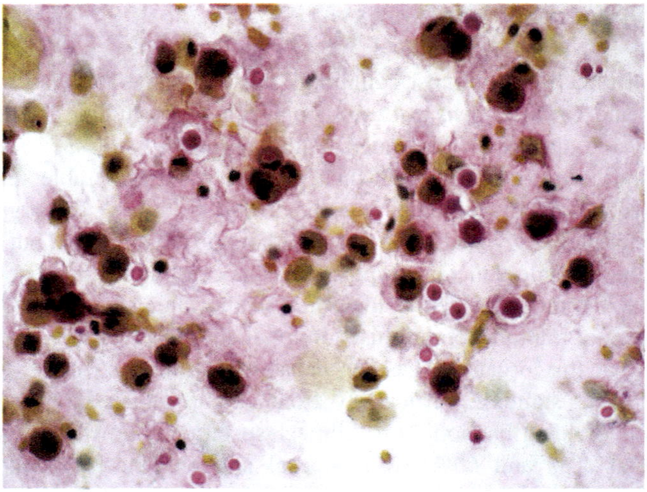

Fig. 4.14 Stains for mucin, such as mucicarmine and alcian blue, may highlight the capsule in cases where cryptococcal infection is suspected. Capsule-deficient organisms may demonstrate faint or absent staining using these methods. Shown here is a bronchoalveolar lavage specimen demonstrating prominent bright red staining of *Cryptococcus neoformans* with mucicarmine. 600× magnification

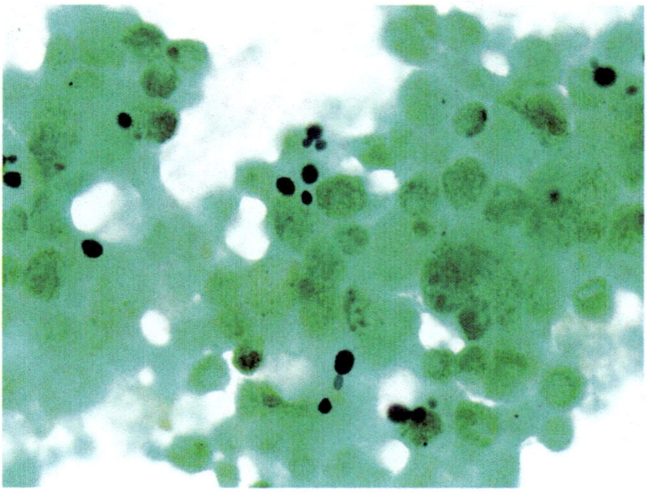

Fig. 4.15 Gomori methenamine silver stain of bronchoalveolar lavage fluid demonstrating *Cryptococcus* species. The prominent capsule that is easily visualized on most other stains is not typically apparent using fungal silver staining methods. Note, however, that the typical size variation remains present. 1000× magnification

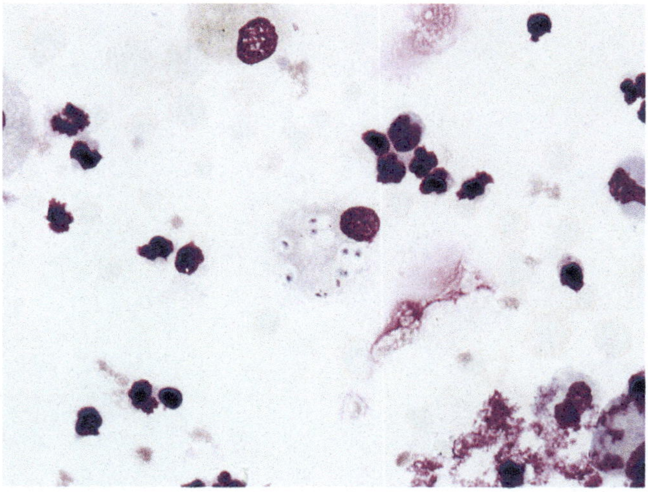

Fig. 4.16 Intracellular cryptococcal yeast. Prominent capsules can be seen even when engulfed in phagocytic cells. Giemsa stain, 1000× magnification

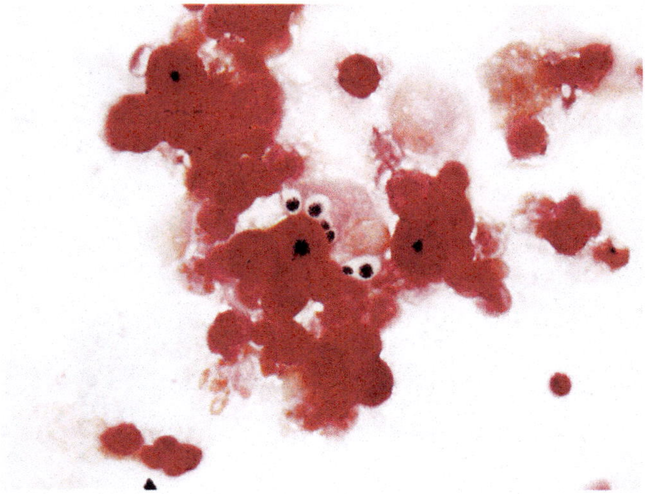

Fig. 4.17 Gram stain of intracellular *Cryptococcus* from a bronchoalveolar lavage specimen. Note that like *Candida* species, *Cryptococcus* retains the crystal violet stain, although typically to a lesser extent, appearing to have beaded or granular staining. Capsules surrounding the organisms are usually readily apparent. 1000× magnification

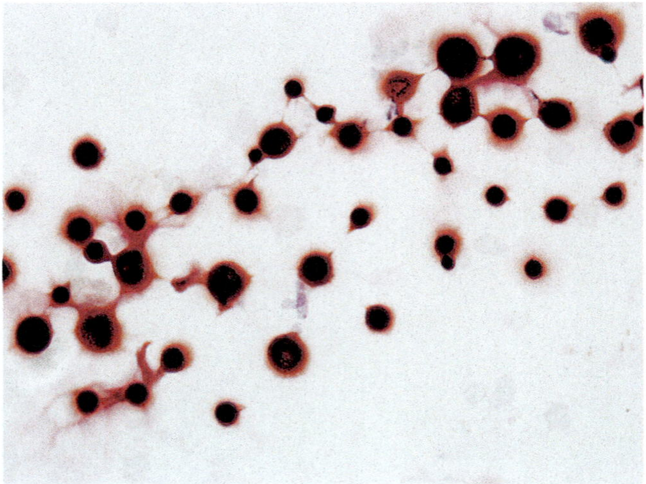

Fig. 4.18 Gram stain of cerebrospinal fluid demonstrating *Cryptococcus neoformans*. Note the significant size variability and partial retention of the crystal violet stain. Threadlike connections between the yeast cells can be seen, particularly in cerebrospinal fluid specimens, which represent retention of the safranin stain by mucoid capsular material. 1000× magnification

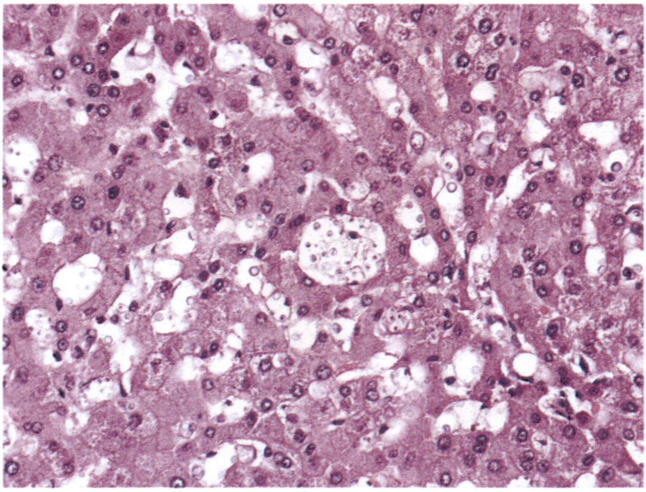

Fig. 4.19 Cryptococcal infection of the liver. As previously mentioned, *Cryptococcus* species can infect nearly any body site, with the liver perhaps being the most frequent behind pulmonary and central nervous system infections. In this case, the characteristic size variation and prominent capsules are present. H&E, 400× magnification

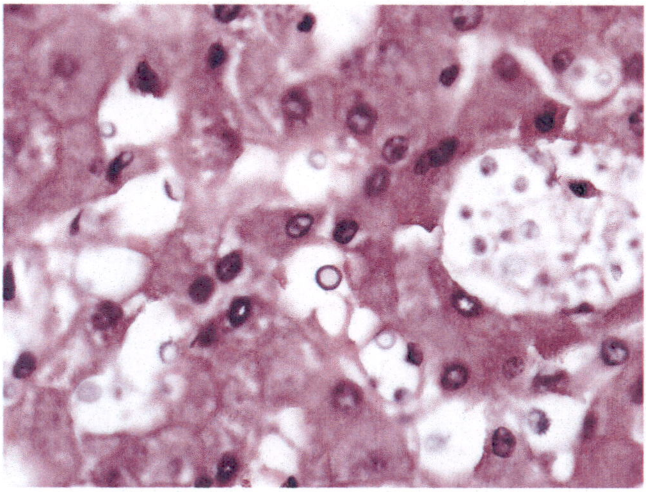

Fig. 4.20 In a higher magnification image from the case demonstrated in Fig. 4.19, *Cryptococcus* species may sometimes demonstrate a thick wall reminiscent of *Blastomyces* species. Significant size variation not usually seen in *Blastomyces* infections as well as the presence of a capsule in the majority of infections should provide evidence for identification of one genus over the other despite some overlap in size between the organisms

4.4 *Pneumocystis jirovecii*

Pneumocystis jirovecii (formerly *Pneumocystis carinii*) is a yeast-like fungal pathogen that was originally thought to be a protozoan parasite. It is most commonly seen as a cause of pneumonia in patients infected with human immunodeficiency virus but was first identified in malnourished children. The organism may colonize both immunocompetent and immunocompromised people and as such, when it is present in low numbers consideration must be given to the possibility that the organisms may not be the cause of disease. Cyst forms are best visualized in fungal stains such as Gomori methenamine silver, while trophozoite (or trophic) forms are best seen using Romanowsky stains such as Giemsa and Diff-Quik. The terms cyst and trophozoite are holdovers from the previous classification as a protozoan parasite, but they do denote that there is a poorly understood replicative phase (trophozoite) of *Pneumocystis* that develops, at least in part, inside of a protective shell (cyst). As the organism cannot be routinely grown using standard laboratory methods, essentially requiring a living host for growth, identification requires microscopic findings or the use of molecular assays. Although classified as a fungus, *P. jirovecii* is not susceptible to traditional antifungal agents. Treatment instead relies on predominantly antibacterial agents such as trimethoprim/sulfamethoxazole or pentamidine (Figs. 4.21, 4.22, 4.23, 4.24, 4.25, 4.26, 4.27, and 4.28).

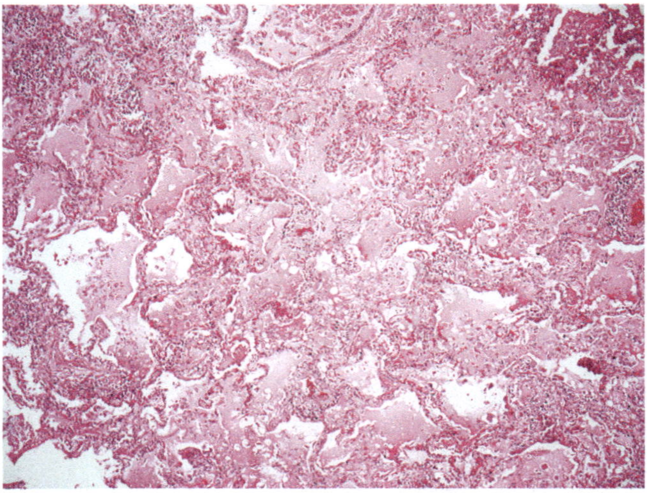

Fig. 4.21 Low magnification image of lung tissue demonstrating the characteristic pattern of pneumocystis pneumonia. Note the eosinophilic, proteinaceous casts that nearly fill the alveolar spaces in a diffuse pattern. Note also that alveolar proteinosis may have a similar appearance, but fungal stains such as Gomori methenamine silver can be used to definitively identify *P. jirovecii*. H&E, 100× magnification

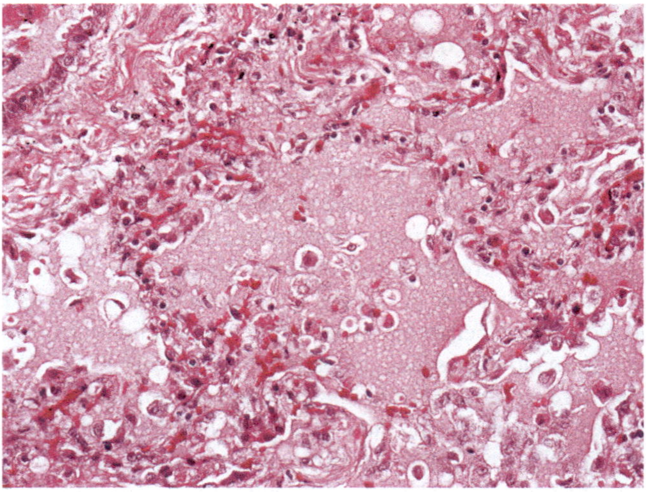

Fig. 4.22 Higher magnification image demonstrating the intra-alveolar proteinaceous casts associated with pneumocystis pneumonia. The casts are often described as having a foamy or "cotton-candy" appearance. H&E, 400× magnification

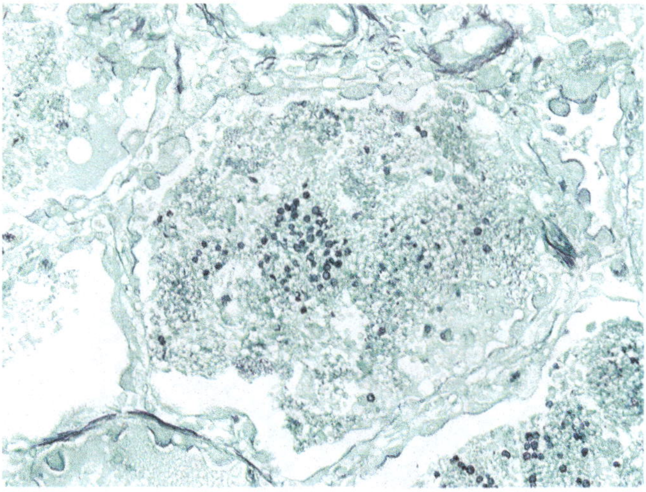

Fig. 4.23 Gomori methenamine silver staining of the case illustrated in the previous two figures. On staining, the cyst forms of *P. jirovecii* are highlighted, measuring approximately 6–8 microns in diameter and demonstrating a characteristic "teacup and saucer" appearance, or, as the author prefers, a "crushed ping-pong ball" appearance. Not highlighted by the stain are the trophozoite forms intermingled with the cysts. 400× magnification

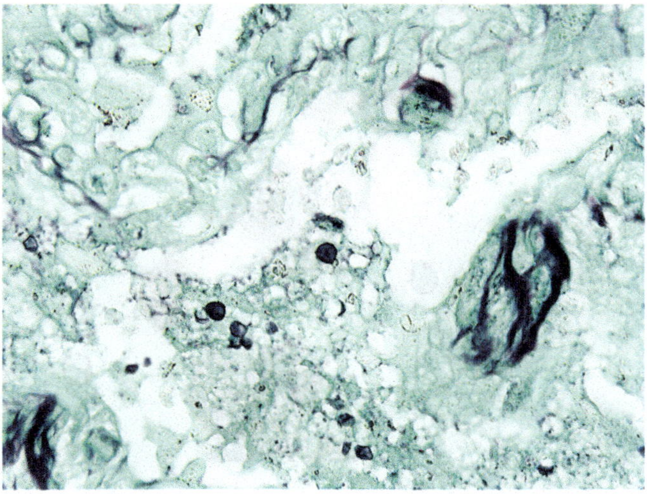

Fig. 4.24 On Gomori methenamine silver staining, two comma-shaped intracystic bodies may occasionally be seen within the cyst forms (*center of image*). These often coalesce into a centrally located dark spot, which may give the cyst form a "target" shape. 1000× magnification

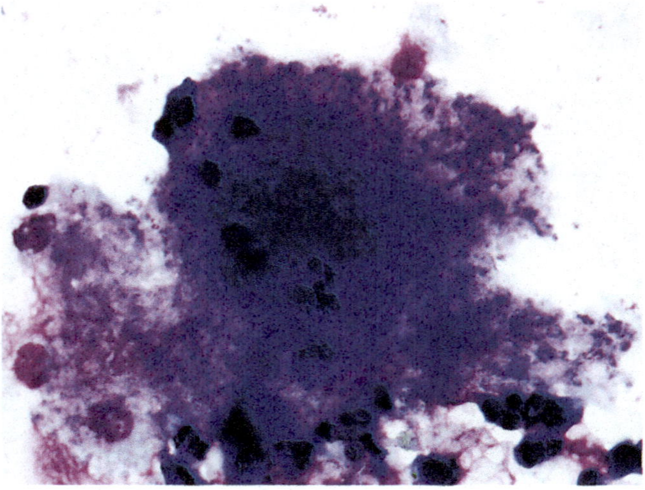

Fig. 4.25 On cytologic touch and fluid preparations such as bronchoalveolar lavage, seen here, the proteinaceous casts frequently retain their shape. Romanowsky stains such as Giemsa most prominently demonstrate purple, dot-like, nuclear staining of the trophozoite forms of pneumocystis. Giemsa stain, 1000× magnification

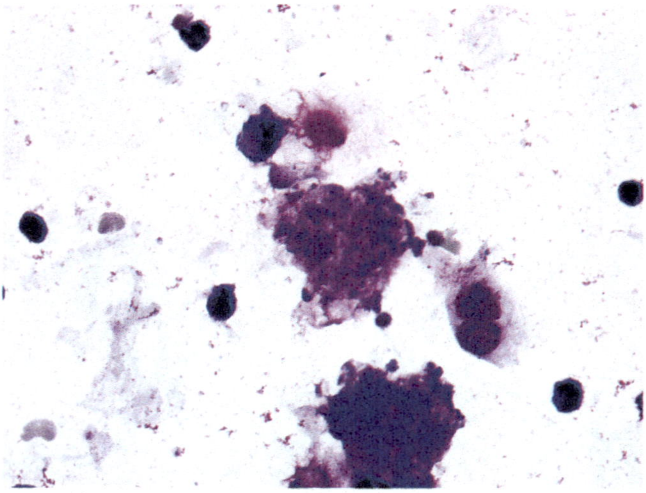

Fig. 4.26 On Giemsa staining, the cyst forms of *P. jirovecii* can sometimes be identified as pale staining or "negative image" bodies intermixed with trophozoite forms. Giemsa stain, 1000× magnification

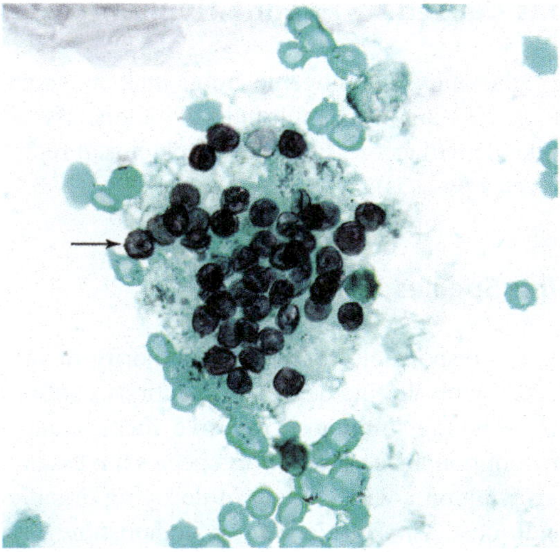

Fig. 4.27 Gomori methenamine silver staining demonstrating a cluster of *P. jirovecii* cyst forms in a bronchoalveolar lavage specimen. Note the "crushed ping-pong ball" appearance and the presence of several target forms (*one of which is denoted by the arrow*). 1000× magnification

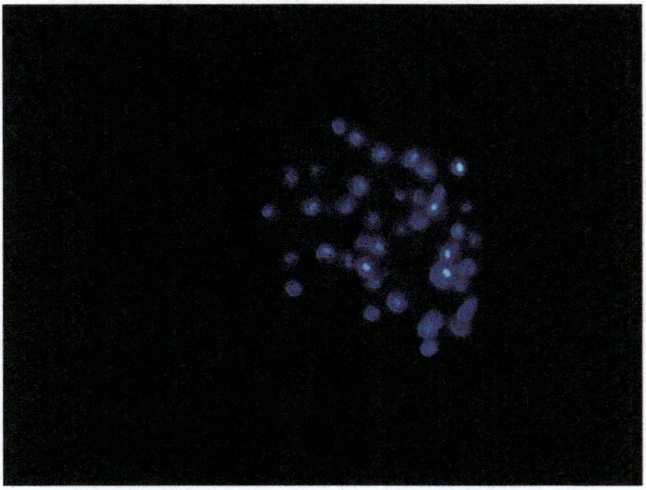

Fig. 4.28 Calcoflour white staining (CFW) of *P. jirovecii* demonstrates the characteristic outline of the cyst forms against a dark background. Bright fluorescence of two comma-shaped intracystic bodies is seen in some of the cysts and allows for definitive identification of *P. jirovecii*. CFW staining typically produces a great deal of background fluorescence if attempted in tissue sections. However, its use in respiratory fluids usually provides good contrast and allows for visualization of these distinguishing features. 600× magnification

4.5 Infections Caused by Hyaline Hyphomycetes

Hyaline (meaning "glass-like") pathogenic fungi include *Aspergillus*, *Fusarium*, and *Scedosporium* species among a multitude of others. By definition, they are nonpigmented (unlike dematiaceous fungi) and lack closed reproductive structures (which the zygomycetes possess).

4.5.1 *Aspergillus* Species Infections

Aspergillus species are responsible for the vast majority of infections caused by hyaline hyphomycetes, with the incidence of infections continually increasing as medical treatments including immunosuppressive therapy and organ transplants have become more commonplace. *Aspergillus* species are essentially ubiquitous in the environment, growing on a wide variety of decaying organic material and in a wide range of conditions. *Aspergillus* species demonstrate septate hyphae with parallel walls, generally 2–6 microns in width and branching at predominantly acute angles. However, it should be noted that other hyaline hyphomycetes, such as *Fusarium* and *Scedosporium* species, may also have overlapping characteristics. In the absence of "fruiting bodies" of *Aspergillus* or characteristic conidia of other genera, definitive identification by microscopy is unreliable, and other common hyaline fungi should be considered. The reader is also cautioned that under the varying conditions present within the human body, growth of hyphae through tissues, exposure to antifungals, and a multitude of other factors, fungal hyphae identified in histopathologic sections often do not obey the rules of morphology seen in optimal laboratory cultures. As a result, identification by morphology alone is further complicated, and therefore culture is recommended for definitive identification whenever possible (Figs. 4.29, 4.30, 4.31, 4.32, 4.33, 4.34, 4.35, 4.36, 4.37, 4.38, 4.39, and 4.40).

4.5.2 Infections with Other Hyaline Fungi (Figs. 4.41, 4.42, 4.43, 4.44, 4.45, 4.46, 4.47, 4.48, 4.49, 4.50, 4.51, 4.52, and 4.53)

4.6 Infections Caused by Zygomycetes

The zygomycetes are hyaline, filamentous fungi that are infrequent pathogens of humans, particularly affecting the immunocompromised patient. While often tied to immunosuppression resulting from organ or stem cell transplantations, another important predisposing factor relates to patients in the midst of or recovering from diabetic ketoacidosis. Zygomycete infections tend to demonstrate wider hyphae, generally 7–15 microns or more, with wide or variable angle branching

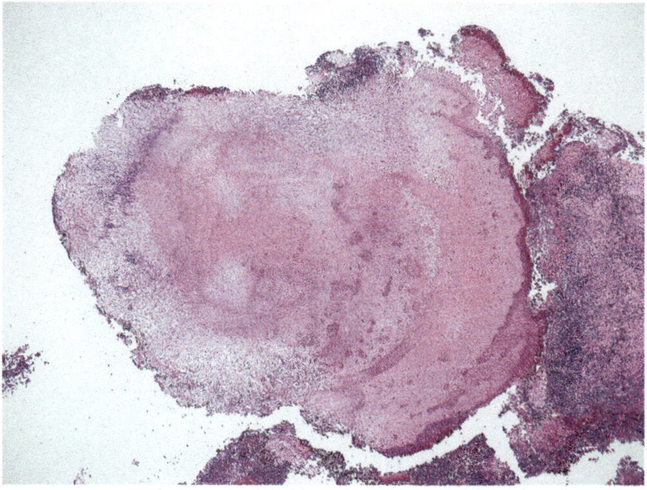

Fig. 4.29 At low magnification, clusters of *Aspergillus* may demonstrate a layered appearance very similar to that of a sulfur granule produced by an actinomycete. Lung, H&E, 40× magnification

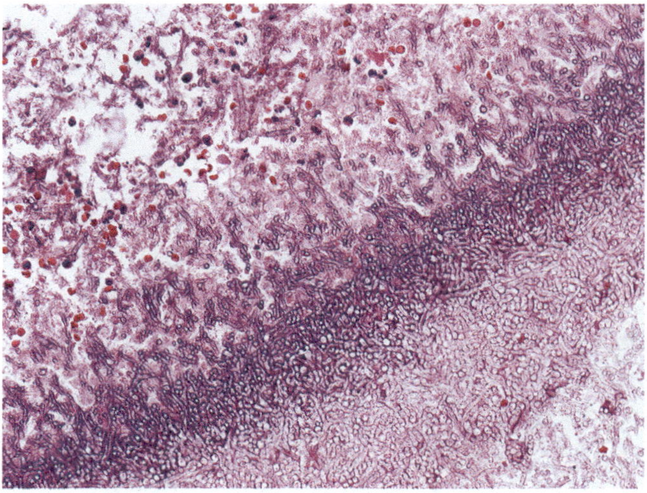

Fig. 4.30 At higher magnification, mats of hyphae much wider than typical bacterial elements are evident. Note that the typical acute or 45-degree angle branching of the hyphae associated with *Aspergillus* species is difficult to discern. In fact, when found in the body, *Aspergillus* often does not adhere to this commonly accepted rule for identification. H&E, 400× magnification

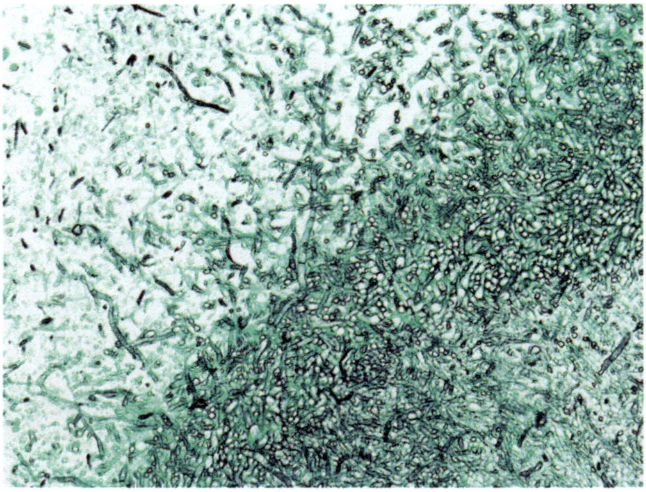

Fig. 4.31 Gomori methenamine silver staining of aspergillosis of the lung. Note mats of hyphae with frequent septations. This is the most common appearance of *Aspergillus* infection. Although *Aspergillus* is the most common pathogenic hyaline hyphomycete, the characteristic fruiting bodies of the species are infrequently found in real world tissue specimens, rendering definitive identification of the fungal organism impossible from microscopy alone. 400× magnification

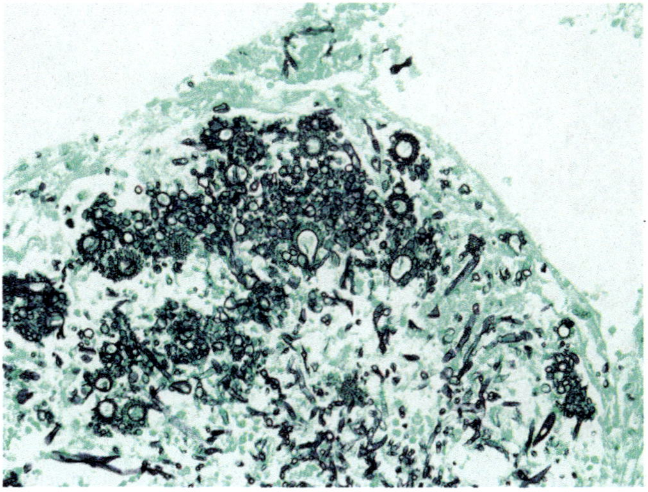

Fig. 4.32 Only rarely can conidiophores or fruiting bodies of *Aspergillus* be seen, allowing for definitive identification of the fungal pathogen to genus level. Gomori methenamine silver, lung biopsy, 400× magnification

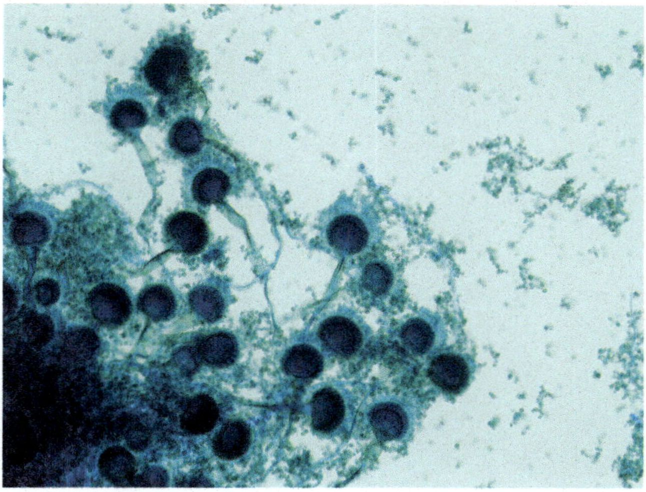

Fig. 4.33 Lactophenol cotton blue tape preparation of an *Aspergillus fumigatus* colony grown from fungal culture. Note the characteristic fruiting bodies. The conidiophores, phialides, and conidia of the many *Aspergillus* species demonstrate different characteristics, allowing them to be speciated on culture preparations such as those shown here. Identification beyond genus level by the examination of histologic sections is very unreliable and should be left to determination by fungal culture. 400× magnification

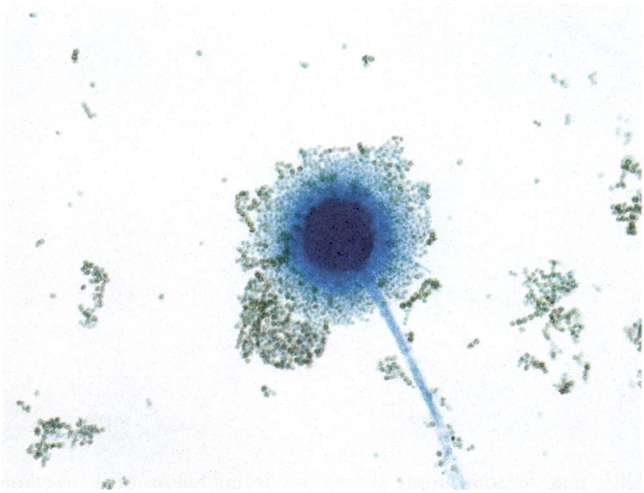

Fig. 4.34 For example, *Aspergillus flavus*, probably the second most prevalent pathogen of the *Aspergillus* species, usually demonstrates a larger fruiting body than *A. fumigatus*, with a rough-appearing conidiophore or "stalk" and conidia bearing phialides that typically surround the vesicle. Lactophenol cotton blue, 400× magnification

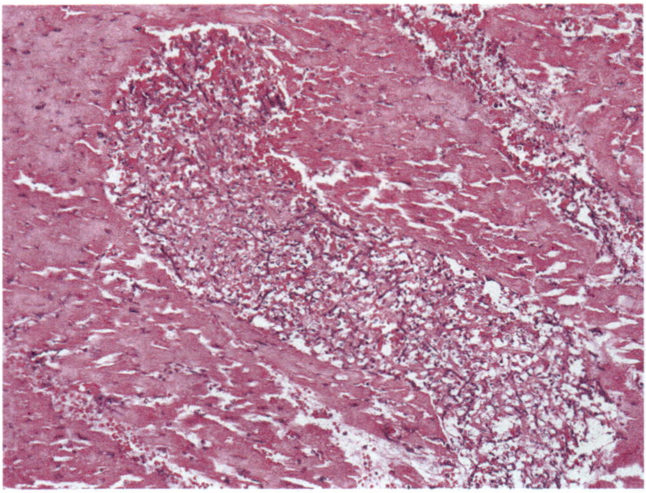

Fig. 4.35 While primarily a respiratory pathogen, it is important to note that *Aspergillus* species can invade every organ system. Seen here is invasion of the cardiac muscle identified at autopsy. H&E, 200× magnification

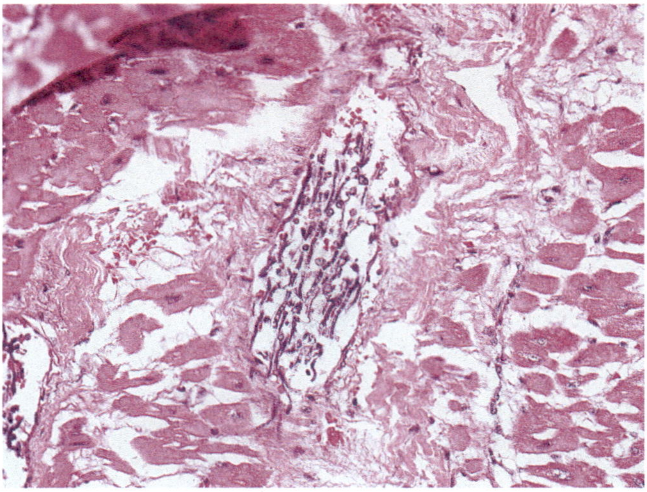

Fig. 4.36 Higher magnification image demonstrating infiltration of *Aspergillus* species into cardiac blood vessels. *Aspergillus* species can be angioinvasive, particularly in immunocompromised individuals. H&E, 400× magnification

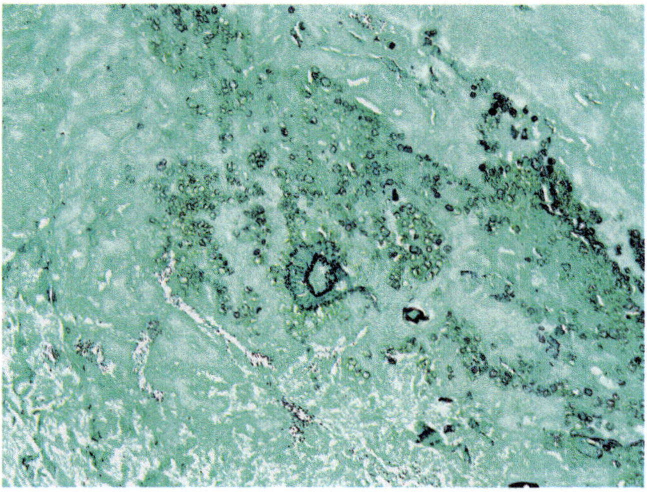

Fig. 4.37 Seen here is a fruiting body of *Aspergillus* species and multiple conidia, later identified by culture as *A. fumigatus*, from a biopsy of a nasal fungus ball. As previously stated, fruiting bodies are infrequently identified in tissue sections. Gomori methenamine silver stain, 400× magnification

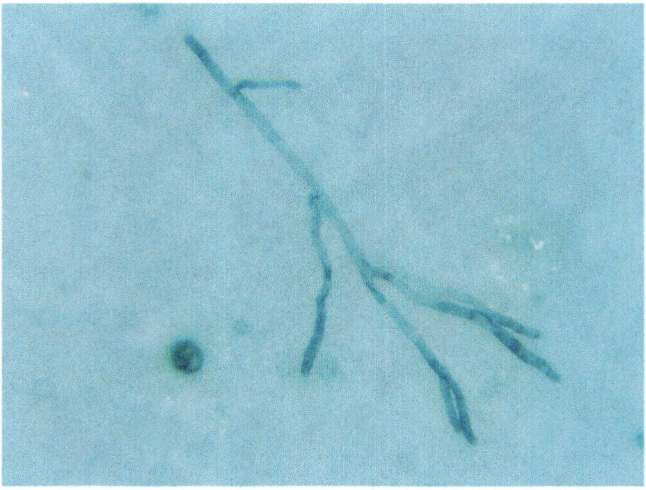

Fig. 4.38 Hyphae of *Aspergillus* species as seen on Gomori methenamine silver stain of brochoalveolar lavage fluid. Note the septate hyphae with parallel walls and acute angle branching. 400× magnification (Image courtesy of Dr. Timothy Walls)

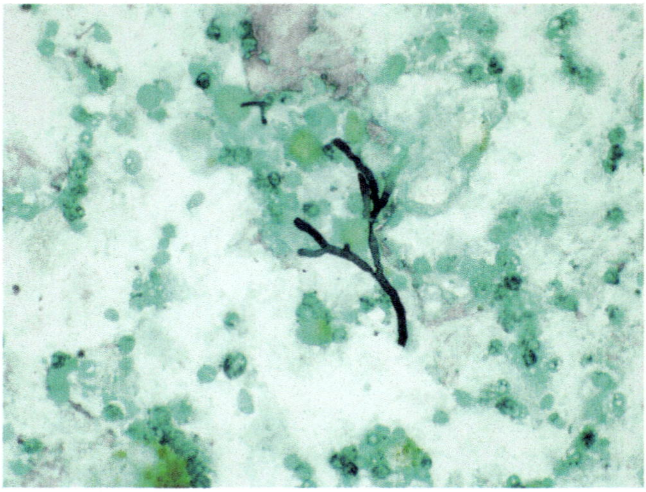

Fig. 4.39 Another example of *Aspergillus* hyphae seen on Gomori methenamine silver staining. Note acute angle branching and septate hyphae. Some species of *Aspergillus*, notably *A. flavus,* can demonstrate significant hyphal size and shape variation and may even appear pauciseptate, features associated with the zygomycetes, necessitating the need for culture to allow for definitive identification. 600× magnification

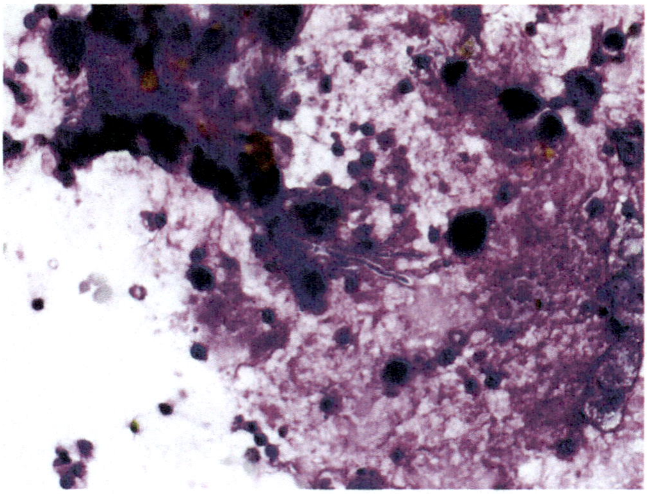

Fig. 4.40 Hyphae can also be visualized using traditional Romanowsky staining methods, such as the Diff-Quik stain shown here on a bronchoalveolar lavage specimen. 600× magnification

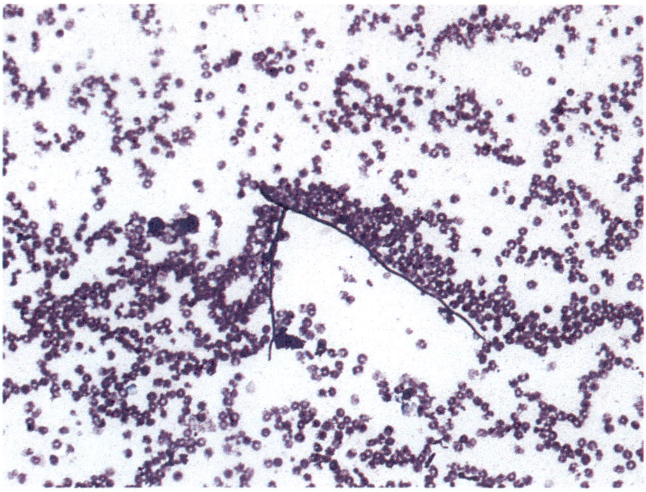

Fig. 4.41 *Fusarium* species is likely the most common, nondimorphic, hyaline fungal pathogen behind *Aspergillus* species. It is often implicated in ocular infections, as is *Aspergillus* species, but it may cause disease in virtually any organ system. Notably, invasive infections with *Fusarium* may sometimes result in positive blood cultures from which the organism can be grown, which is a rare finding among other fungal pathogens, with the notable exceptions of *Candida* species and *Histoplasma capsulatum*. While branching patterns tend to be more variable, like other hyaline fungi definitive identification without visualization of characteristic conidia is impossible. Giemsa stain, blood culture, 400× magnification

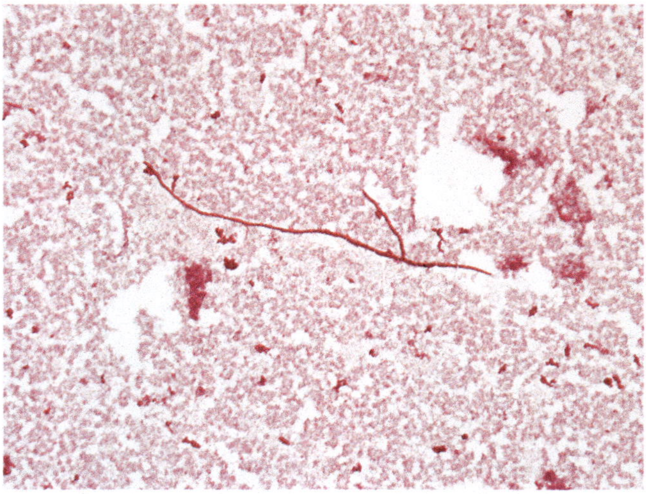

Fig. 4.42 As demonstrated here, most fungal hyphae do not retain the crystal violet stain following decolorization. This feature can be helpful in distinguishing them from hyphal or pseudohyphal elements of *Candida* species. *Fusarium* species, blood culture, Gram stain 400× magnification

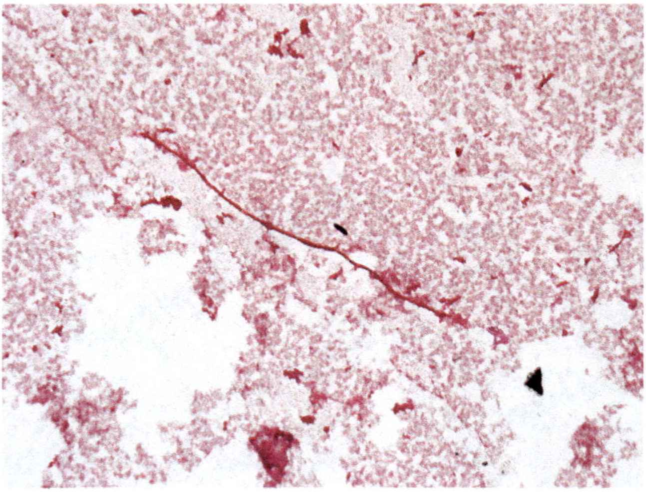

Fig. 4.43 A second Gram stain of *Fusarium* species. Note that while the hyphae do not retain the crystal violet stain, the adjacent characteristic canoe-shaped macroconidia do. The size and characteristic shape of the macroconidia allowed for presumptive identification of *Fusarium* species in this case. Blood culture, 400× magnification

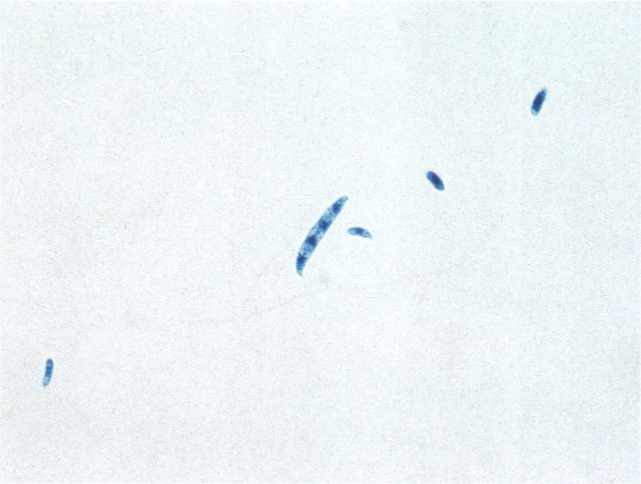

Fig. 4.44 Lactophenol cotton blue preparation from fungal culture demonstrating the characteristic canoe-shaped septate macroconidia of *Fusarium* species. 1000× magnification

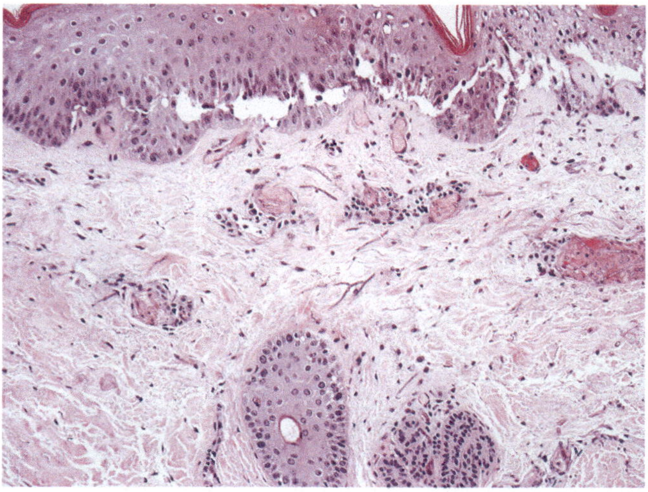

Fig. 4.45 A case of fusariosis that has disseminated to the skin. Hyphae are visible in the upper dermis. H&E, 200× magnification

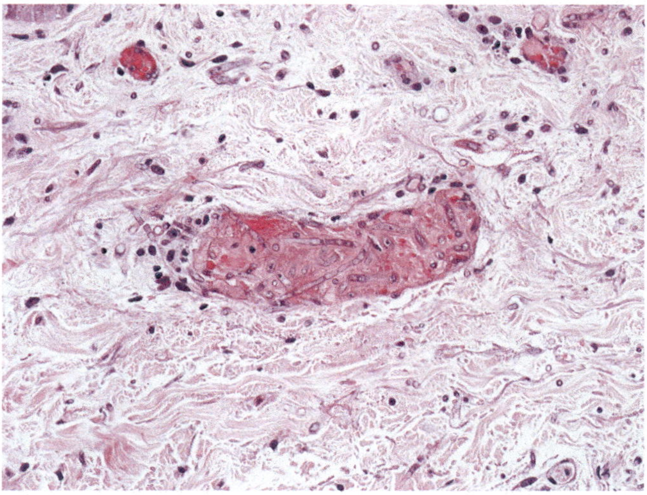

Fig. 4.46 As with many other hyaline hyphomycetes, vascular invasion is commonly seen in cases of disseminated fusariosis. 400× magnification

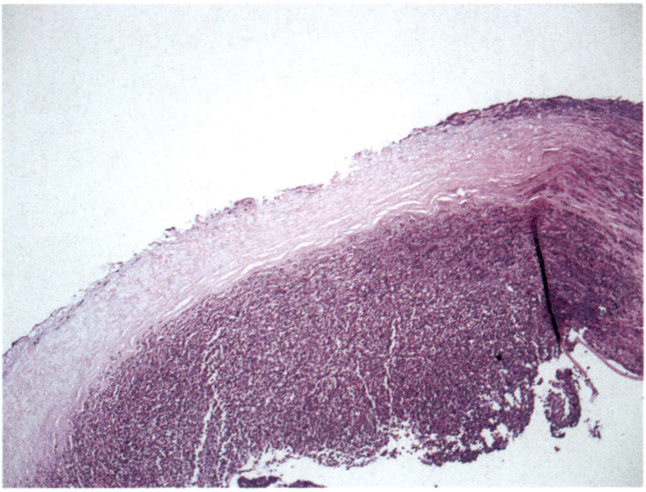

Fig. 4.47 Fungal keratitis caused by *Fusarium* species. Note destruction of the corneal epithelium and an intense acute inflammatory infiltrate. *Fusarium, Aspergillus,* and *Candida* species are the most commonly encountered etiologic agents of fungal keratitis. Dematiaceous fungi, such as *Alternaria,* are also seen with some frequency in certain parts of the world. H&E, 100 magnification

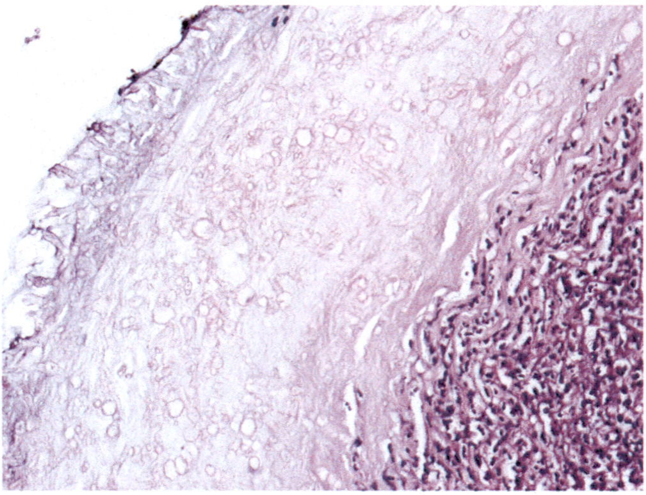

Fig. 4.48 Higher magnification image demonstrating fungal hyphae and accompanying acute inflammation. As in many cases of tissue invasion with fungal hyaline hyphomycetes, they tend to take on bizarre shapes, sometimes producing swollen-appearing chlamydoconidia-like structures. H&E, 400× magnification

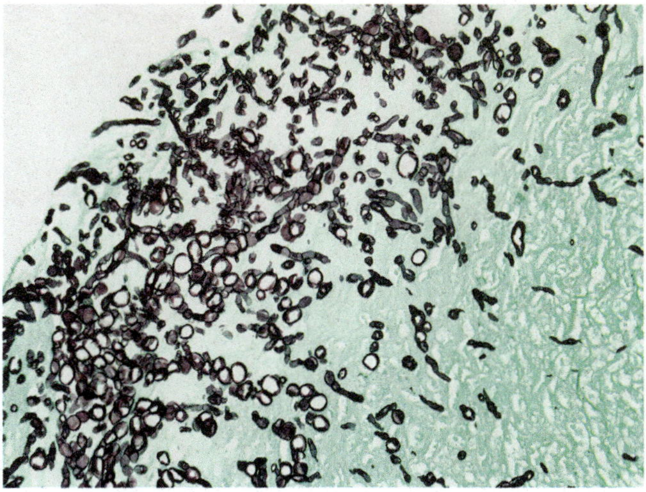

Fig. 4.49 Gomori methenamine silver staining of the same case from the previous two figures highlighting irregular-appearing fungal hyphae and chlamydoconidia-like structures. 400× magnification

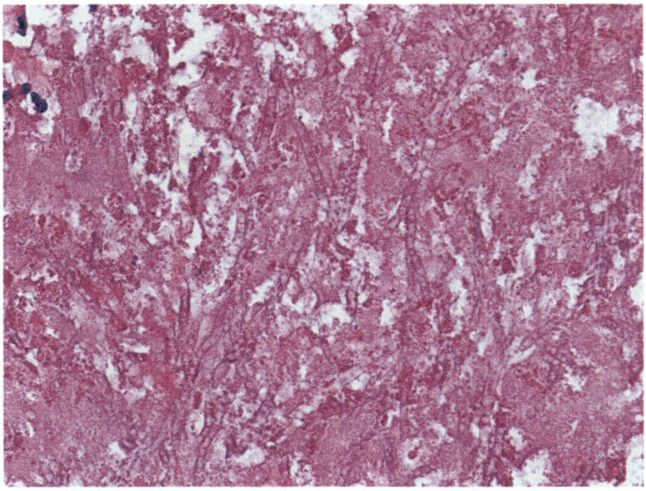

Fig. 4.50 Septate hyphae exhibiting predominantly acute angle branching seen in sections of thrombus obtained from an aortic arch thrombectomy. These findings were originally attributed to fungal endocarditis caused by *Aspergillus* species; however, fungal cultures grew *Scopulariopsis brevicaulis,* illustrating that hyaline fungi in tissues cannot be accurately distinguished by hyphal features alone. H&E, 400× magnification (Image courtesy of Dr. Timothy Walls)

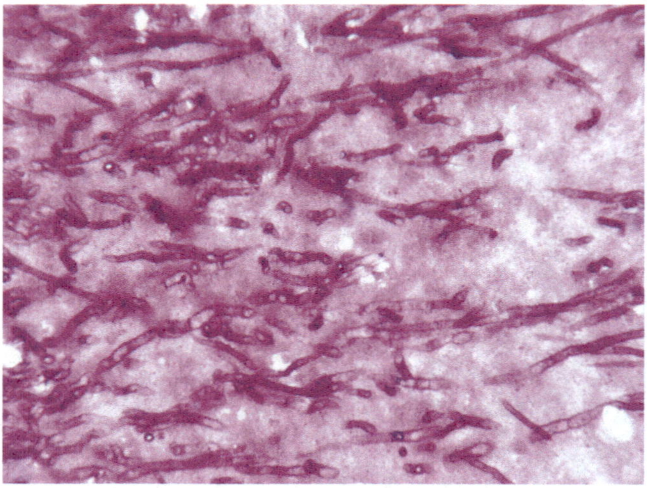

Fig. 4.51 Periodic acid–Schiff staining appearance of *Scopulariopsis brevicaulis* from the same case. Note septate hyphae with predominantly acute angle branching and parallel walls very similar to what would be expected to be seen in *Aspergillus* species. 400× magnification (Image courtesy of Dr. Timothy Walls)

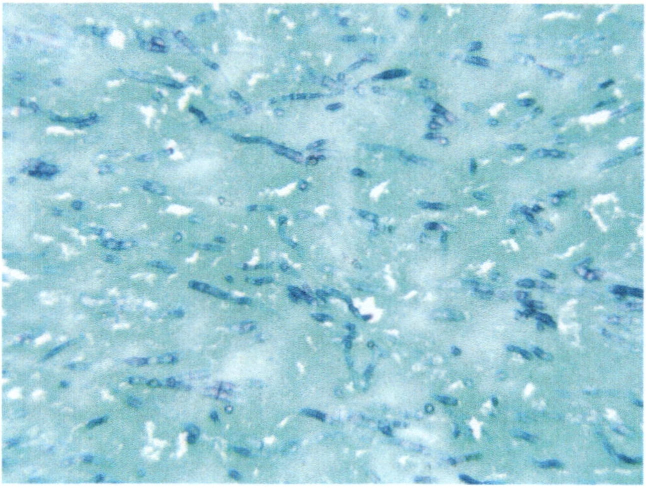

Fig. 4.52 Gomori methenamine silver staining of *Scopulariopsis brevicaulis* from the previously discussed case. Again, note the similarities in the hyphal appearance between *Aspergillus* species and other hyaline fungi. 400× magnification (Image courtesy of Dr. Timothy Walls)

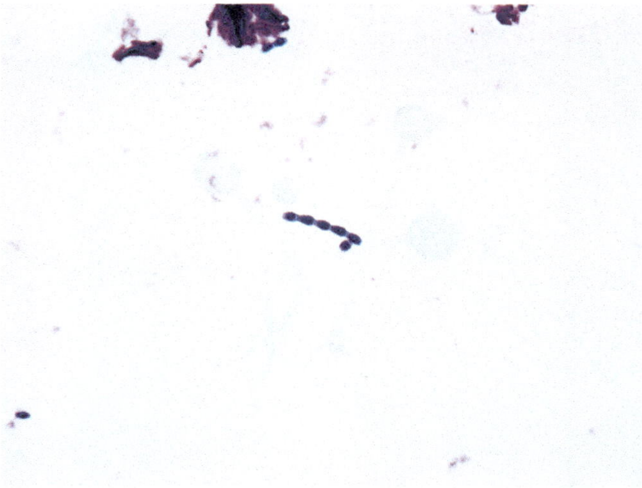

Fig. 4.53 A chain of "light-bulb" shaped conidia suggestive of *Scopulariopsis* species demonstrated on a corneal scraping. As with almost every pathogenic hyaline mold, characteristic structures such as these are nearly always absent on histopathologic sections. Giemsa stain, 1000× magnification

and nonparallel walls. The hyphae are often described as twisting or ribbon-like. Older texts often describe zygomycete hyphae as aseptate, but the term "pauciseptate" describes the appearance of the hyphae more accurately. Like the hyaline hyphomycetes, characteristic reproductive structures are rarely seen in tissue sections. Therefore definitive identification usually depends on obtaining a proper specimen for culture. Differentiation from other hyaline fungi is often an emergency, particularly in cases of rhinocerebral disease because the zygomycetes tend to behave in a more aggressive fashion, requiring extensive and emergent debridement for a successful patient outcome (Figs. 4.54, 4.55, 4.56, 4.57, 4.58, 4.59, 4.60, 4.61, 4.62, 4.63 and 4.64).

4.7 Infections Caused by Dimorphic Fungi

The dimorphic fungi typically demonstrate yeast forms when grown under human body conditions, and mold forms when they are grown under environmental conditions; hence the term dimorphic. Because of this, the yeast forms are easily the most commonly identified morphology on histopathologic sections. Most of the fungi classically defined as dimorphic are "thermally dimorphic," with the form seen depending mostly on temperature. A notable exception is *Coccidiodes* species, which appears to depend mostly on carbon dioxide concentrations in determining whether the yeast or mold form (or a combination of the two) is present. Unlike most hyaline fungi, most of the pathogenic fungi classified as dimorphic are geographically restricted. The most commonly encountered dimorphic fungi are

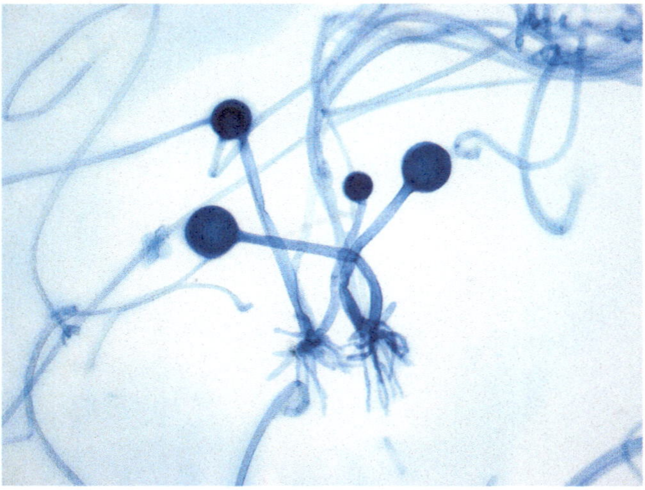

Fig. 4.55 Lactophenol cotton blue preparation of *Rhizopus* species from fungal culture. Zygomycetes demonstrate sporangia that are usually round, enclosed structures, containing asexually produced spores. This is a major feature that differentiates them from most other pathogenic molds, which will typically demonstrate unenclosed "fruiting" bodies or conidia. Like conidia however, these structures are only rarely seen on histopathologic sections. 200× magnification

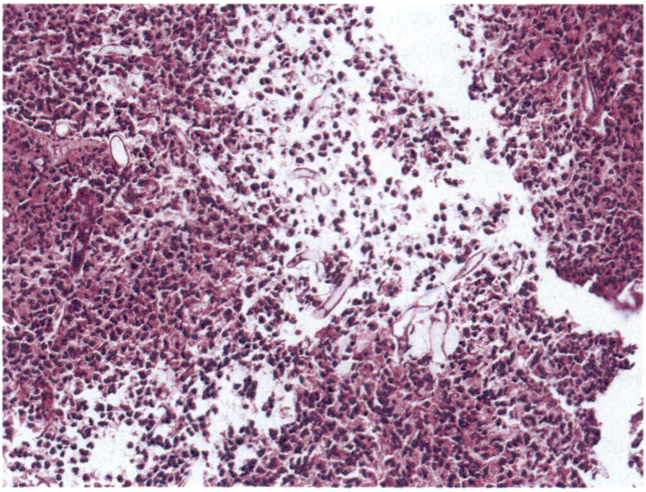

Fig. 4.54 *Rhizopus* species in nasal sinus currettings from a case of rhinocerebral zygomycosis. Zygomycetes usually have much wider, pauciseptate, variably sized hyphae with nonparallel walls. They are often described as "ribbon-like" or "twisting." Note also the accompanying intense acute inflammatory infiltrate. H&E, 400× magnification

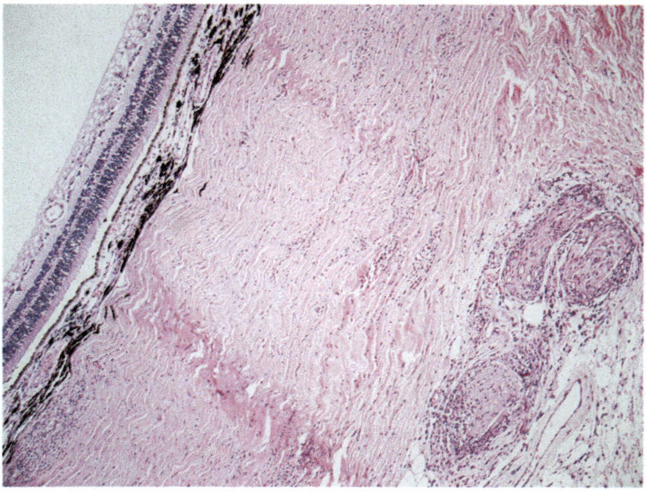

Fig. 4.56 These images were taken from sections of an enucleated eye from a patient with rhinocerebral zygomycosis that had spread to the orbit. Rhinocerebral zygomycosis is rapidly progressive, and treatment involves aggressive debridement followed by antifungal therapy. Note neural invasion by wide, ribbon-like hyphae in the lower right of the image. H&E, 100× magnification

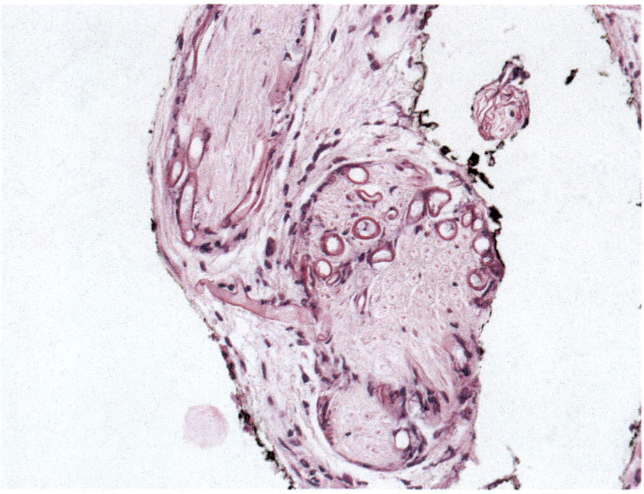

Fig. 4.57 A higher magnification image demonstrating invasion of the surrounding nerves with wide, pauciseptate, ribbon-like hyphae. H&E, 400× magnification

discussed here. Usually grouped with the dimorphic pathogens but rarely encountered, *Talaromyces marneffei* (formerly *Penicillium marneffei*) is an important cause of morbidity and mortality in certain areas of Southeast Asia but is not discussed in this chapter. The reader is referred to other sources if this pathogenic fungus is under consideration in the differential diagnosis.

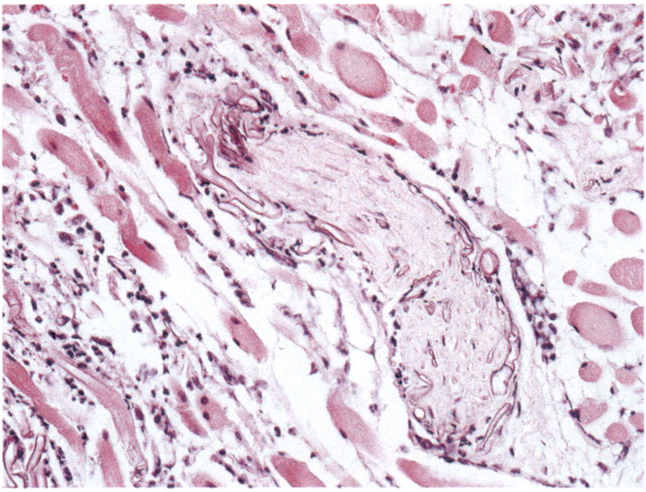

Fig. 4.58 Invasion of nerves and surrounding soft tissue of the orbit by a zygomycete. Note the acute inflammatory response within the surrounding soft tissue. H&E, 400× magnification

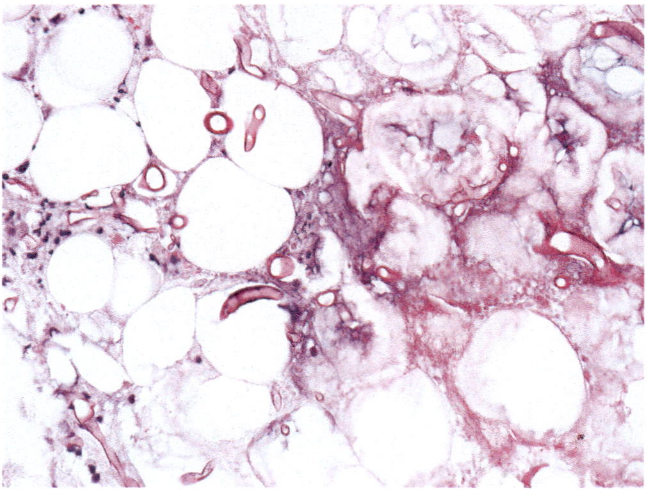

Fig. 4.59 Invasion into the surrounding periorbital fat from the previously discussed case. Extensive fat necrosis and a sparse acute inflammatory infiltrate were seen. This extensive invasion into a variety of tissues can present great difficulty in securing clear surgical margins. H&E, 400× magnification

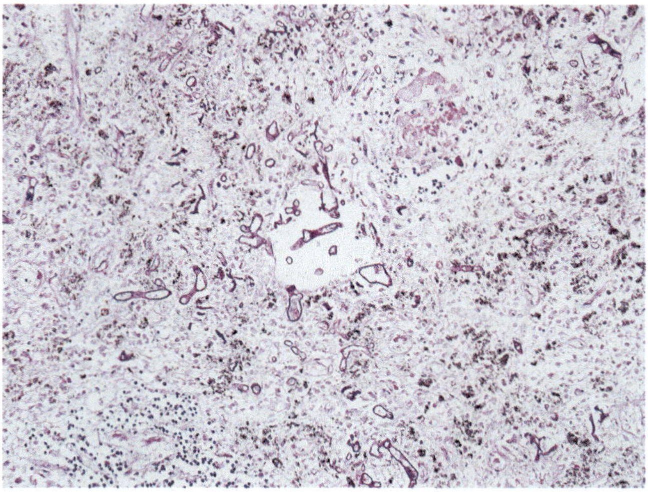

Fig. 4.60 Lymph node invasion is commonly seen with some zygomycete species. Here, invasion of a mediastinal lymph node is demonstrated in a case of primary pulmonary disease. Periodic acid–Schiff stain, 200× magnification

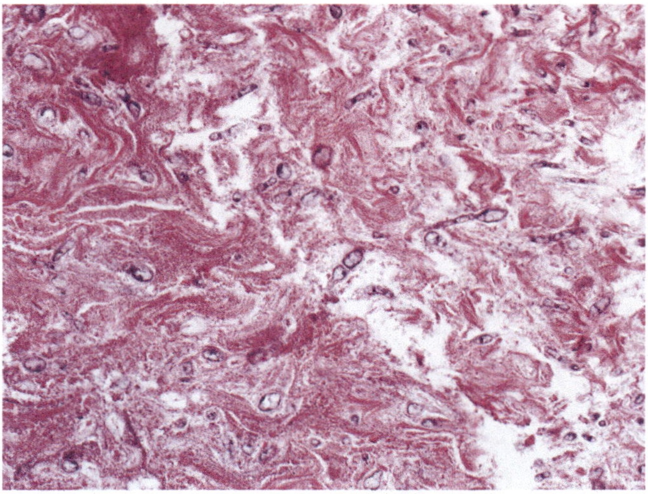

Fig. 4.61 In addition to diabetic and immunosuppressed patients, burn victims are at great risk for soft tissue infections with zygomycetes. Poor staining and seemingly sparse hyphae are seen here infiltrating through necrotic tissue obtained from the lower extremity in a burn patient. H&E, 400×

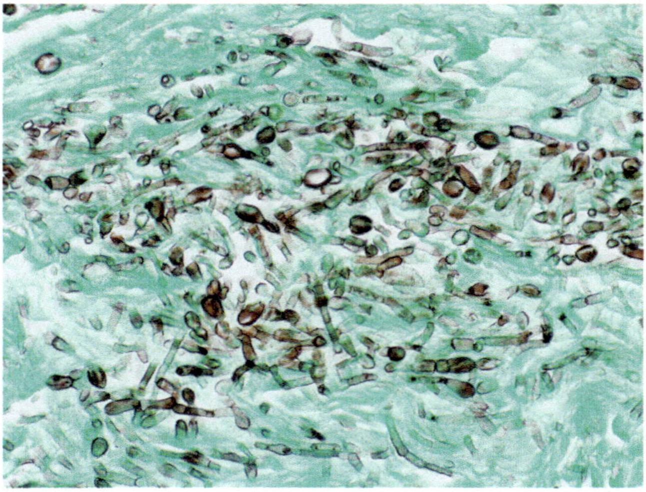

Fig. 4.62 Gomori methenamine silver staining of the same region demonstrated in Fig. 4.61. Note that the staining reveals extensive infiltration of fungal hyphae. Note also that the hyphae are very irregular in appearance and are not very wide, most being 3–4 microns in width. Perhaps most striking is the presence of frequent septations. This originally led to the erroneous conclusion that the pathogen was likely an *Aspergillus* species. Cultures later grew *Rhizomucor* species. 400× magnification

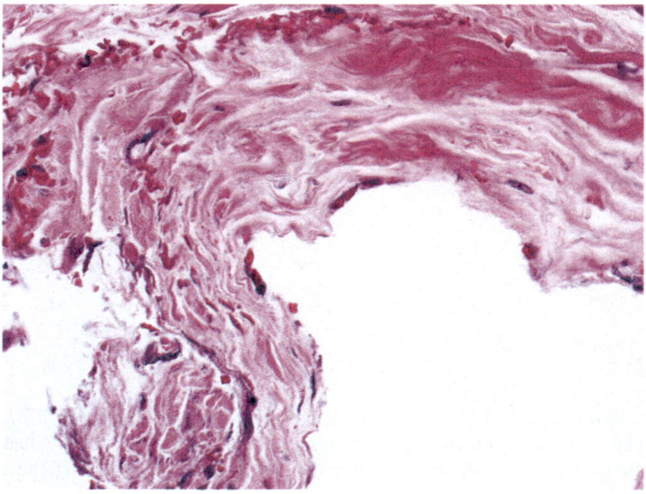

Fig. 4.63 Angioinvasion is a common feature of zygomycete infections. Again note that the presence of hyphae may be difficult to detect on H&E stained sections. Stains such as Gomori methenamine or periodic acid–Schiff fungus stain may be more helpful in detecting this feature. 400× magnification

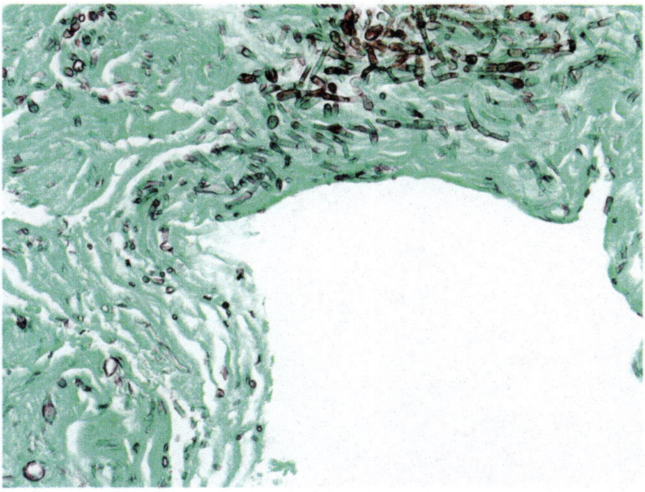

Fig. 4.64 Gomori methenamine silver staining of the same area seen in Fig. 4.63 demonstrating numerous hyphae within the vessel wall. Again note the atypical appearance in that this example of an infection with *Rhizomucor* has predominantly thin hyphae with frequent septations. These findings emphasize the importance of obtaining proper fungal cultures for definitive identification. 400× magnification

4.7.1 Blastomyces Species

Blastomyces dermatiditis is found in the United States and Canada, most frequently in areas surrounding the Ohio and Mississippi river valleys. While primarily a localized disease found in these areas, *B. dermatiditis* has also infrequently been implicated as a cause of disease in parts of Africa, the Middle East, and India. Recently a morphologically identical but novel species – *Blastomyces gilchristii* sp. nov – has also been identified as a cause of blastomycosis. *Blastomyces* species are thermally dimorphic, with the yeast forms generally measuring 8–12 microns in diameter and demonstrating classically broad-based budding. The yeast tend to have thick double refractile walls that bend the light differently when shifting planes of focus. Pulmonary infections are most common, with many being subclinical; however, infections of nearly every body site have been reported, with a particular predilection for skin and bone. Note that dermatologic infections may be primary following trauma; however, if cutaneous disease is encountered, a primary pulmonary site of infection should be considered (Figs. 4.65, 4.66, 4.67, 4.68, 4.69, 4.70, 4.71, 4.72, 4.73, 4.74, 4.75, 4.76, 4.77, 4.78, and 4.79).

4.7.2 Histoplasma Species

Histoplasma capsulatum has a major endemic region very similar to *B. dermatiditis,* being found most commonly in the Mississippi and Ohio river valleys of the United States and Canada, but it has an essentially overall worldwide

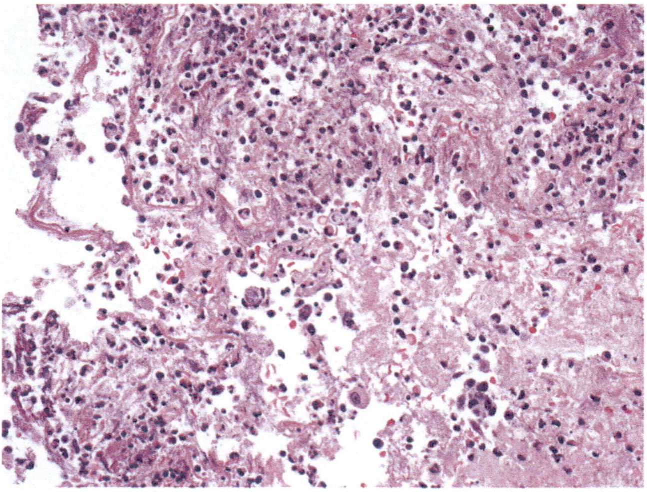

Fig. 4.65 An example of *Blastomyces* infection of the lung on H&E staining. These infections present in a wide variety of different patterns but usually as a mixture of predominantly acute and both necrotizing and non-necrotizing granulomatous inflammation. The yeast forms may be difficult to identify at first glance if they are not initially suspected. Performance of a Gomori methenamine silver stain is recommended to highlight the organism. Note generally round yeast forms with thick double refractile walls. Broad-based budding may not be readily evident on H&E staining. 400× magnification

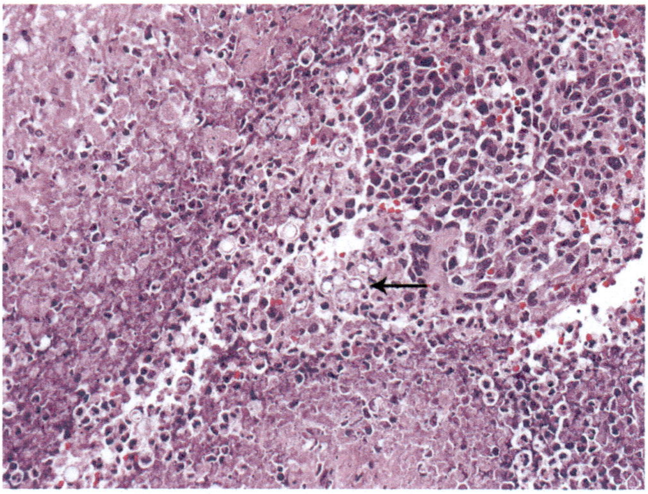

Fig. 4.66 Another example of the H&E appearance of *Blastomyces* infection of the lung. In this area, there is a mixture of acute and chronic inflammation as well as surrounding necrosis. Many yeast cells, some exhibiting broad-based budding (arrow), are scattered throughout. 400× magnification

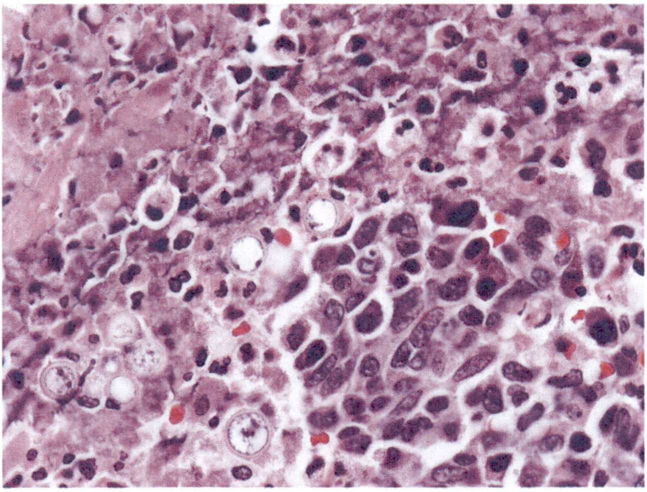

Fig. 4.67 Higher magnification of the area demonstrated in Fig. 4.66 demonstrating round, relatively consistently sized yeast forms of *B. dermatiditis*. Note the thick walls and broad-based budding. Focusing in different planes highlights the refractile nature of the walls

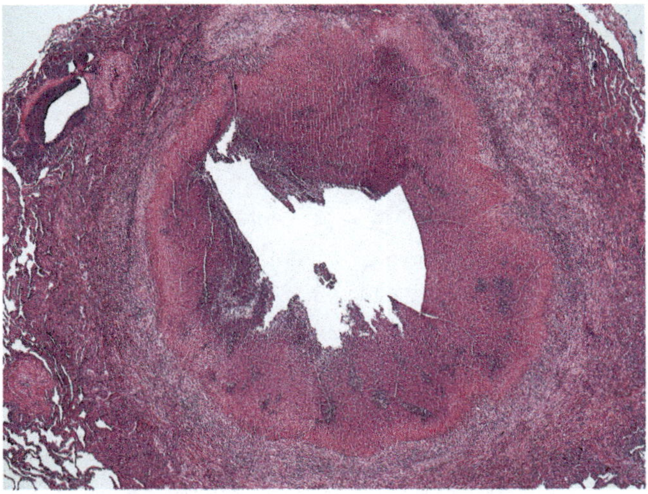

Fig. 4.68 A well-circumscribed necrotic granuloma of the lung in a patient with primary pulmonary *B. dermatiditis* infection. H&E, 40× magnification

distribution. This fungus is thermally dimorphic, with yeast forms being small, generally 2–4 microns, and usually demonstrating single terminal buds with characteristic narrow-based budding. Small *Candida* species such as *Candida glabrata* may at times resemble the yeast cells of *Histoplasma*, particularly because

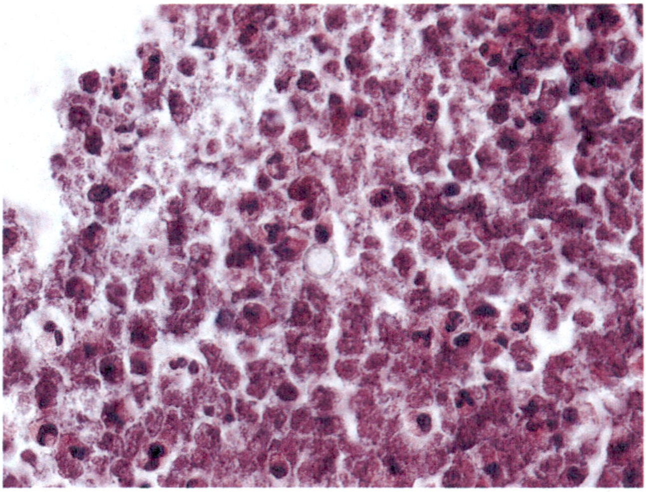

Fig. 4.69 A higher magnification image demonstrating a solitary, thick-walled, round yeast cell of *B. dermatiditis* within the central portion of the granuloma demonstrated in Fig. 4.68. As they do not particularly highlight with H&E staining, comparison with Gomori methenamine silver or other fungal stains is recommended. 1000× magnification

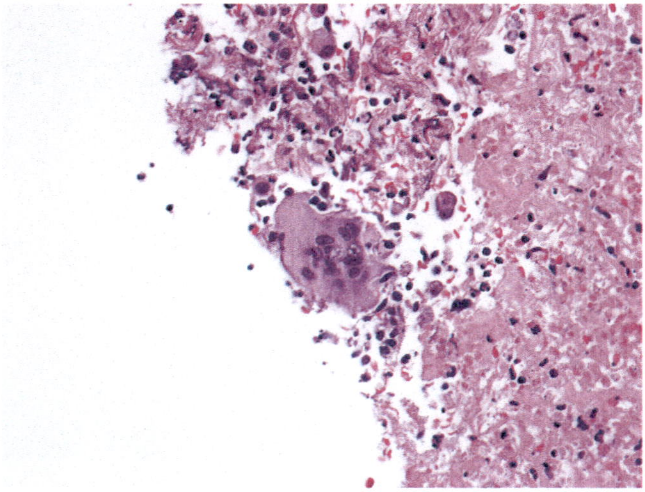

Fig. 4.70 Blastomyces yeast forms can also frequently be found engulfed within multinucleated giant cells. H&E, 400× magnification

C. glabrata does not produce pseudohyphae. The fact that *Candida* species usually retain the crystal violet on Gram staining can be helpful, since *Histoplasma* species do not. The typically more random budding patterns of *Candida* species may also be helpful. Like most dimorphic fungi, primary pulmonary infections are the most

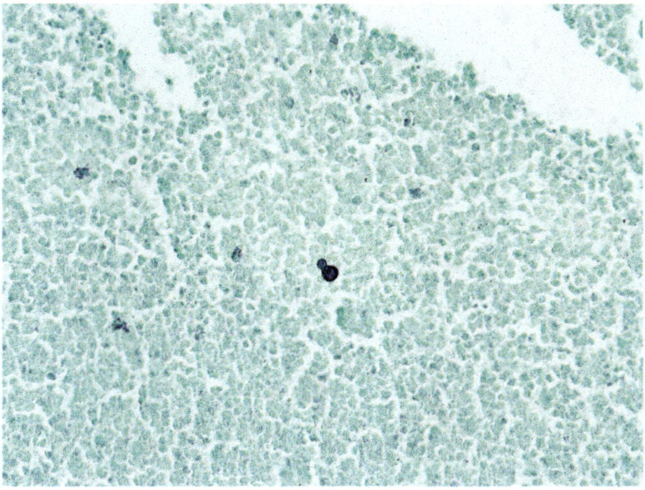

Fig. 4.71 Gomori methenamine silver stain of mother and daughter yeast cells of *B. dermatiditis* demonstrating classic broad-based budding. This pattern is often difficult to distinguish on H&E staining. The Gomori stain usually allows for significant contrast with the counterstained background so as to easily visualize the budding patterns of dimorphic fungi and other pathogenic yeast. 400× magnification

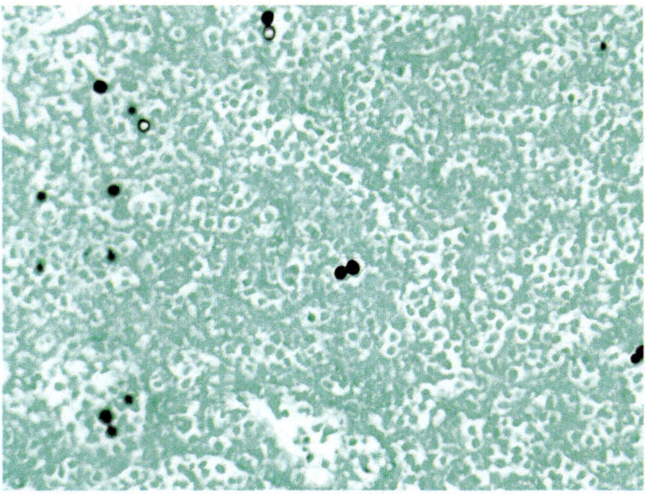

Fig. 4.72 Gomori methenamine silver stained sections frequently demonstrate a central clearing within the yeast cells, but depending on the plane of section and other factors, the yeast may appear entirely black. 400× magnification

commonly seen, but *Histoplasma* may also frequently disseminate to hilar and mediastinal lymph nodes, spleen, liver, adrenals, and bone marrow. The yeast cells are frequently found clustered within macrophages but resist destruction. This feature is thought to actually assist in the spread of the organism throughout the

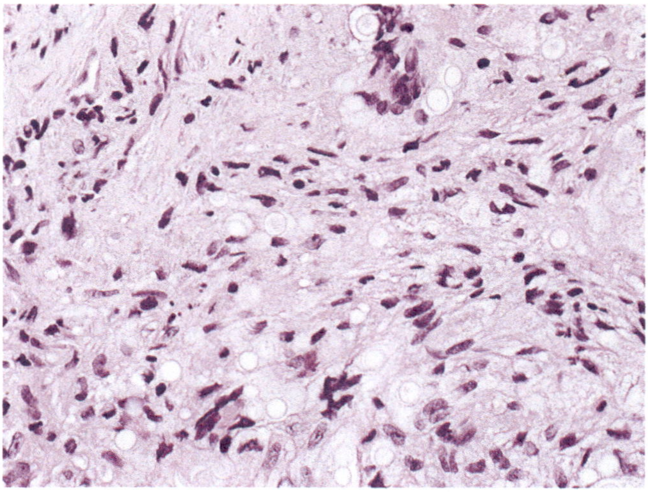

Fig. 4.73 Rarely, *Blastomyces* species may demonstrate some retraction artifact owing to fixation that may resemble the capsule of *Cryptococcus* species. This is especially problematic in the case illustrated here, in which the yeast also appears to demonstrate significant size variation. While notable size variation is another characteristic of *Cryptococcus* species, here that appearance is largely due to differing planes of section. Subcarinal lymph node, H&E, 600× magnification

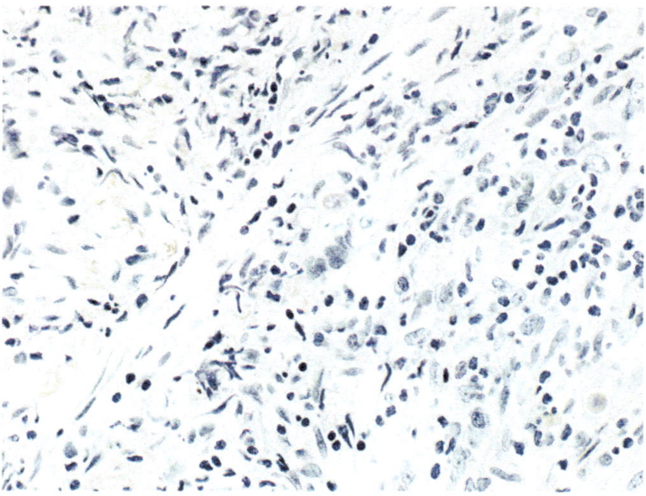

Fig. 4.74 In cases such as demonstrated in Fig. 4.73, a negative mucicarmine stain as well as ancillary patient *Blastomyces* antigen testing may assist in arriving at the correct identification. Fungal culture is recommended for definitive diagnosis but is not universally successful. Polymerase chain reaction testing from formalin-fixed paraffin-embedded tissue is also available at some institutions. 600× magnification

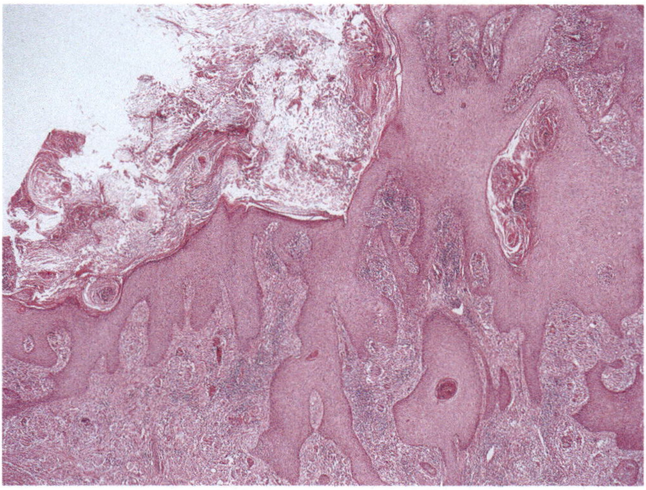

Fig. 4.75 Dermatologic manifestations of cutaneous blastomyces infections usually begin as a papule or nodule, which may become keratinized or wart-like. Superficial ulceration is common. Histopathologically, pseudoepitheliomatous hyperplasia is a hallmark feature. Underlying acute and granulomatous inflammation may be seen. H&E, 40× magnification

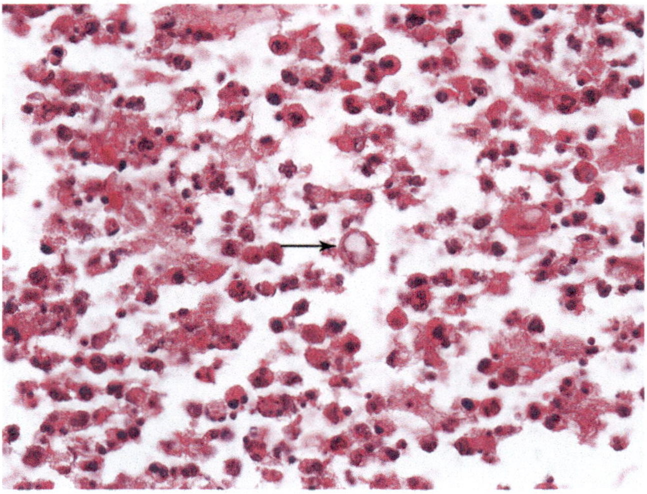

Fig. 4.76 In skin infections with *Blastomyces dermatiditis,* yeast cells may be found scattered throughout; these may be most easily identified within giant cells and areas of necrotizing granulomatous inflammation. Note that the walls (*arrow*) can stain slightly eosinophilic, slightly basophilic, or not at all, often blending in with the surrounding necrosis or tissue. Changing planes of focus as you search may help to reveal the double refractile walls. H&E, 1000× magnification

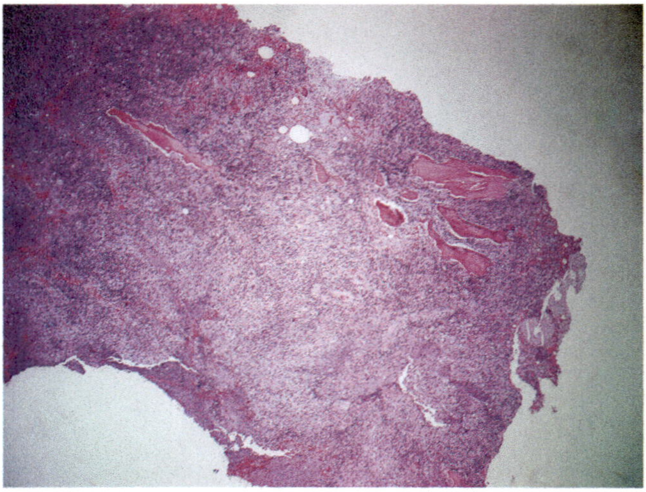

Fig. 4.77 Dissemination to bone in systemic *Blastomyces* infections is also seen on an infrequent basis. The lower extremities, particularly locations around the knee joint, are the most common sites. Illustrated here is a section of tibia that presented as a mass concerning for an osteosarcoma. Note the destruction of the bone and replacement with necrotic tissue, granulomatous inflammation, and giant cells. H&E, 40× magnification

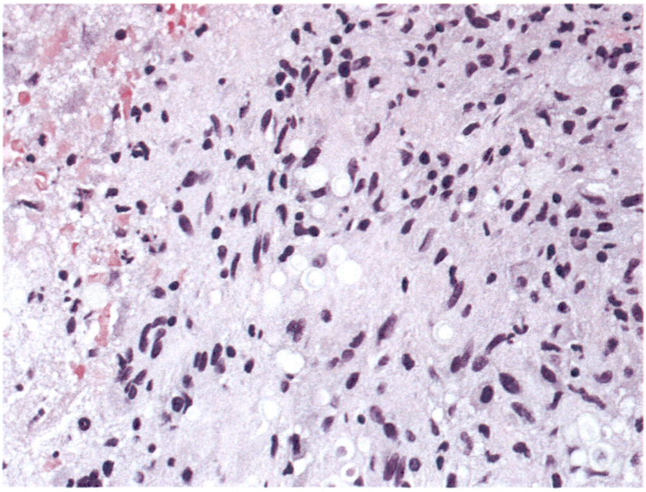

Fig. 4.78 Higher magnification demonstrating many characteristic broad-based budding yeast of *Blastomyces dermatiditis* scattered throughout. 600× magnification

reticuloendothelial system. *Histoplasma* is also a known cause of fungal meningitis, in which it typically presents as basilar meningeal enhancement radiologically. *Histoplasma* infection of the mediastinal lymph nodes is thought to be a cause of fibrosing mediastinitis, a hyperimmune response to *H. capsulatum* that may present

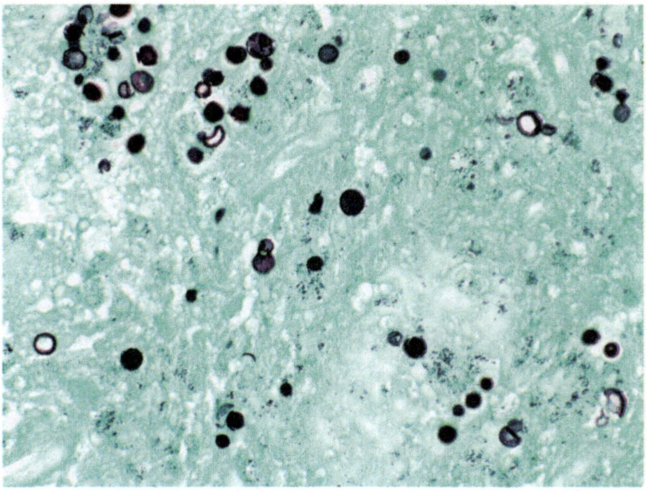

Fig. 4.79 Gomori methanimine silver staining of bone tissue from the previously discussed case. 600× magnification

with superior vena cava syndrome and a variety of other symptoms. *Histoplasma* antigen testing may be a useful adjunct test to determine if there is disseminated disease present, with the caveat that there is significant cross-reactivity with *Blastomyces* and vice versa. This issue can be problematic because there is significant overlap in the major endemic regions of these pathogens. Fortunately, the treatment for these two dimorphic fungi is similar and usually involves a combination of long-term therapy with amphotericin B and/or itraconazole (Figs. 4.80, 4.81, 4.82, 4.83, 4.84, 4.85, 4.86, 4.87, 4.88, 4.89, 4.90, 4.91, 4.92, and 4.93).

4.7.3 Coccidiodes Species

Coccidiodes species are typically classified as dimorphic fungi, but it is important to note that while other classic dimorphic pathogens are more precisely thermally dimorphic, the dimorphism of *Coccidiodes* species relies more heavily on concentrations of carbon dioxide. Two pathogenic species exist, *C. immitis*, which is thought to be geographically limited to the San Joaquin Valley and northern Mexico, and *C. posadasii,* which has a wider range of distribution including California, Arizona, Nevada, Texas, Utah, and parts of Mexico and South America. These two species are microscopically indistinguishable, and differentiation at this time is only useful for epidemiologic purposes. For this reason, the identification is frequently reported as *Coccidiodes immitis/posadasii* by mycology laboratories.

On histopathologic examination, the hallmark feature of coccidiodomycosis is the presence of large, generally 20–120 micron spherules that contain numerous endospores. The growing spherules eventually rupture, releasing the endospores

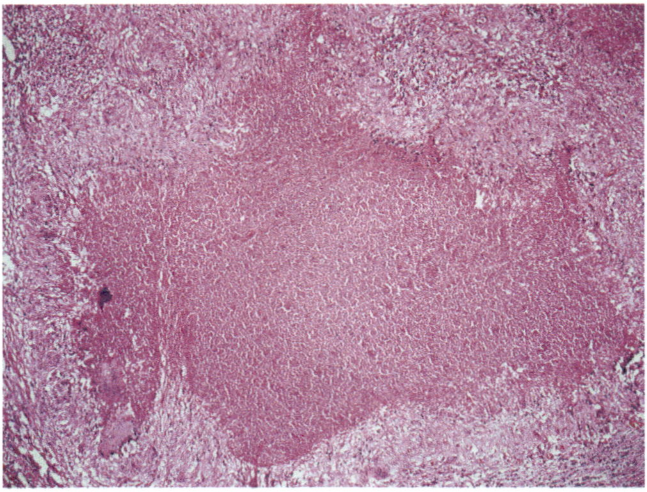

Fig. 4.80 A typical necrotizing granuloma associated with pulmonary infection with *H. capsulatum*. In immunocompetent hosts, a mixture of necrotic and non-necrotic granulomas may be seen. The patterns seen in immunocompromised hosts may be variable since their capacity to form granulomas may be compromised. H&E, 100× magnification

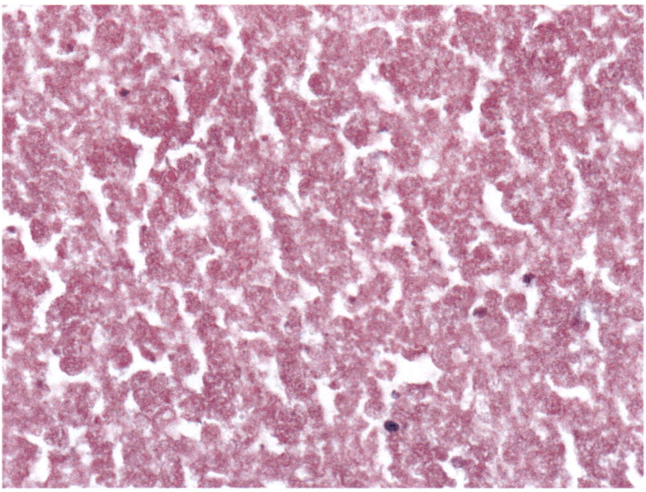

Fig. 4.81 Higher magnification image of the necrotic area demonstrated in Fig. 4.80. *H. capsulatum* is usually not readily apparent on H&E staining as shown here, necessitating the use of special stains such as Gomori methenamine silver. 1000× magnification

into the surrounding tissue, where they begin to develop into spherules themselves, perpetuating the cycle. While the endospores typically range in size from 4 to 8 microns, once released they continually mature into spherules, resulting in significant size variation. Because of this, endospores of *Coccidiodes* species may

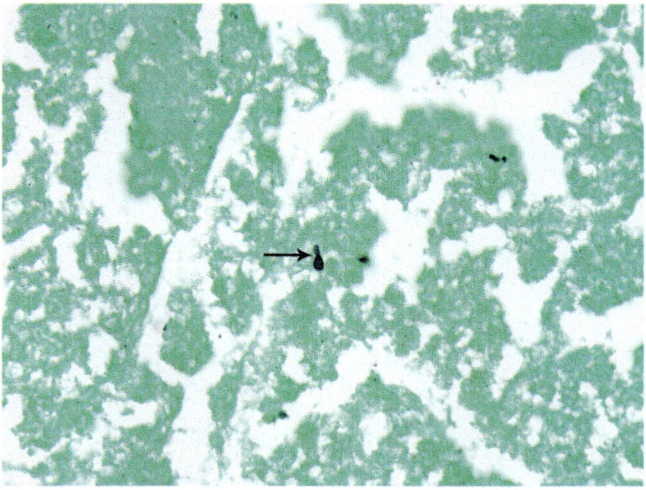

Fig. 4.82 Gomori methenamine silver stain demonstrating classic narrow-based budding (*arrow*) of *H. capsulatum* within a necrotizing granuloma. Note the presence of the bud at the terminal tip of the organism. Also demonstrated here is the "sesame-seed" shape that often characterizes *H. capsulatum*. The opposite end of the yeast appears slightly wider, tapering toward the terminal end. 100× magnification

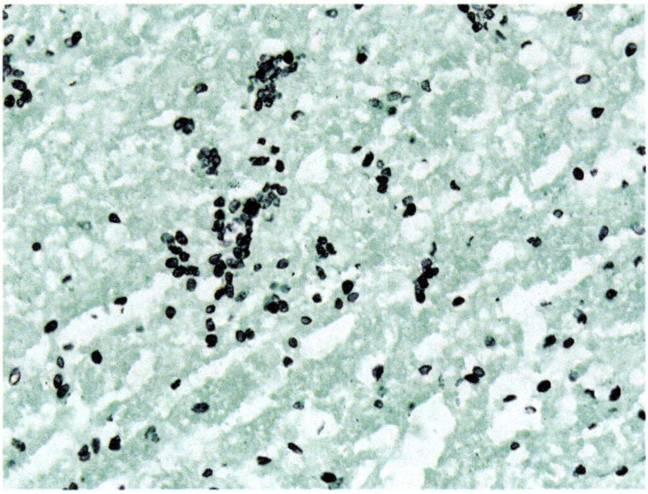

Fig. 4.83 Hyalinized lung nodule containing numerous *H. capsulatum* yeast forms. Small, well-circumscribed and partially calcified granulomas are frequent findings at autopsy of patients who lived or have previously lived in endemic areas. Similar nodules may also be found in the liver or spleen amongst other sites. As the yeast have in many cases been encased in granulomas for years, they are often inactive or dead. Note that many of these forms appear cracked or broken and not the typical round to oval shape. While the staining will still highlight these organisms, culture in many cases will not yield viable growth. Gomori methenamine silver stain, 1000× magnification

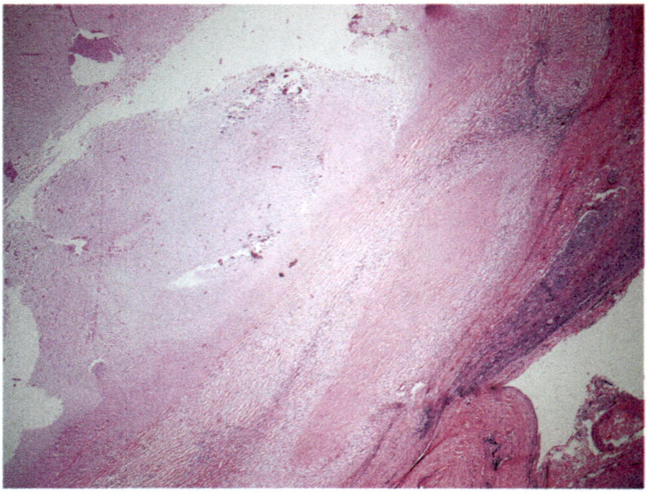

Fig. 4.84 A partially calcified, "old" granuloma within a hilar lymph node. These findings are typical in walled-off Histoplasma. Note the fibrotic wall of the nodule with remnant lymphoid tissue at the periphery. H&E, 40× magnification

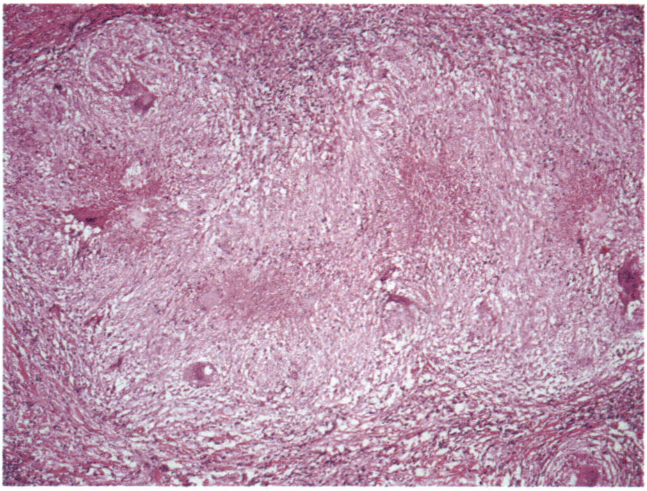

Fig. 4.85 Mediastinal lymph node. Local lymph node invasion by *Histoplasma* is common and demonstrates similar patterns of mixed necrotizing and non-necrotizing granuloma formation similar to that that seen in primary pulmonary infection. Giant cells may also be frequently seen. H&E, 100× magnification

be mistaken for pathogenic yeast, particularly those of *Blastomyces* species. This is especially problematic if accompanying spherules or spherule remnants are not readily apparent. Additionally, there may be significant overlap in size range with *Blastomyces* species (typically 8–12 microns), and endospores in close proximity

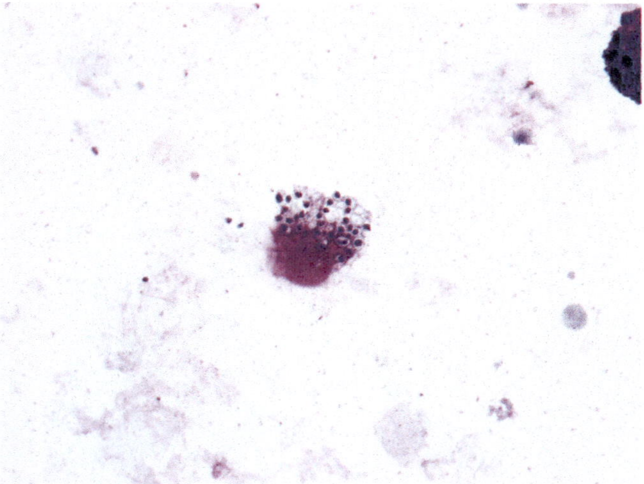

Fig. 4.86 Giemsa stain of bronchoalveolar lavage fluid demonstrating the small intracellular yeast of *H. capsulatum*. While a single yeast can be identified in these specimens, *H. capsulatum* is often seen clustered inside of pulmonary macrophages. Note eccentric purple staining nuclear material and bluish cytoplasm as well as the thin halo around the organisms representing the "pseudocapsule" that is sometimes seen. The amastigotes of *Leishmania* species also tend to cluster inside of macrophages and are very similar in size and morphologic appearance. *Leishmania* species, however, should exhibit a purple staining, bar-shaped kinetoplast, although at times it may be difficult to visualize. While not usually found in the lung, specimens from other sites, such as the spleen, bone marrow, or skin, may introduce leishmaniasis into the differential. Gomori methenamine silver staining, which is positive in histoplasmosis and negative in leishmaniasis, may be helpful in making an identification. 1000× magnification

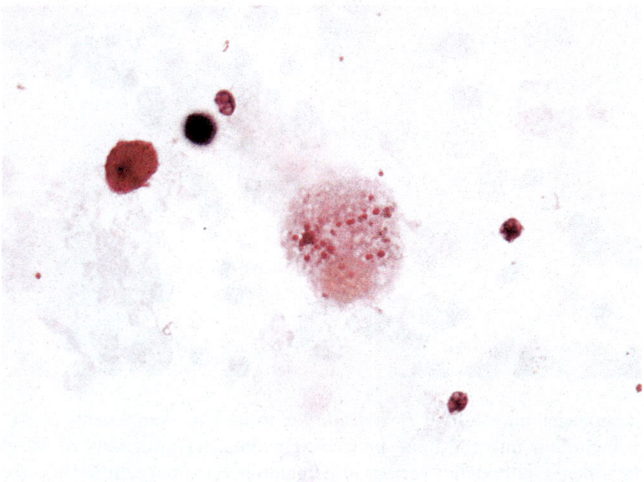

Fig. 4.87 Gram stain of bronchoalveolar lavage fluid demonstrating the appearance of intracellular *H. capsulatum*. These yeast are of a similar size and shape to some *Candida* species, in particular *C. glabrata*. However, note that *H. capsulatum* does not retain the crystal violet stain and will either pick up the safranin stain, appearing *pink* or *red*, or will stain clear, demonstrating a negative image. *Candida* species, with a properly performed Gram stain, will appear purple owing to the retained crystal violet. 1000× magnification

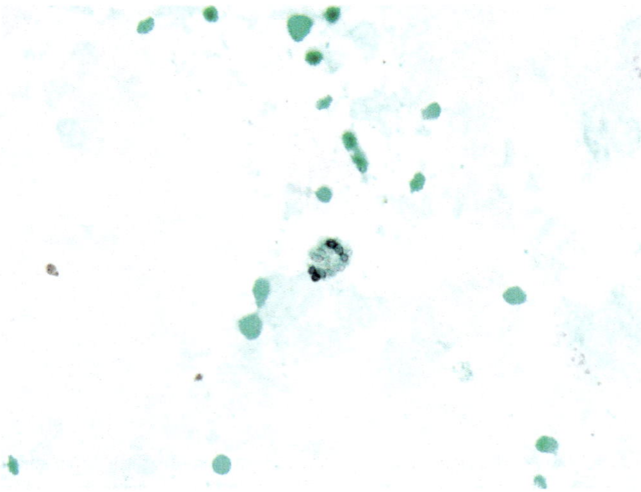

Fig. 4.88 Gomori methenamine silver staining of bronchoalveolar lavage fluid demonstrating the typical appearance of intracellular yeast of *H. capsulatum*. 1000× magnification

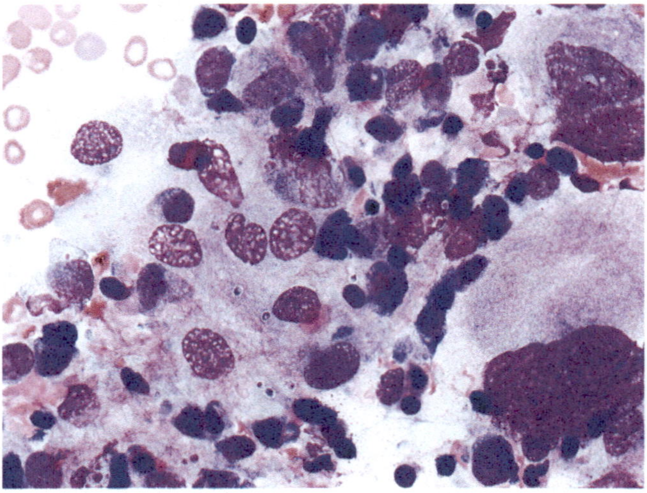

Fig. 4.89 Macrophages may deliver *H. capsulatum* to various components of the reticuloendothelial system, including into the bone marrow. Histoplasma infections of the bone typically present as pancytopenia, although a variety of hematopoietic abnormalities have been described. Note that, in contrast to *B. dermatiditis* infections involving bone, *H. capsulatum* does not usually present as an outwardly destructive lesion. Small round to oval yeasts with pseudocapsules are seen here in a bone marrow aspirate. Again, visceral leishmaniasis may also present in a similar fashion and must be considered if the patient lives in or has visited a region where this infection is common. Giemsa stain, 1000× magnification

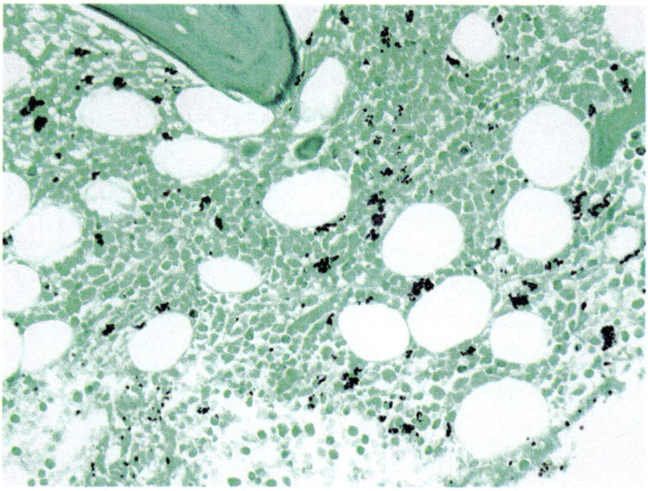

Fig. 4.90 Gomori methenamine silver stained bone marrow biopsy section taken from the same patient illustrated in Fig. 4.89. Note that there are multiple clusters of positive staining organisms present, representing intracellular organisms as well as a few scattered single yeasts. 400× magnification

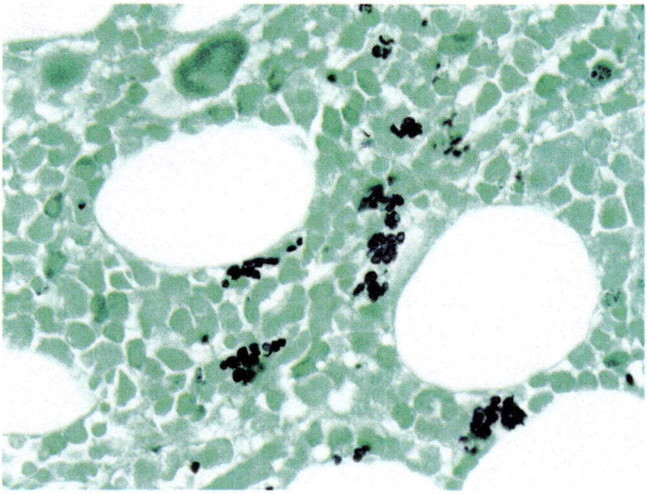

Fig. 4.91 Higher magnification image demonstrating the small, 2–4 micron, round to oval yeast forms of *H. capsulatum* in a bone marrow biopsy. Gomori methenamine silver stain, 1000× magnification

may also suggest broad-based budding. A careful history and/or additional sections may be helpful in cases that are difficult to distinguish (Figs. 4.94, 4.95, 4.96, 4.97, 4.98, 4.99, 4.100, 4.101, 4.102, 4.103, 4.104, and 4.105).

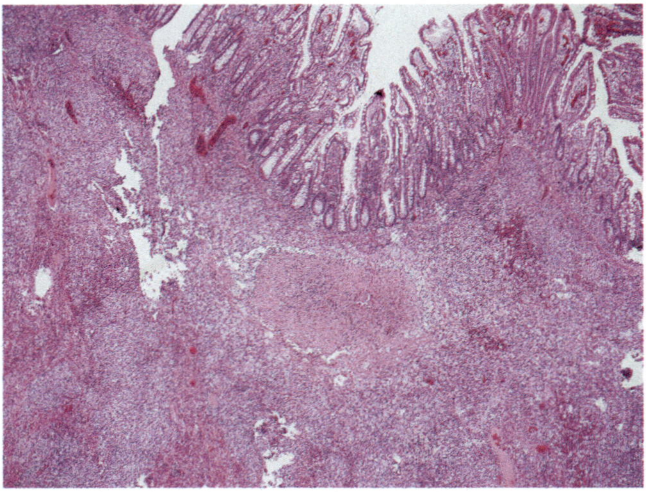

Fig. 4.92 Like many dimorphic fungi, *Histoplasma* has the ability to disseminate to any organ system. In this unusual case, it has disseminated to the small bowel. The mucosal surface is well preserved with intact and seemingly unaffected villi. However, note granulomatous inflammation with necrotic granuloma formation just below the mucosal layer. H&E, 40× magnification

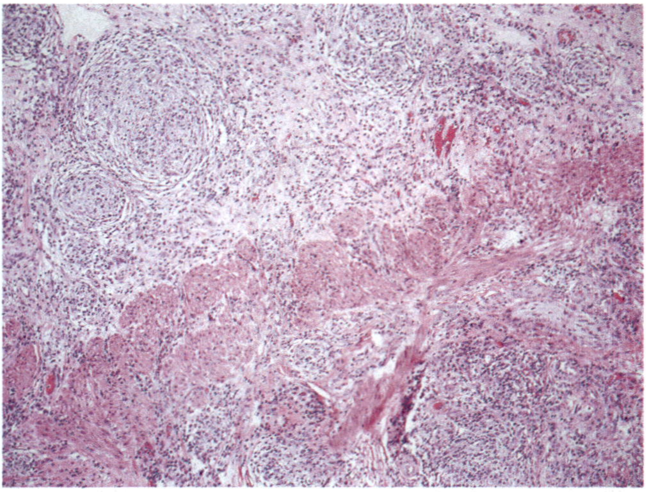

Fig. 4.93 In addition to necrotic granuloma formation, non-necrotizing granulomas are present throughout the muscularis propria as well as a diffuse acute inflammatory response. H&E, 100× magnification

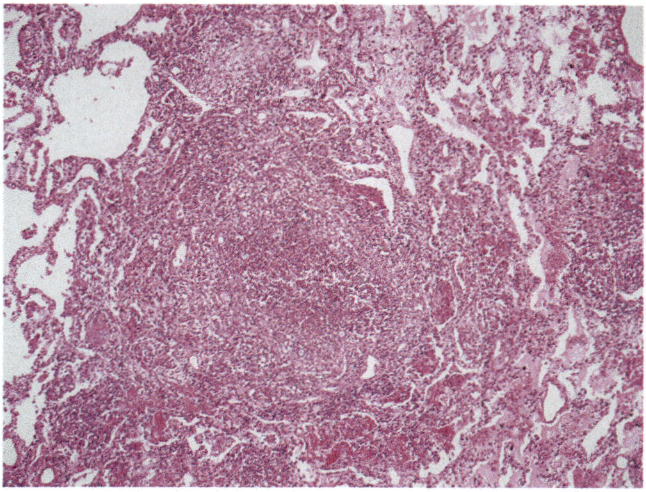

Fig. 4.94 A section of lung demonstrating the typical appearance of coccidioidomycosis. Granulomatous inflammation intermixed with areas of acute inflammation is typically seen. Larger spherules may be visible at low magnification. H&E, 100× magnification

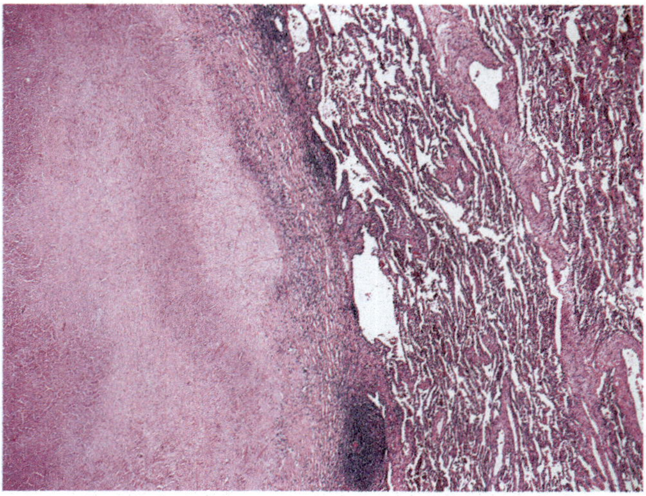

Fig. 4.95 An older, large granuloma caused by *Coccidiodes* species infection of the lung to the *left* of the image. The nodule in this case is well circumscribed with a thick fibrotic capsule and a necrotic center. A lymphocytic infiltrate is apparent around the periphery of the nodule. H&E, 40× magnification

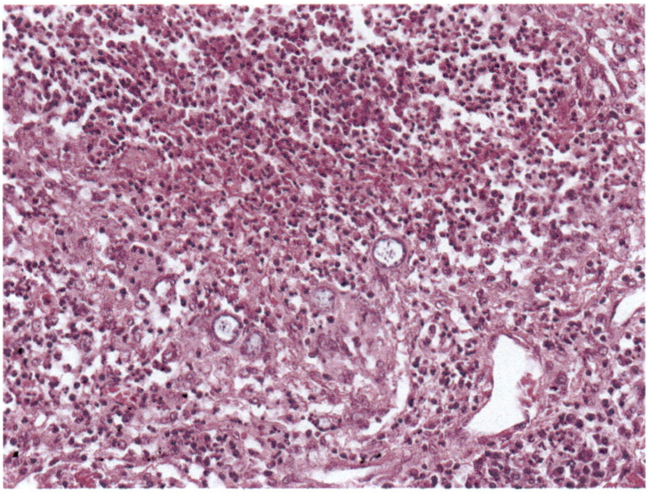

Fig. 4.96 Higher magnification image of the spherules of *Coccidiodes* species. Scattered endospores are also seen. Note the large size and relatively thick wall of the spherules. Abundant acute inflammation is present and is typically associated with the response to the release of endospores. H&E, 400× magnification

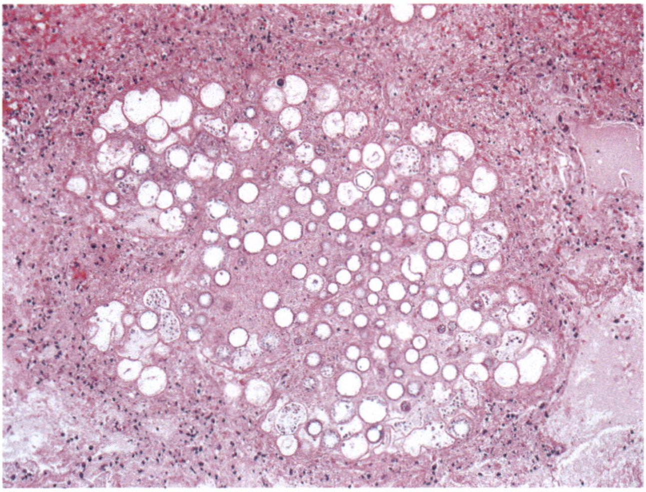

Fig. 4.97 Clusters of spherules can be seen infrequently. This image demonstrates many spherules in various stages of development. Some demonstrate endospores, but others demonstrate the more frequently encountered empty-appearing forms. Note the massive variability in size and the presence of endospores in some but not all spherules. H&E, 200× magnification

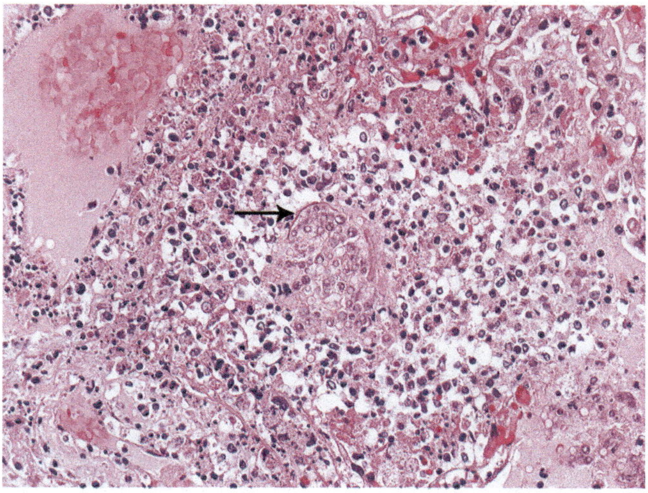

Fig. 4.98 A ruptured spherule. Note the spilling of endospores into the surrounding lung tissue and the mixed predominantly acute inflammatory response. The remainder of the spherule wall is identified by the *arrow*. H&E, 400× magnification

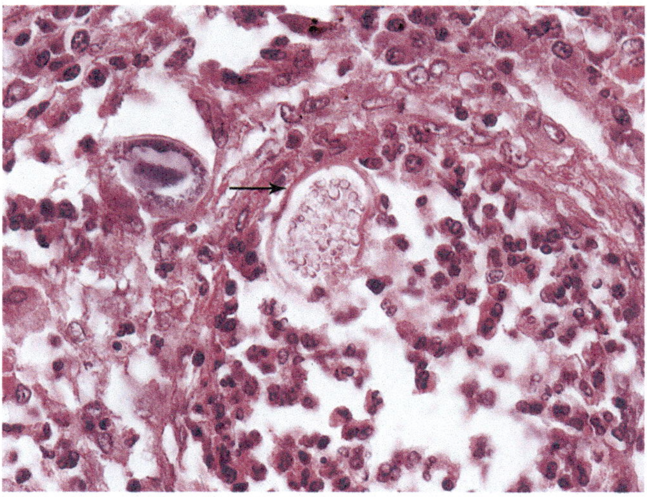

Fig. 4.99 Higher magnification of a ruptured spherule. Note that the normally round spherule wall has begun to collapse as the endospores empty into the surrounding tissue accompanied by abundant acute inflammation. The remaining spherule wall (*arrow*) can often be identified by an eosinophilic "glassy" appearance. H&E, 1000× magnification

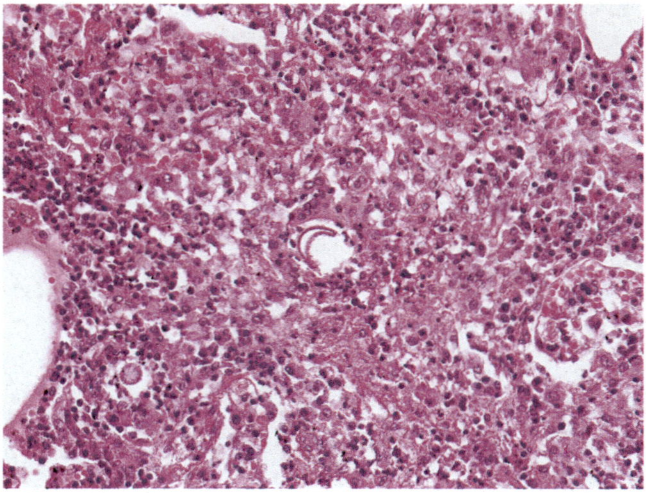

Fig. 4.100 A collapsed and empty shell of a ruptured spherule is seen here. Often, particularly in cases where few endospores are seen, the presence of empty spherules may be the best indication that the fungal pathogen is in fact a *Coccidiodes* species. H&E, 400× magnification

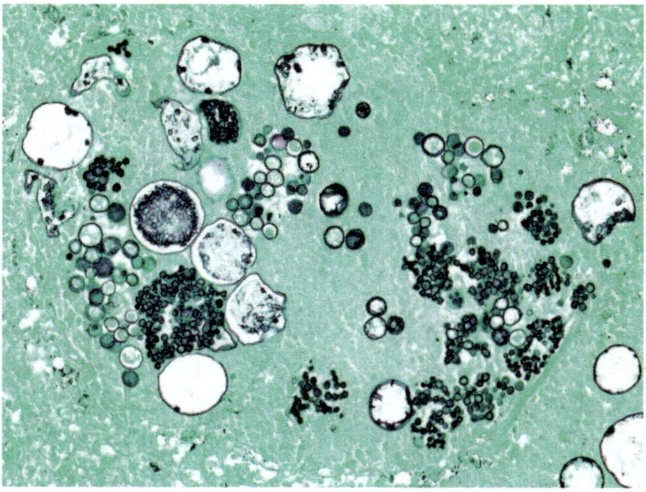

Fig. 4.101 Spherules and endospores of *Coccidiodes* species in various stages of development. Note the tremendous size variation. Gomori methenamine silver stain, 400× magnification

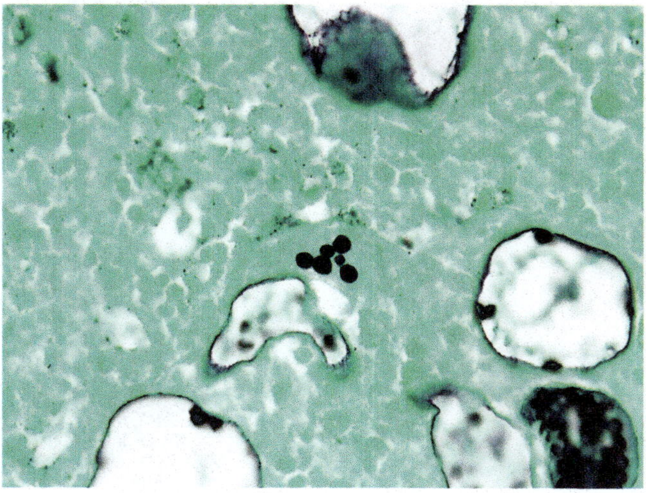

Fig. 4.102 Endospores of *Coccidiodes* species may have an appearance and size similar to that of *Blastomyces* species, and when lying in close proximity to each other may give the false appearance of broad-based budding. In this case, ruptured and intact spherules are present in the background. Gomori methenamine silver stain, 1000× magnification

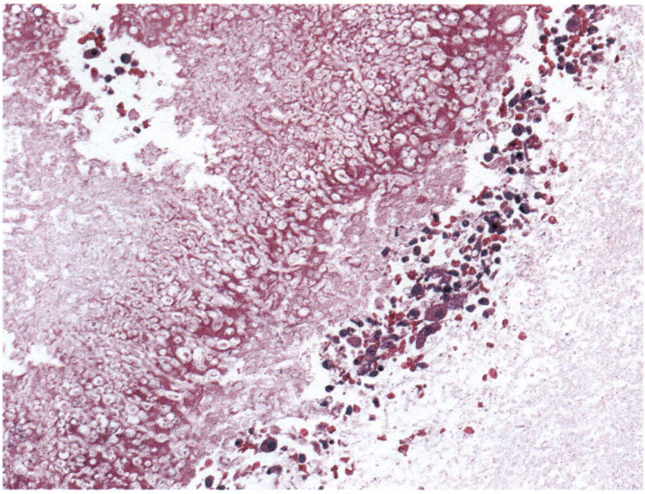

Fig. 4.103 While the "yeast" forms of dimorphic fungi are far and away the most frequently encountered on histopathologic examination, variations in temperatures as well as other factors can lead to the growth of hyphal forms. Perhaps because of their reliance on carbon dioxide concentration rather than on temperature, hyphal forms are relatively commonly seen in *Coccidiodes* infections. These are usually intermixed with spherules and endospores but may be the predominant form, sometimes overwhelmingly so, making definitive diagnosis from microscopic sections difficult. H&E, 400×

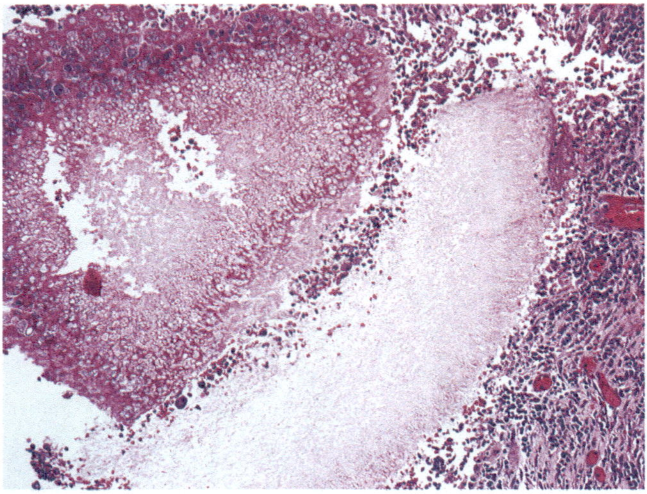

Fig. 4.104 Another example of hyphal forms of *Coccidiodes* in the lung. Note the additional presence of spherules in the *upper left* portion of the image. H&E, 200× magnification

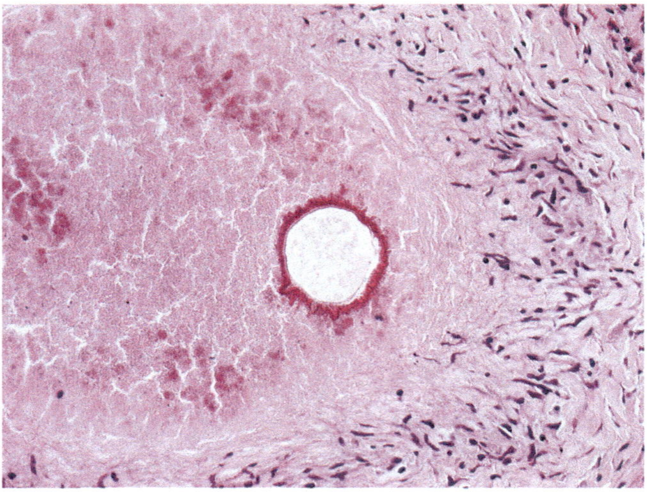

Fig. 4.105 Splendore-Hoeppli phenomenon in a case of coccidiomycosis of the lung. This phenomenon can be seen in a variety of different infectious disease etiologies. Illustrated here is a particularly stunning case, demonstrating a "starburst" pattern of eosinophilic material representing deposition of immunoglobulin surrounding a spherule of *Coccidiodes* species. H&E, 400× magnification

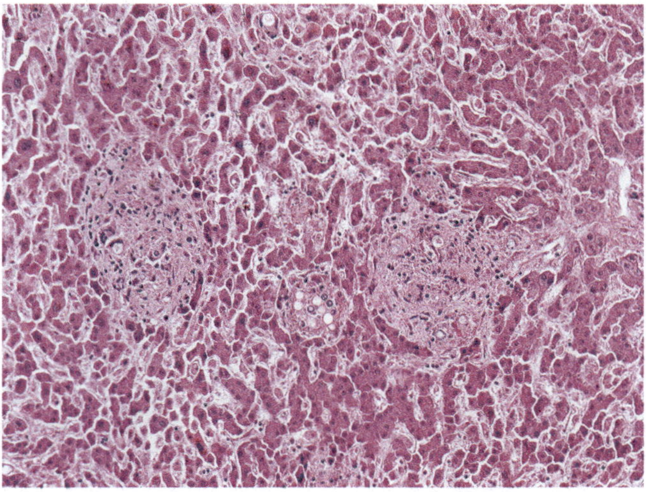

Fig. 4.106 Paracoccidioidomycosis of the liver. At first glance, the yeast cells may resemble the spherules of *Coccidiodes* species, demonstrating significant variation in size. The daughter cells characteristic of *Paracocciddiodes* species are often not initially evident on H&E staining. H&E, 200× magnification

4.7.4 Paracoccidiodes Species

Paracoccidiodes brasiliensis is the causative agent of a disease sometimes referred to as South American blastomycosis. Cases of paracoccidioidomycosis are relatively geographically restricted to Brazil, where it is most commonly found, as well as Venezuela and Colombia. Characteristically, the yeast forms appear as a "mariner's wheel" with centrally located mother cells measuring 10–20 microns in diameter and multiple surrounding spherical buds representing the handles of the wheel. Like many infections caused by dimorphic fungi, the pulmonary system is a frequent primary site of infection. However, the oral mucosa and nasal sinuses are also frequently seen as the first identified sites. This entity is also frequently found to infiltrate the lymphoid system as well as skin and bone (Figs. 4.106, 4.107, 4.108, 4.109, and 4.110).

4.7.5 *Sporothrix shenckii*

The thermally dimorphic fungi belonging to the *Sporothrix schenkii* complex are found worldwide, with greater frequency in tropical and temperate regions. Residing in soil or decaying vegetation, the typical route of infection is traumatic inoculation. Although classically associated with a rosebush thorn, leading to the name "rose gardener's disease," traumatic implantation leading to sporotrichosis can happen by any number of mechanisms. The organism characteristically spreads

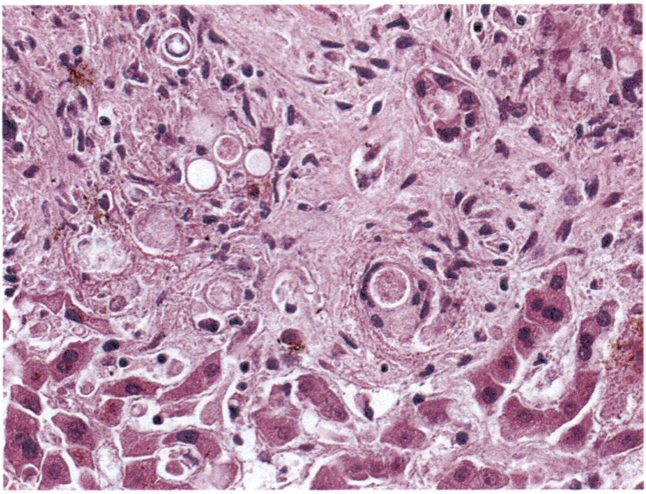

Fig. 4.107 On higher magnification, the large yeast forms of *P. brasiliensis* do not demonstrate discrete endospores, as would be seen in *Coccidiodes* infections. Again, note that the characteristic daughter yeast cells are often not readily apparent on H&E staining. 600× magnification

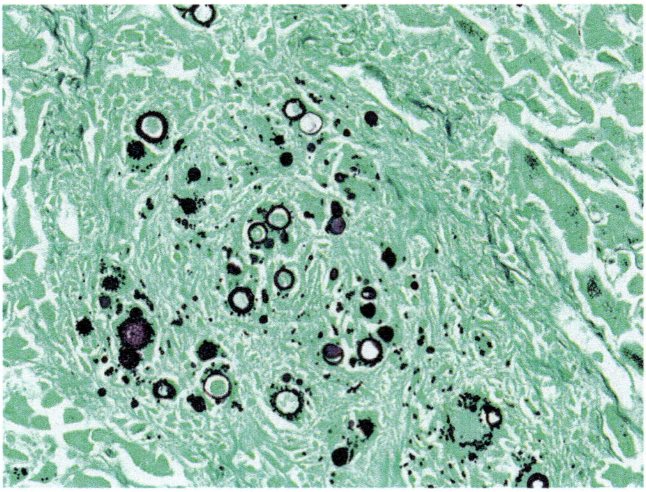

Fig. 4.108 Gomori methenamine silver stain demonstrating variably sized yeast cells, many of which also feature multiple and typically smaller cells surrounding the periphery. These findings are characteristic of *Paraccoccidiodes* species and can sometimes resemble a "mariner's wheel." Gomori methenamine silver stain, 400× magnification

proximally from the initial site of inoculation, most often the upper extremity, through the lymphatics. This leads to localized lymphadenopathy, which may demonstrate overlying cutaneous ulceration or draining sinus formation. Primary pulmonary infections have occurred through inhalation of the fungus, and disseminated disease may occur in immunocompromised patients. Zoonotic

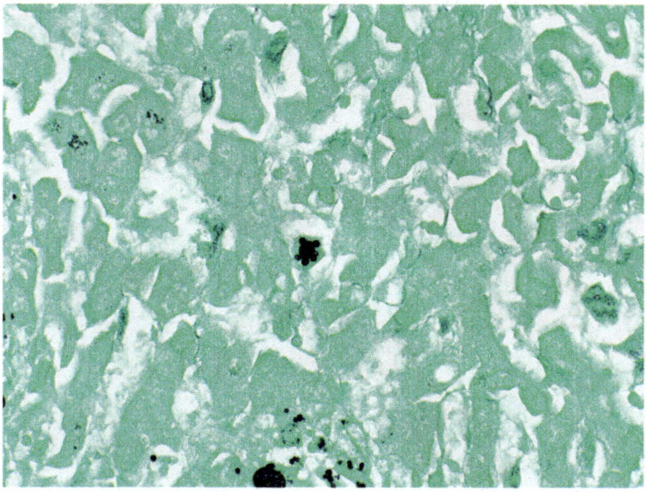

Fig. 4.109 Higher magnification image suggesting the mariner's wheel of *Paracoccidodes* species. 600× magnification

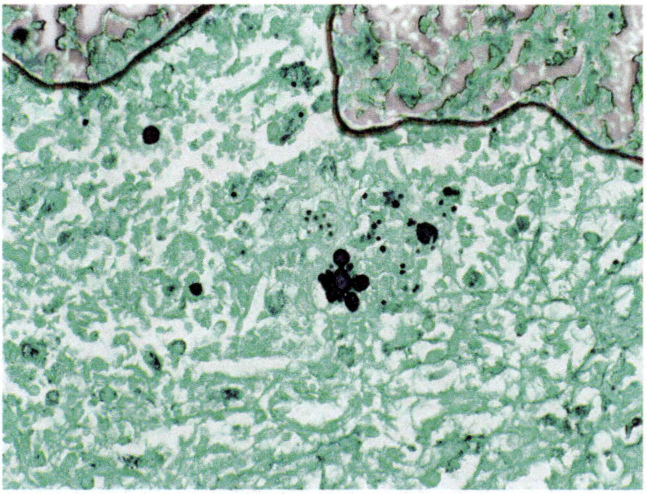

Fig. 4.110 An additional example or the mariner's wheel morphology. Note significant variability in the size of the daughter yeast cells, some of which approximate the size of the mother cells. 600× magnification

infections, particularly through scratches from infected cats, which are prone to heavy infections, are also a well-recognized cause of transmission. Most often, variably sized yeast forms 2–6 microns in length are seen. Round to oval yeast forms are usually present. However, elongated, typically crystal violet retaining "cigar bodies" are characteristic and should raise suspicion for sporotrichosis (Figs. 4.111 and 4.112).

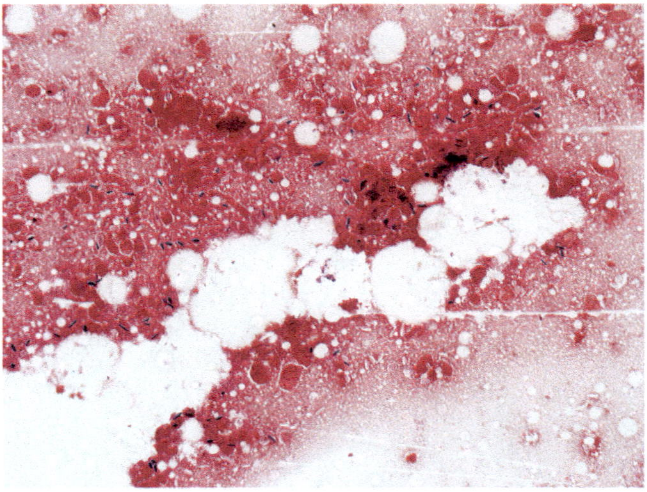

Fig. 4.111 Gram stain of a lymph node aspirate from the forearm of a patient with sporotrichosis. Note many "cigar-shaped" yeast forms. Unlike other dimorphic fungi, the yeast forms of *Sporothrix schenkii* complex tend to retain the crystal violet stain. 400× magnification

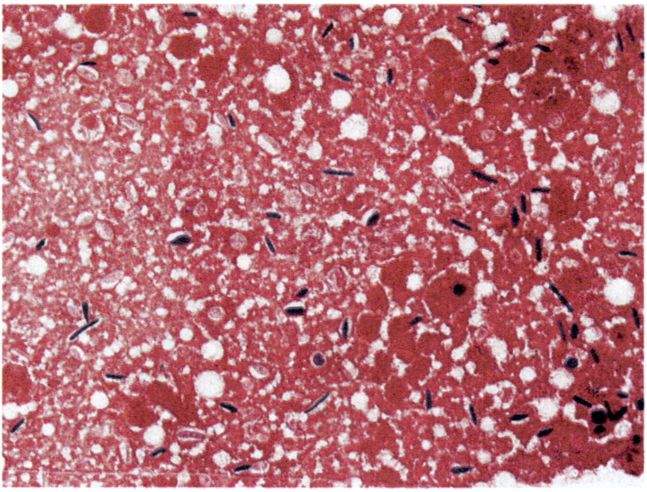

Fig. 4.112 Higher magnification image of the previously illustrated case demonstrating intermixed round and cigar-shaped forms. On careful observation, in addition to many "purple staining" forms, many pink-staining yeast forms are also evident in the background. 1000× magnification

4.8 Infections Caused by Dematiaceous Fungi

Dematiaceous fungi produce darkly pigmented colonial growth on fungal cultures, typically both on the forward (front of plate) and the reverse (back of plate). This is usually through the production of melanin or melanin-like pigment. Important for the anatomic pathologist, microscopic examination of histopathologic sections may demonstrate heavy, faint, or apparently absent pigmentation. In cases in which a dematiaceous fungus is the suspected pathogen, melanin stains, such as Fontana Masson, can be of use. Of note, there are many other fungal pathogens that are known to produce melanin, such as *Cryptococcus* species and *Sporothrix schenkii* complex, which are traditionally placed in other categories.

4.8.1 Phaeohyphomycosis

Phaeohyphomycosis is a loose term applied to infections of potentially any site caused by infection with dematiaceous fungi with over 100 species having been identified as pathogens. Cutaneous phaeohyphomycosis as well as chromoblastomycosis, to be discussed further on, are the most commonly seen infections with dematiaceous fungi worldwide and are caused by traumatic inoculation of the fungi. Cerebral phaeohyphomycosis is the most serious form of the disease and is most frequently caused by *Cladophialophora bantiana*, *Wangiella dermatitidis*, and *Rhinocladiella mackenziei*. Cerebral phaeohyphomycosis is most frequently the result of spread from the paranasal sinuses, although development of disease from traumatic inoculation or hematogenous spread from other sites has been known to occur. While most fungal central nervous system infections occur in severely immunocompromised patients, approximately half of reported cases of cerebral phaeohyphomycosis occur in apparently immunocompetent individuals (Figs. 4.113, 4.114, 4.115, 4.116, 4.117, 4.118, 4.119, and 4.120).

4.8.2 Black Grain Mycetoma

Black grain mycetoma, otherwise known as Madura foot or maduromycosis, is caused by eumycotic dematiaceous fungi, most frequently *Madurella* species. This entity primarily affects the extremities, favoring the legs and feet (hence the name Madura foot), but it may be found in any area of the body following traumatic inoculation. Like subcutaneous phaeohyphomycosis and chromoblastomycosis, this disease can be found worldwide, but it is most frequently seen in tropical or subtropical climates. Occupational injury, often in agricultural workers, is the most frequently identified route of infection. The lesions develop slowly, often over years, tend to be large and fungating, and frequently demonstrate sinus tracts that discharge black, grainy fluid (Figs. 4.121, 4.122, and 4.123).

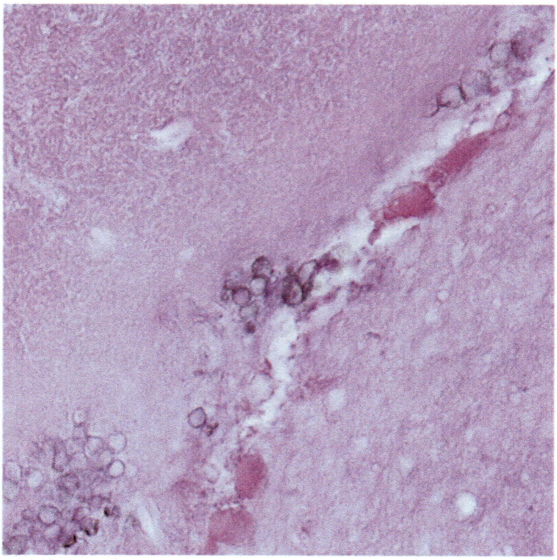

Fig. 4.113 Invasive pulmonary phaeohyphomycosis. The appearance of dematiaceous fungi on histopathologic sections are myriad. In this particular case, darkly pigmented chlamydoconidia-like structures are seen within an area of necrosis. Hyphae are frequently poorly staining and may not be readily apparent. 1000× magnification

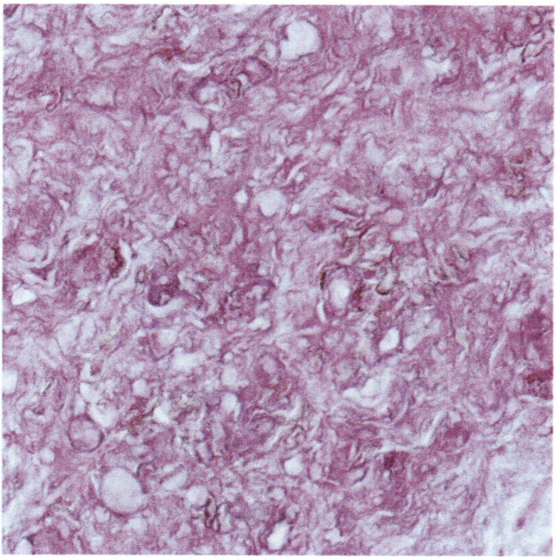

Fig. 4.114 Mats of irregular fungal hyphae were also seen in the case illustrated in Fig. 4.113. Note that dark pigmentation is frequently present in patches and may not be regularly dispersed throughout. 1000× magnification

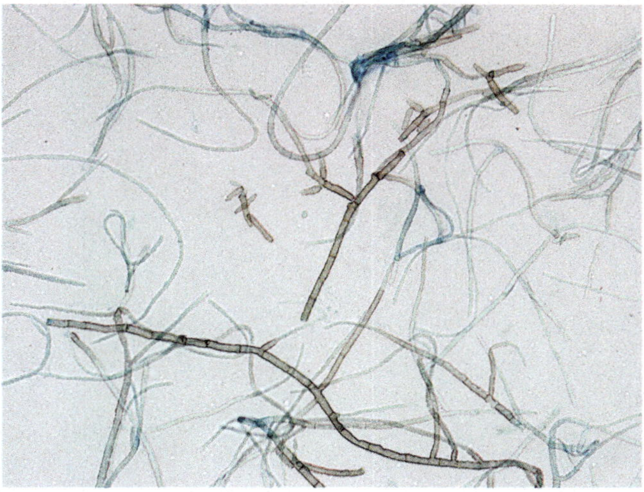

Fig. 4.115 Shown here, for purposes of illustration, is the typical appearance of the darkly pigmented hyphae of a dematiaceous fungus (in this case *Cladosporium* species) on a lactophenol cotton blue tape preparation from colonial growth. In addition to the pigment production evident in this image, dematiaceous molds are also classified in the mycology laboratory according to their reproductive structures, colony features, and growth characteristics. 400× magnification

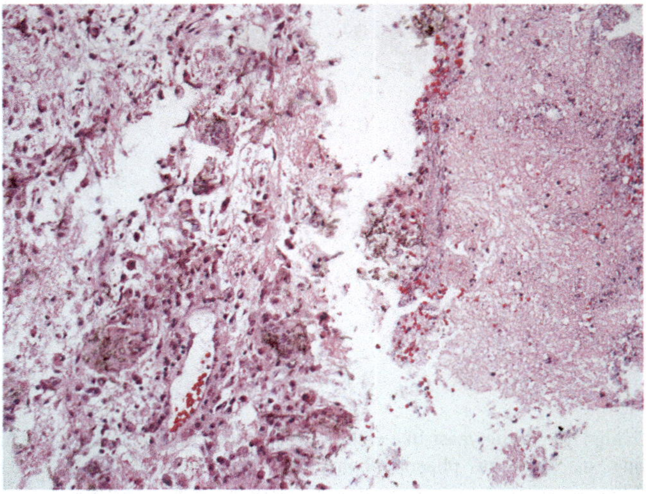

Fig. 4.116 Cerebral phaeohyphomycosis caused by infection with *Cladophialophora bantiana* identified in brain biopsy tissue. Areas of necrosis as well as reactive gliosis are identified. Darkly pigmented fungal hyphae are evident. H&E, 100× magnification

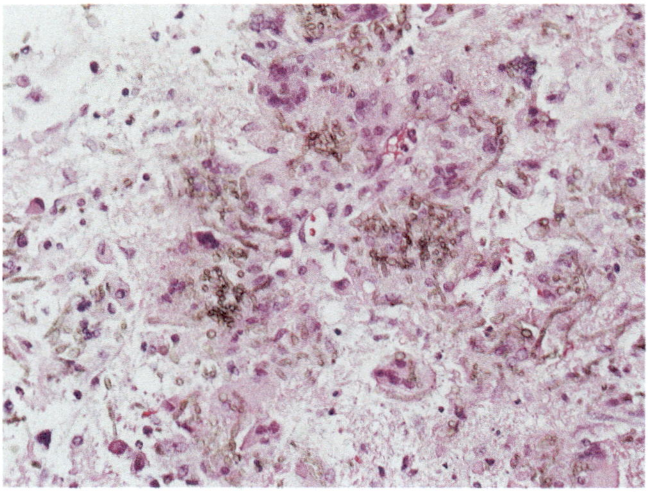

Fig. 4.117 In other areas of the brain biopsy, pigmented hyphae are seen, scattered throughout the brain parenchyma and within multinucleated giant cells. H&E, 400× magnification

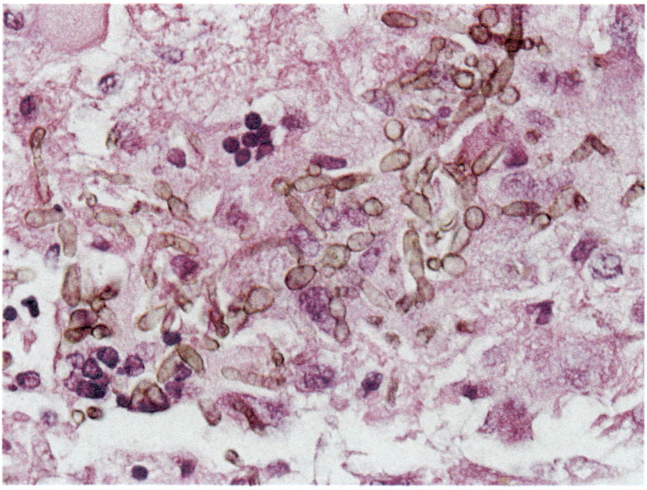

Fig. 4.118 Chains of budding yeast-like cells were also seen throughout the specimen and are a frequent finding in cases of phaeohyphomycosis regardless of location. H&E, 1000× magnification

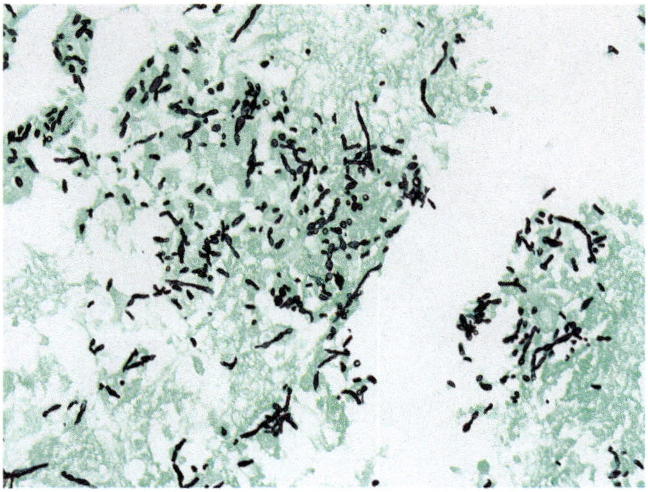

Fig. 4.119 Gomori methenamine silver stain of cerebral phaeohypomycosis demonstrating chains of budding, yeast-like cells and irregular-appearing hyphae. Note that pigmentation cannot be discerned on GMS-stained tissues, thereby requiring careful correlation with H&E or other stains. 400× magnification

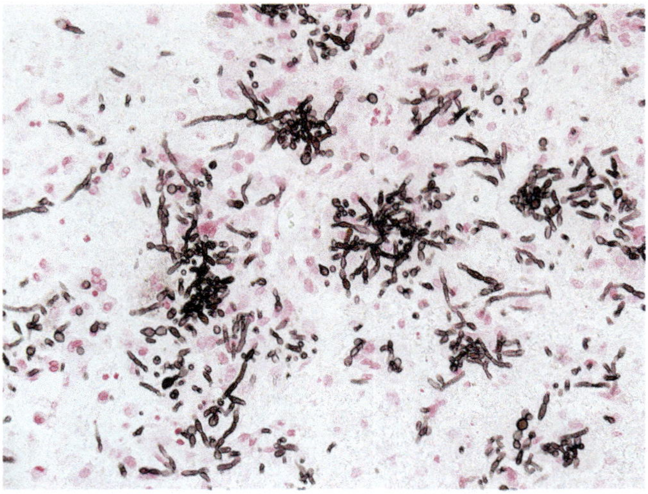

Fig. 4.120 Fontana Masson stain highlighting the melanized hyphae in the previously illustrated case. While melanin production is readily evident here, in some cases of infection with dematiaceous fungi, melanin may be difficult to visualize on standard H&E staining. Specific stains for melanin, such as Fontana Masson, may be helpful in these situations. 400× magnification

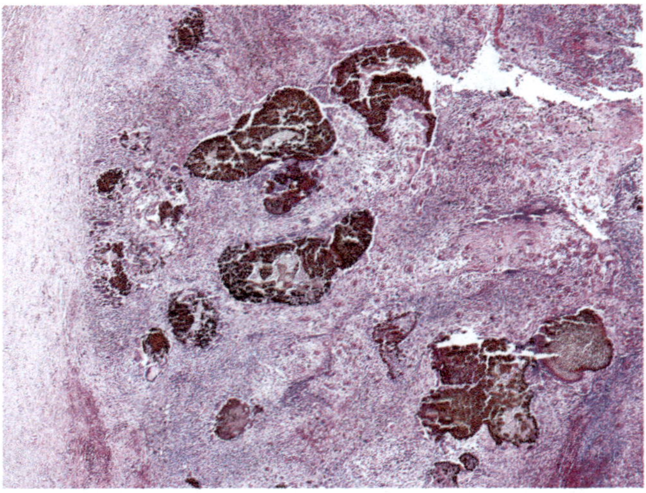

Fig. 4.121 An example of black grain mycetoma from a lower extremity tissue resection. Note the granular, darkly pigmented nodules surrounded by granulation tissue and abundant, predominantly chronic inflammation and multinucleated giant cells. Actinomycotic mycetoma may have a very similar low-power appearance, but the granules will be nonpigmented. H&E, 40× magnification

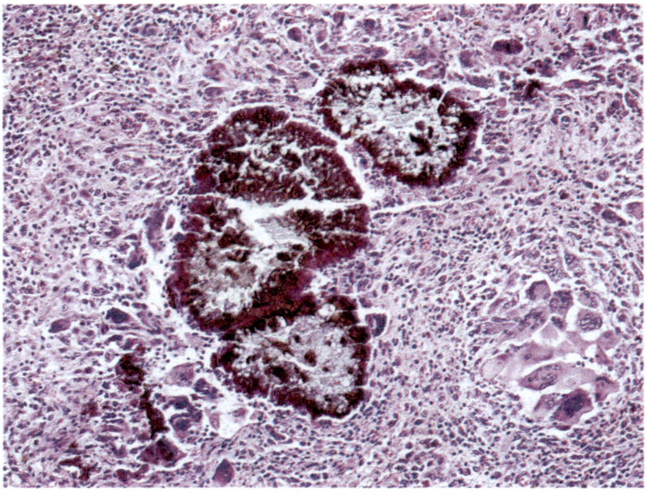

Fig. 4.122 Higher magnification of the previously illustrated case. Note the prominent, darkly pigmented hyphae as well as the predominantly chronic inflammatory cell infiltrate and multinucleated giant cells. H&E, 200× magnification

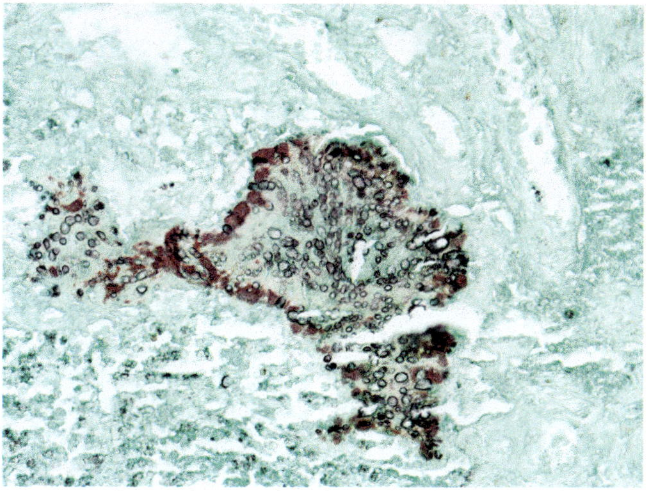

Fig. 4.123 In cases in which a non-eumycotic mycetoma, such as may be caused by *Actinomyces* species, is part of the differential, a Gomori methenamine silver stain may be helpful in outlining the much larger fungal elements as opposed to the thin (1 micron or less) bacteria. 400× magnification

4.8.3 Chromoblastomycosis

Chromoblastomycosis is a chronic infection of the skin and subcutaneous tissues by dematiaceous fungi. Note that subcutaneous phaeohyphomycosis, which consists predominantly of hyphal forms, is considered a separate entity. Chromoblastomycosis is defined as infection with dematiaceous fungi manifesting characteristic 5–12 micron, darkly pigmented muriform bodies, also referred to by a variety of other names including Medlar bodies, fumagoid cells, sclerotic bodies, or "copper pennies." The overlying epidermis characteristically demonstrates pseudoepitheliomatous hyperplasia with hyperkeratosis and parakeratosis. Microabscesses, along with a chronic inflammatory infiltrate and multinucleated giant cells, may be present. Like typical phaeohyphomycosis, these infections are most often seen in tropical or subtropical climates and are most often associated with traumatic inoculation in association with vegetation or soil (Figs. 4.124, 4.125, and 4.126).

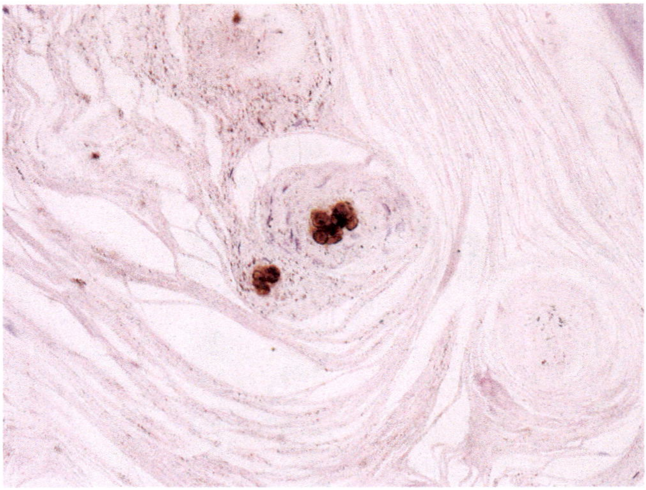

Fig. 4.124 Classic, darkly pigmented, muriform bodies present within the stratum corneum. Note the generally round appearance, along with the dark pigmentation that is reminiscent of "copper pennies." H&E, 400× magnification

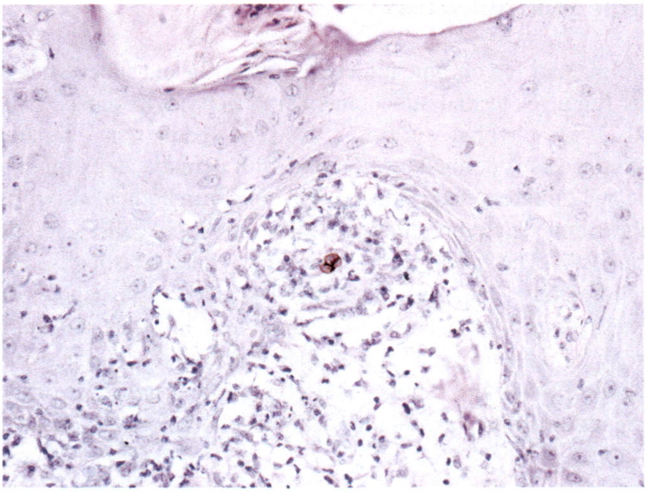

Fig. 4.125 Muriform bodies often demonstrate intersecting septations caused by fungal organisms reproducing by fission rather than budding. They may be frequently found within microabscesses but can also be freely dispersed throughout the affected tissue. H&E, 400× magnification

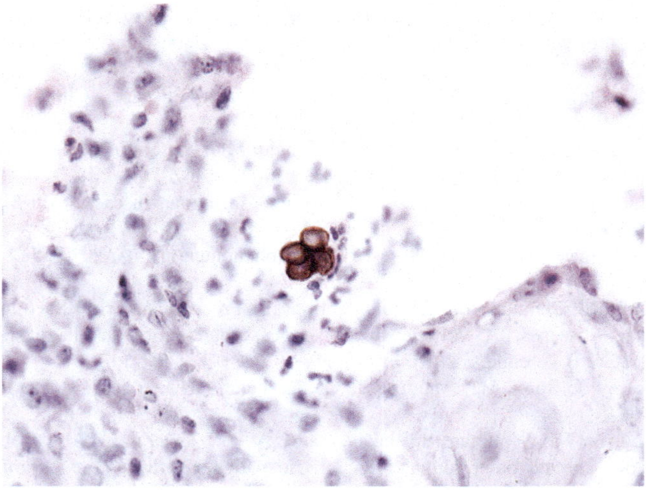

Fig. 4.126 Higher magnification image demonstrating the thick outer cell wall commonly seen with the muriform bodies of chromoblastomycosis. Note also the appearance of intersecting septations. H&E, 1000× magnification

Suggested Reading

Azar MM, Relich RF, Schmitt BH, Spech RW, Hage CA. Cutaneous blastomycosis masquerading as pyoderma gangrenosum. J Clin Microbiol. 2014;52:1298–300.

Dankner WM, Spector SA, Fierer J, Davis CE. Malassezia fungemia in neonates and adults: complication of hyperalimentation. Rev Infect Dis. 1987;9:743–53.

Frater JL, Hall GS, Procop GW. Histologic features of zygomycosis: emphasis on perineural invasion and fungal morphology. Arch Pathol Lab Med. 2001;125:375–8.

Guarner J, Brandt ME. Histopathologic diagnosis of fungal infections in the 21st century. Clin Microbiol Rev. 2011;24(2):247–80.

Jain R, Singh K, Lamzabi I, Harbhajanka A, Gattuso P, Reddy VB. Blastomycosis of bone: a clinicopathologic study. Am J Clin Pathol. 2014;142:609–16.

Kradin RL, Mark EJ. The pathology of pulmonary disorders due to *Aspergillus* spp. Arch Pathol Lab Med. 2008;132:606–14.

Li DM, de Hoog GS. Cerebral phaeohyphomycosis – a cure at what lengths? Lancet Infect Dis. 2009;9:376–83.

López Martínez R, Méndez Tovar LJ. Chromoblastomycosis. Clin Dermatol. 2007;25:188–94.

Marques SA. Paracoccidioidomycosis: epidemiological, clinical, diagnostic and treatment up-dating. An Bras Dermatol. 2013;88(5):700–11.

Morris A, Norris KA. Colonization by *Pneumocystis jirovecii* and its role in disease. Clin Microbiol Rev. 2012;25:297–317.

Nucci M, Anaissie E. Fusarium infections in immunocompromised patients. Clin Microbiol Rev. 2007;20:695–704.

Pfaller MA, Diekema DJ. Epidemiology of invasive candidiasis: a persistent public health problem. Clin Microbiol Rev. 2007;20:133–63.

Procop GW, Haddad S, Quinn J, Wilson ML, Henshaw NG, Reller LB, et al. Detection of *Pneumocystis jiroveci* in respiratory specimens by four staining methods. J Clin Microbiol. 2004;42:3333–5.

Quintella LP, Passos SR, do Vale AC, Galhardo MC, Barros MB, Cuzzi T, et al. Histopathology of cutaneous sporotrichosis in Rio de Janeiro: a series of 119 consecutive cases. J Cutan Pathol. 2011;38:25–32.

Revankar SG, Sutton DA. Melanized fungi in human disease. Clin Microbiol Rev. 2010;23:884–928.

Revankar SG, Patterson JE, Sutton DA, Pullen R, Rinaldi MG. Disseminated phaeohyphomycosis: review of an emerging mycosis. Clin Infect Dis. 2002;34:467–76.

Ribes JA, Vanover-Sams CL, Baker DJ. Zygomycetes in human disease. Clin Microbiol Rev. 2000;13:236–301.

Rodig SJ, Dorfman DM. Splendore-Hoeppli phenomenon. Arch Pathol Lab Med. 2001;125:1515–6.

Schmitt BH, Pritt BS. Dematiaceous fungal infections. In: Procop GW, Pritt BS, editors. Pathology of infectious diseases, A volume in the series: foundations in diagnostic pathology. Philadelphia: W.B. Saunders; 2015. p. 516–30.

Shah CP, McKey J, Spirn MJ, Maguire J. Ocular candidiasis: a review. Br J Ophthalmol. 2008;92:466–8.

Shibuya K, Coulson WF, Wollman JS, Wakayama M, Ando T, Oharaseki T, et al. Histopathology of cryptococcosis and other fungal infections in patients with acquired immunodeficiency syndrome. Int J Infect Dis. 2001;5:78–85.

Sobonya RE, Yanes J, Klotz SA. Cavitary pulmonary coccidioidomycosis: pathologic and clinical correlates of disease. Hum Pathol. 2014;45:153–9.

Sokulska M, Kicia M, Wesołowska M, Hendrich AB. *Pneumocystis jirovecii* – from a commensal to pathogen: clinical and diagnostic review. Parasitol Res. 2015;114:3577–85.

Wheat LJ. Antigen detection, serology, and molecular diagnosis of invasive mycoses in the immunocompromised host. Transpl Infect Dis. 2006;8:128–39.

Wheat LJ, Azar MM, Bahr NC, Spec A, Relich RF, Hage C. Histoplasmosis. Infect Dis Clin N Am. 2016;30:207–27.

Wojewoda C, Procop GW. Infections with yeast and yeastlike fungi. In: Procop GW, Pritt BS, editors. Pathology of infectious diseases, A volume in the series: foundations in diagnostic pathology. Philadelphia: W.B. Saunders; 2015. p. 531–72.

Parasitic Infections

5

Bryan H. Schmitt

While this chapter details many of the most frequently encountered parasites in anatomic pathology, it is by no means an exhaustive treatment of the subject. Additionally, certain regions of the world may be endemic for parasites not frequently encountered in pathology practices of the United States. For the identification of these less frequently encountered organisms, many extensive medical parasitology texts are available. In addition, the CDC DPDx website (http://www.cdc.gov/DPDx) is an excellent resource as well as a provider of authoritative consulting services.

5.1 Helminth Infections

Helminths encompass the parasitic worms. They are typically large and visible to the naked eye, unlike most other infectious agents. As such, identification is often more easily accomplished by gross observation rather than by histologic section. If a specimen is identifiable as a worm when received in the gross room, it is advisable to forward the organism to the microbiology lab as the first line for identification, with follow-up sections as needed. Parasitic helminths, particularly those that inhabit the gastrointestinal tract, also have characteristic eggs that may be expressed from the organism and identified in microbiology. On histopathologic examination, eggs are frequently present within or around the worms and may also provide valuable information regarding the identity of the organism; therefore many of the common egg morphologies are also discussed in this chapter.

B.H. Schmitt (✉)
Department of Pathology and Laboratory Medicine, Indiana University School of Medicine, Indianapolis, IN, USA
e-mail: bhschmit@iupui.edu

B.H. Schmitt (ed.), *Atlas of Infectious Disease Pathology*,
Atlas of Anatomic Pathology, DOI 10.1007/978-3-319-54702-2_5

5.1.1 Cestode Infections

Cestodes are more commonly known as "tapeworms," generally having ribbon-like bodies consisting of a scolex, or head, of the organism, a neck, and multiple proglottids containing reproductive structures and eggs. The larger members, such as *Taenia* and *Diphyllobothrium* species, may reach several meters or more in length, consisting almost entirely of a chain of proglottids. Since the proglottids are typically numerous and designed to break off in segments, they are much more likely to be encountered in anatomic pathology rather than the comparatively minute scolex and head structures (Figs. 5.1, 5.2, 5.3, 5.4, 5.5, 5.6, 5.7, 5.8, 5.9, 5.10, 5.11, 5.12, 5.13, 5.14, 5.15, 5.16, 5.17, 5.18, 5.19, 5.20, 5.21 and 5.22).

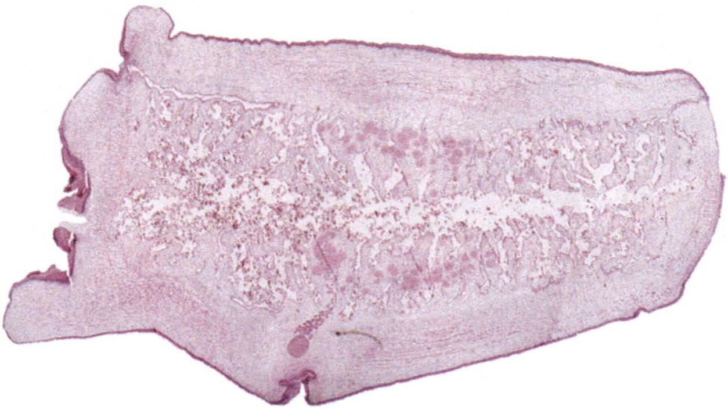

Fig. 5.1 Low magnification of a proglottid of *T. saginata*. Proper mounting of histopathologic specimens in order to demonstrate the uterine branching of *Taenia* species is difficult but was performed very well in this case owing to prior notification. Note that greater than 13 uterine branches (counted off one side only) are seen. *T. solium,* the second most frequently encountered *Taenia* species and cause of cysticercosis, has less than 13 branches. It should also be mentioned that *T. asiatica* will demonstrate greater than 13 uterine branches, similar to *T. saginata*. Infection with *T. asiatica* appears to be geographically restricted to parts of Asia as the name would suggest, and it is currently unclear whether *T. asiatica* is capable of causing cysticercosis. Hematoxylin and eosin (H&E), 20× magnification (Image courtesy of Jean Siders)

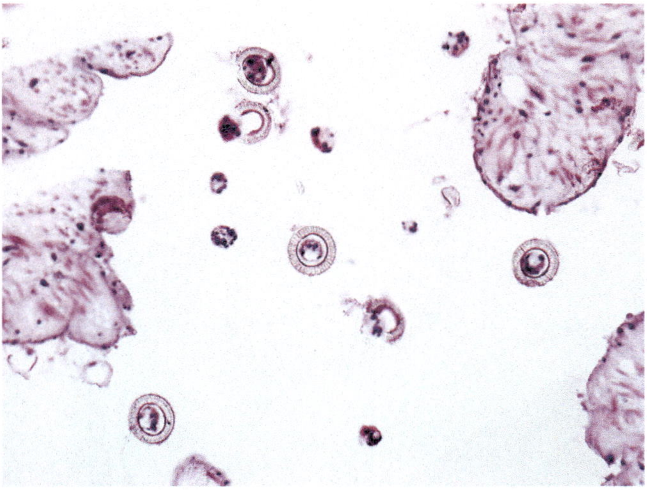

Fig. 5.2 Classic appearance of the eggs of *Taenia* species are seen in this case within the uterine branches. Note the thick shell, which demonstrates characteristic radial striations appearing similar to tightly packed "spokes on a wheel." In mature eggs, refractile hooklets are often visible in the center of the egg. Since eggs of *Taenia* species are essentially indistinguishable, patient history or examination of the uterine branches if possible is essential to making the correct identification. H&E, 400× magnification

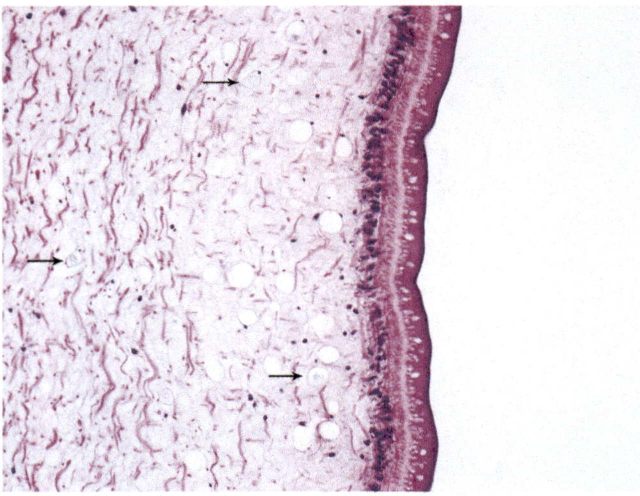

Fig. 5.3 An image of the proglottid wall. Note the thick cuticle, which is a common feature of many helminths. Characteristic for cestodes, however, are the many calcareous corpuscles (*arrows*), which are layered deposits of calcium carbonate often appearing as clear staining or purple laminated bodies within the walls of cestodes or within cestode-associated cyst fluid. H&E, 400× magnification

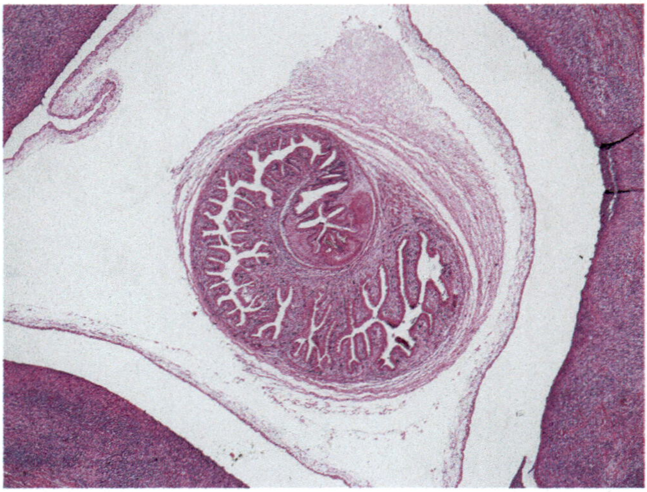

Fig. 5.4 Cysticercosis caused by infection with the larval stage of *T. solium* can manifest in nearly any organ system. However, infection of the central nervous system or "neurocysticercosis" is particularly devastating, leading to seizures and other neural disorders. The eggs of *T. solium* are autoinfectious to humans and may also pose a risk to contacts, whereas ingestion of *T. saginata* eggs does not lead to the development of cysticercosis. Differentiation of the two species may therefore be important for the purpose of treatment of patient contacts. Seen here is the typical appearance of a live *T. solium* cyst demonstrating the invaginated neck and head region of the protoscolex. Brain biopsy. H&E, 40× magnification

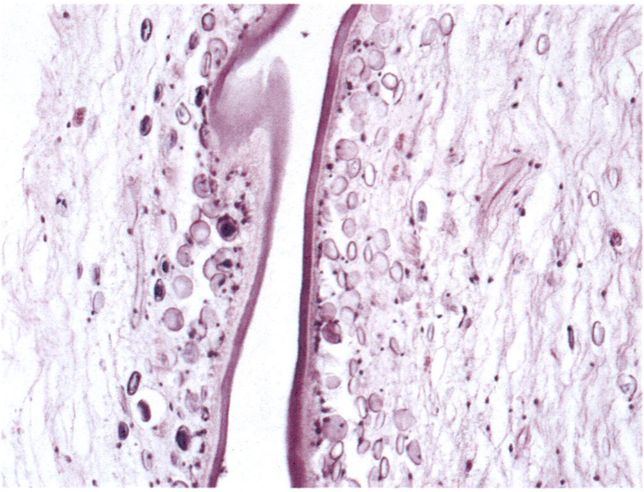

Fig. 5.5 Higher magnification of the cysticercus demonstrates numerous purple staining, calcareous corpuscles that are characteristic for cestode tissue. This finding may be very helpful in the identification of tapeworm parts, when scant tissue is present or if the plane of section does not demonstrate other characteristic structures. H&E, 400× magnification

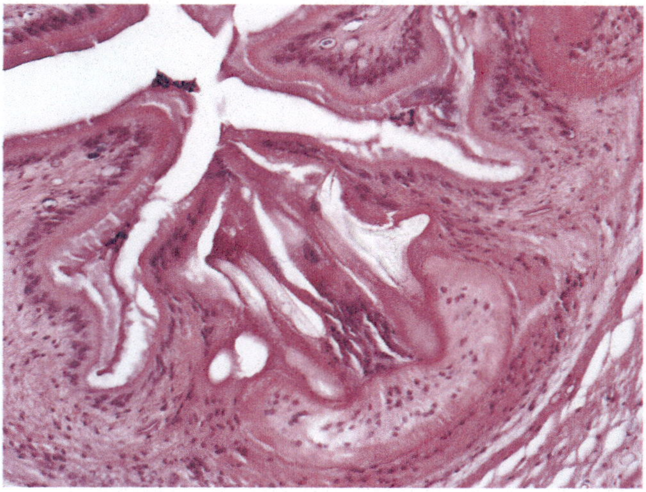

Fig. 5.6 A section of the tissue from the case seen in Fig. 5.4 demonstrating rows of refractile appearing hooklets. Adjustment into differing planes of focus often highlights these structures. H&E, 1000× magnification

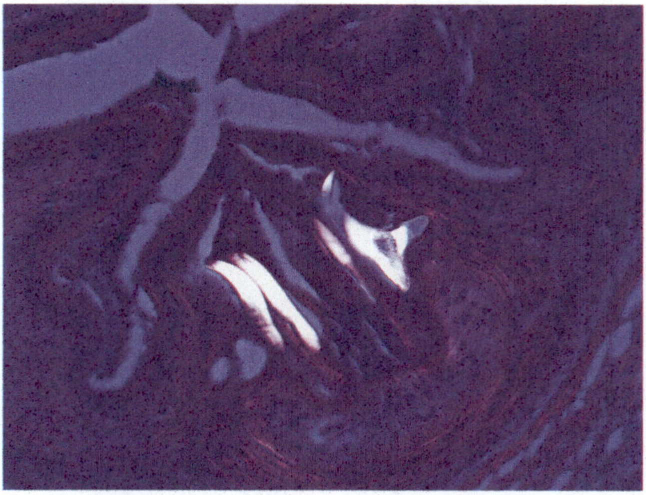

Fig. 5.7 Hooklets of cestodes in general are often birefringent and appear bright under polarized light. H&E, 1000× magnification

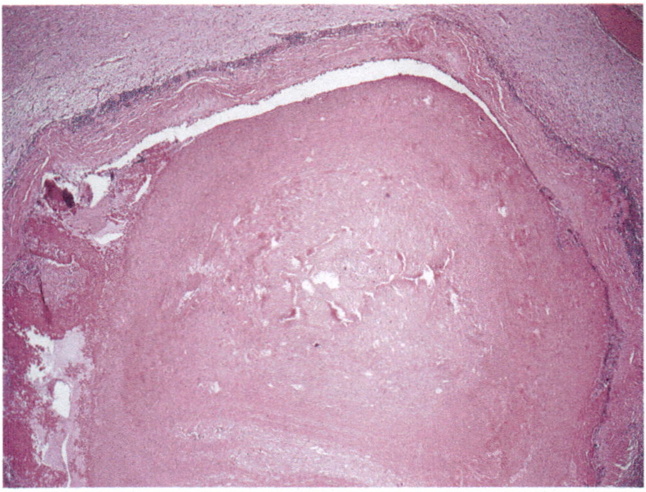

Fig. 5.8 A "dead" cyst in a case of neurocysticercosis identified at autopsy from a patient who had developed seizures, a common complication of neurocysticercosis. The inflammatory host response in reaction to dying cysticerci is significantly greater than when they are live, initially recruiting a dense acute inflammatory infiltrate and eosinophils and later a chronic granulomatous response. Eventually the cyst develops a thick fibrotic wall that may also demonstrate significant calcification. H&E, 40× magnification

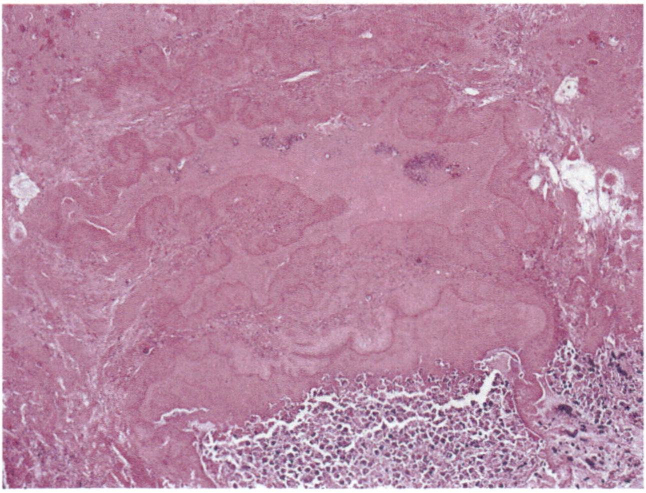

Fig. 5.9 "Ghosted-out" folds or invaginations can still be identified in this specimen. The appearance is similar to that seen in coagulative necrosis. H&E, 200× magnification

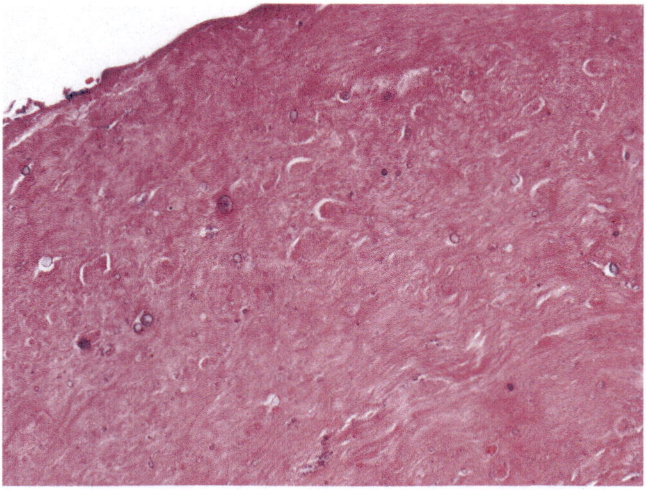

Fig. 5.10 Calcareous corpuscles frequently remain behind in the necrotic cysticercus and may be the only means of identification as a cestode infection. H&E, 400× magnification

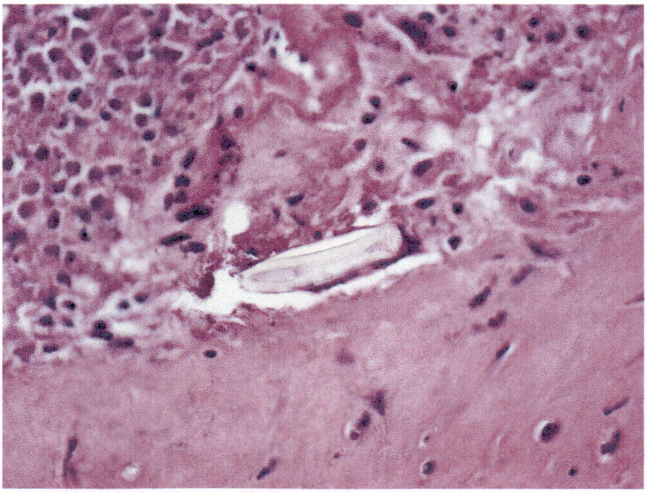

Fig. 5.11 Higher magnification of the case from Figs. 5.8, 5.9 and 5.10. In addition to calcareous corpuscles, refractile hooklets may occasionally be found within the degenerated material. H&E, 600× magnification

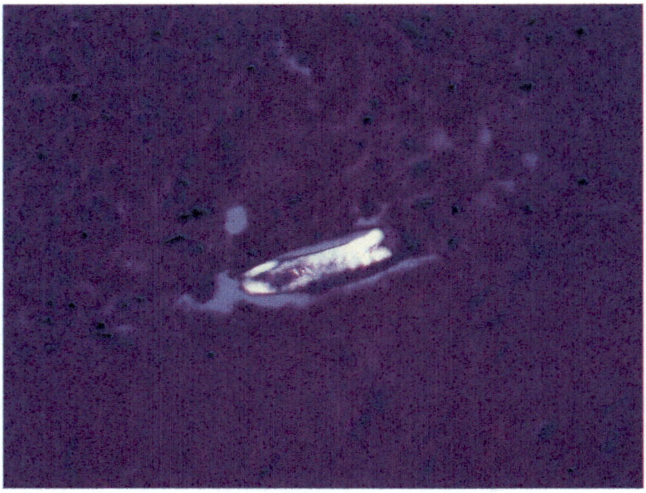

Fig. 5.12 The hooklet demonstrated in Fig. 5.11 under polarized light. This quality may help ascertain if the object is indeed a hooklet or if it is other mineralized material or debris. H&E, 600× magnification

Fig. 5.13 Of the large tapeworms that routinely infect humans, *Diphyllobothrium latum* along with *Taenia* species are likely the most frequently encountered, depending on geographic location. They can be distinguished by the shape of the mature proglottids being broader than long; hence the term "broad fish tapeworm." Note that the uterus has a characteristic "rosette" pattern differing from the branching pattern of *Taenia* species. Carmine stain, 20× magnification

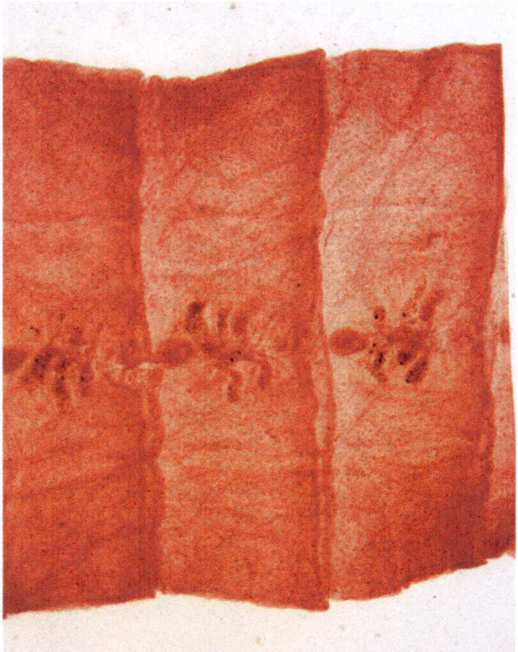

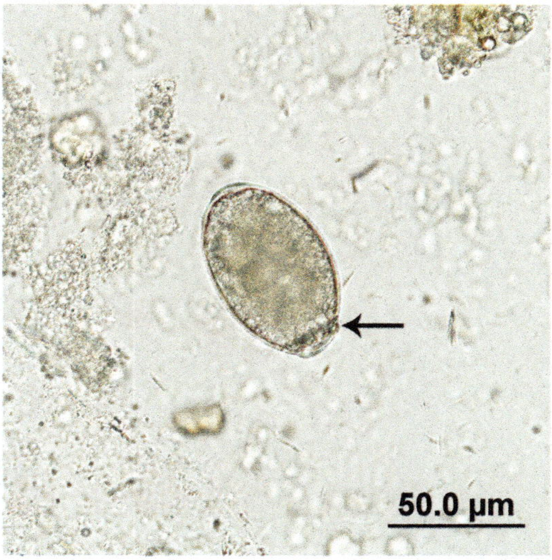

Fig. 5.14 The eggs of *D. latum* are also significantly different in appearance from those of *Taenia* species. The eggs are larger and have a "hatch" at one end (the operculum, denoted by an *arrow*) as well as a subtle abopercular knob or thickening at the opposite end. The eggs may be seen in proglottids but can also be encountered near the luminal surface of lower gastrointestnal tract specimens. Wet mount, 400× magnification (Image courtesy of Dr. Ryan Relich)

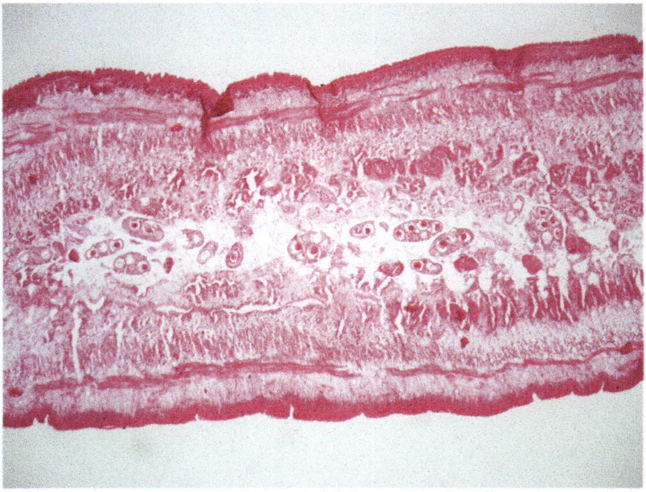

Fig. 5.15 *Dipylidium caninum* most commonly infects dogs and cats but can be transferred to humans through the ingestion of fleas harboring the cysticercoid stage. The proglottids are small, resembling rice grains, and they are often actively moving when freshly passed. Observation of "egg packets" within a sectioned proglottid or gastrointestinal tract specimen is characteristic. H&E, 100× magnification

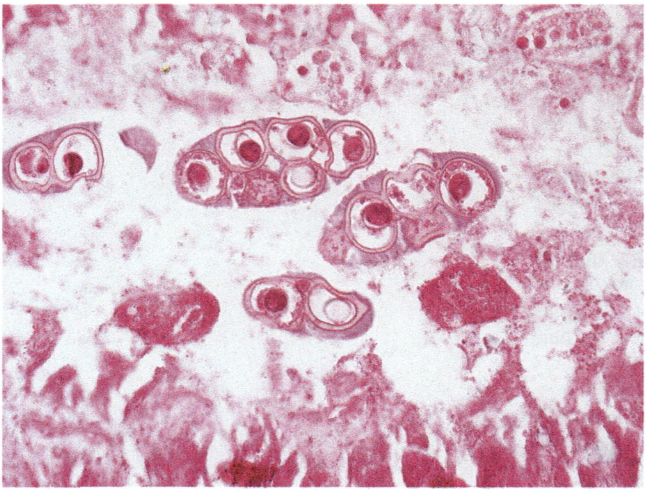

Fig. 5.16 Higher magnification demonstrating eggs clustered together in "packets" surrounded by a thin membrane. More mature eggs may demonstrate sets of internal hooklets. H&E, 400× magnification

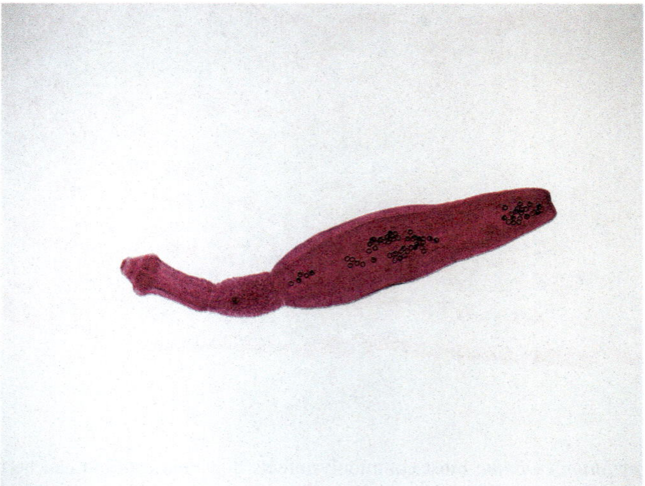

Fig. 5.17 Adult *Echinococcus granulosus*. These cestodes are significantly smaller than the previously discussed species. Adults measure up to 6 mm and demonstrate three proglottids in varying stages of maturation. As canines are the definitive host, adults are not typically encountered as anatomic pathology specimens. Humans act as an intermediate host in which hydatid cyst forms are seen. Whole mount, carmine stain, 40× magnification

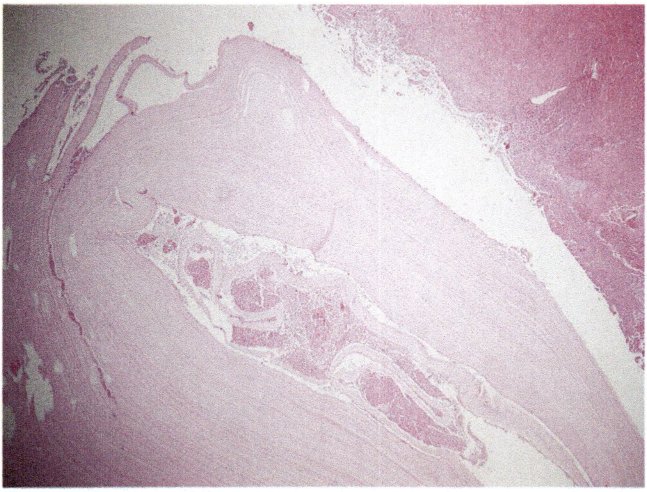

Fig. 5.18 Degenerated hydatid cyst of the liver caused by infection of *E. granulosus*. Note that *E. granulosus* typically produces a thick, unilocular cyst wall that has a prominent laminated appearance. Prior rupture of the cysts resulting from trauma or medical procedures may cause the formation of additional, usually adjacent cysts; however, the laminated appearance should be preserved. H&E, 40× magnification

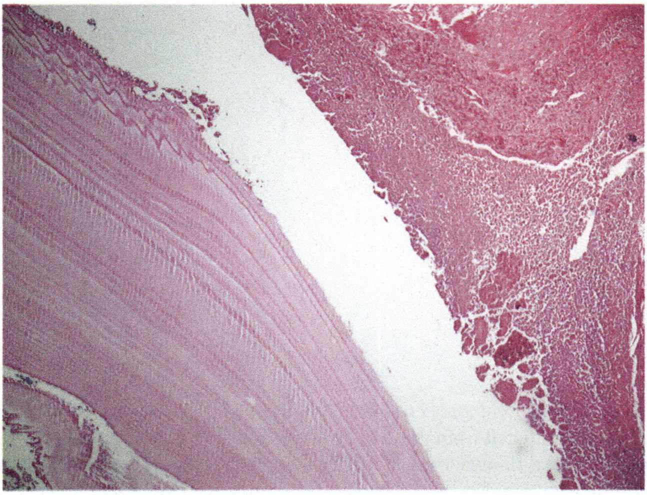

Fig. 5.19 Higher magnification image demonstrating prominent lamination of the cyst wall. H&E, 100× magnification

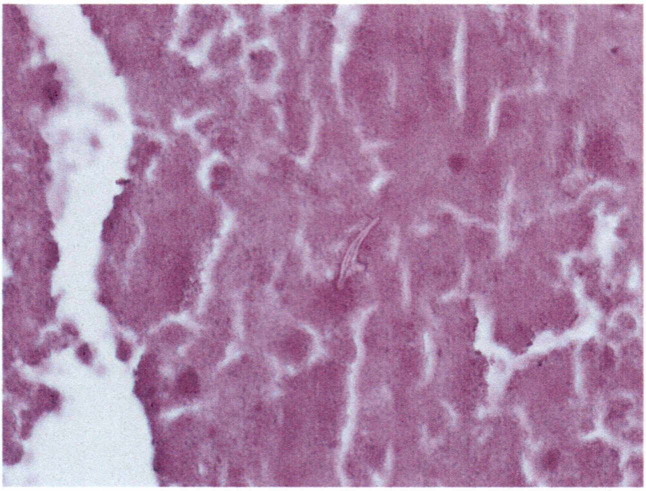

Fig. 5.20 In this particular case, rare refractile hooklets could be found within the degenerating cellular material. H&E, 1000× magnification

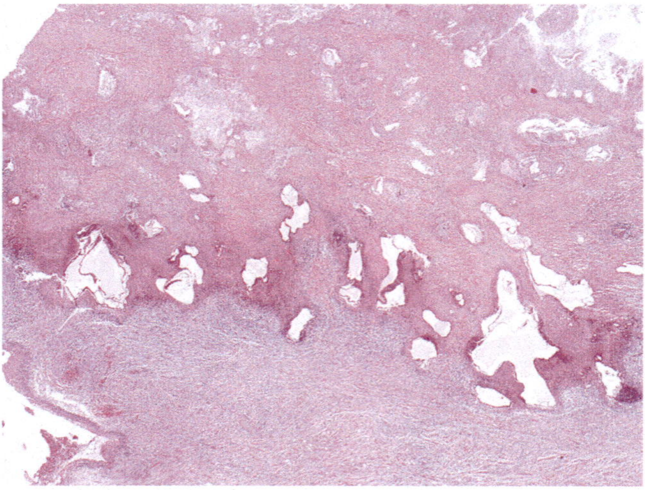

Fig. 5.21 An example of *Echinococcus multilocularis* infection in liver tissue. *E. multilocularis* infections can be differentiated from those of *E. granulosus* in that there are usually multiple thin-walled cysts present that will invade through tissue and may even demonstrate dissemination. The cysts are also often multilocular, as the name would suggest. H&E, 20× magnification (Image courtesy of Dr. Bobbi Pritt)

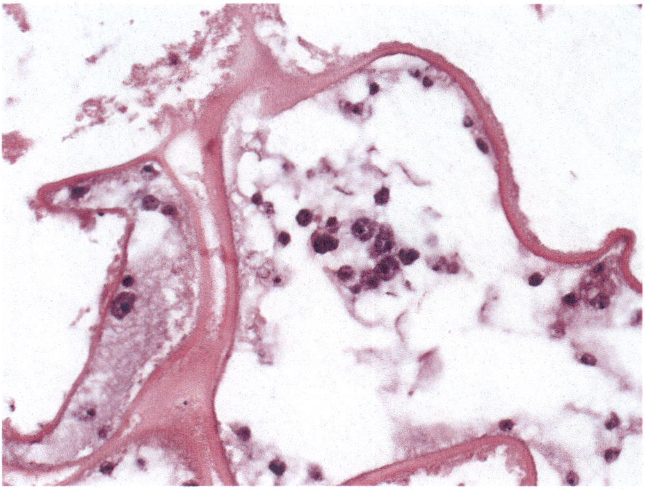

Fig. 5.22 Higher magnification image demonstrating multilocular cysts of *E. multilocularis*. The walls are thinner than those of *E. granulosus*, and while laminations may be present, they are not nearly as prominent. Protoscolices are not usually indentified. H&E, 1000× magnification (Image courtesy of Dr. Bobbi Pritt)

5.1.2 Trematode Infections

The trematodes are a group of parasitic flatworms, more commonly known as flukes. The most well known of this group are the schistosomes, the adults of which inhabit the mesenteric or urinary plexus, depending on species. As these areas are infrequently surgically sampled, schistosome infections are most commonly identified by detection of their eggs in stool, urine, or on biopsy of the lower gastrointestinal tract or urinary bladder. Other trematodes such as *Clonorchis*, *Opisthorchis*, or *Fasciola* species have a predilection for the biliary system, while *Paragonimus* species are most frequently found within pulmonary tissue (Figs. 5.23, 5.24, 5.25, 5.26, 5.27, 5.28, 5.29, 5.30, 5.31, 5.32, 5.33, 5.34, 5.35, 5.36, 5.37, 5.38, 5.39, 5.40 and 5.41).

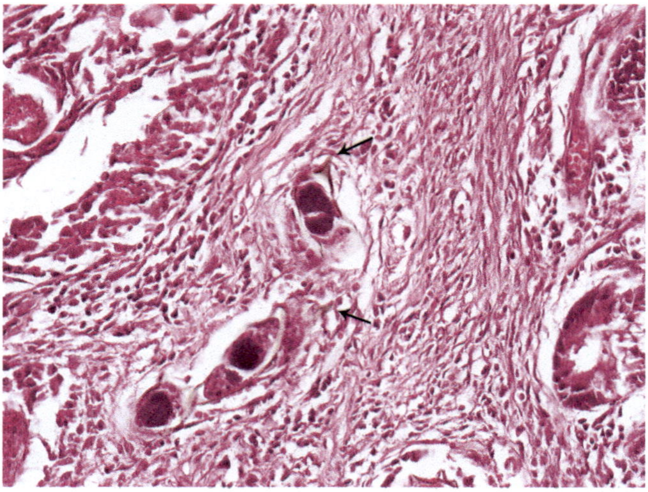

Fig. 5.23 Adult schistosomes are rarely identified in anatomic pathology tissue. Instead, their characteristic eggs are seen. The eggs of *Schistosoma mansoni*, the most well-known of the species, are usually seen in the mucosa of the lower gastrointestinal tract, often causing a polyp-like mass that is biopsied at routine colonoscopy. Shown here is the characteristic appearance of eggs of *S. mansoni,* which demonstrate a large lateral spine. The spines may be very difficult to identify on histopathologic examination because their appearance depends largely on the plane of section. While not seen here, significant calcification of the eggs, particularly in longstanding lesions, may be present. H&E, 400× magnification

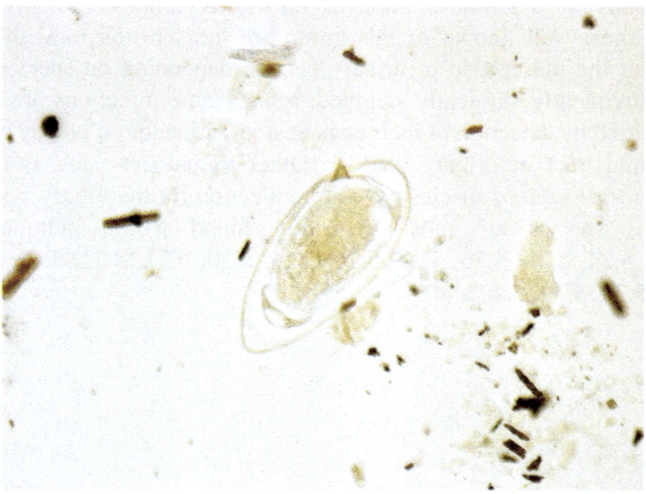

Fig. 5.24 *S. mansoni* egg from an iodine-stained stool microscopic examination demonstrating the classic appearance of the large lateral spine. 400× magnification

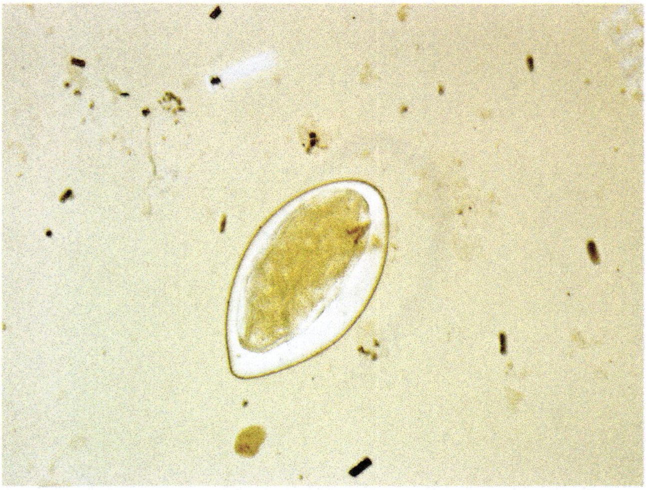

Fig. 5.25 A rotated *S. mansoni* egg from the same preparation. Here the spine is positioned toward the microscopist. A histologic section taken with an egg oriented in this manner likely would not demonstrate the characteristic lateral spine. 400× magnification

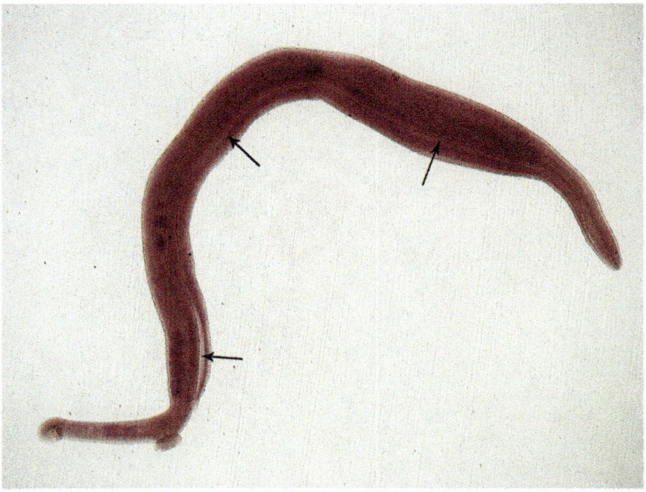

Fig. 5.26 An adult male *S. mansoni* fluke. Note the gynecophoral canal (*arrows*) in which the copulating female fluke resides. Carmine stain, whole mount, 40× magnification

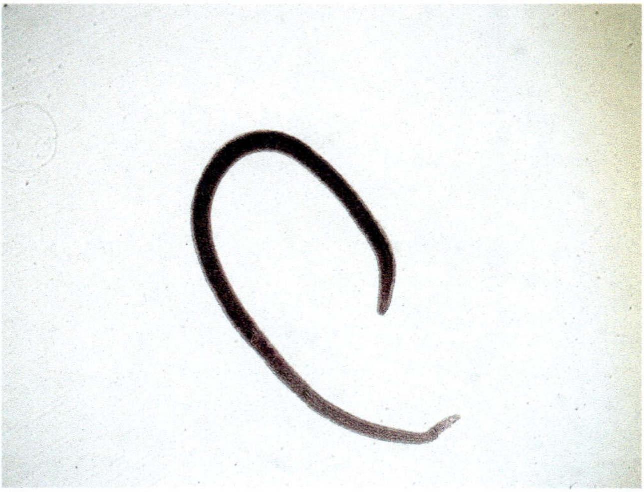

Fig. 5.27 An adult female *S. mansoni* fluke. Unlike the typical "flatworm" appearance of most trematodes, female schistosomes are cylindrical. Carmine stain, whole mount, 40× magnification

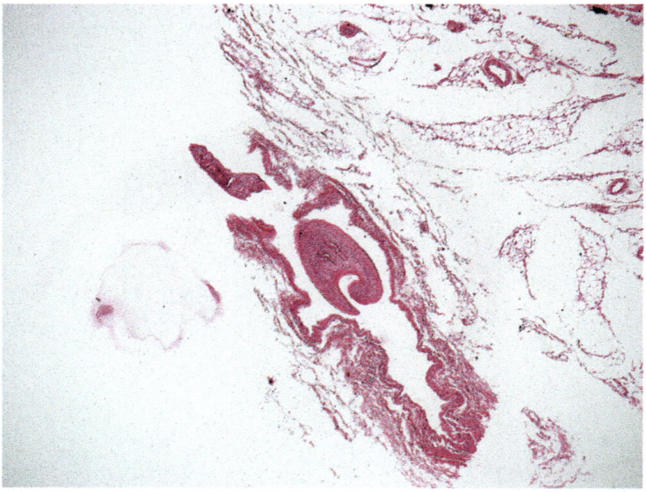

Fig. 5.28 Male *S. mansoni* within a mesenteric vein. Note that a whole mount, such as demonstrated in Fig. 5.26, might give the appearance of a cylindrical worm. Male shistosomes are in fact flat, curling their edges around copulating females. H&E, 40× magnification

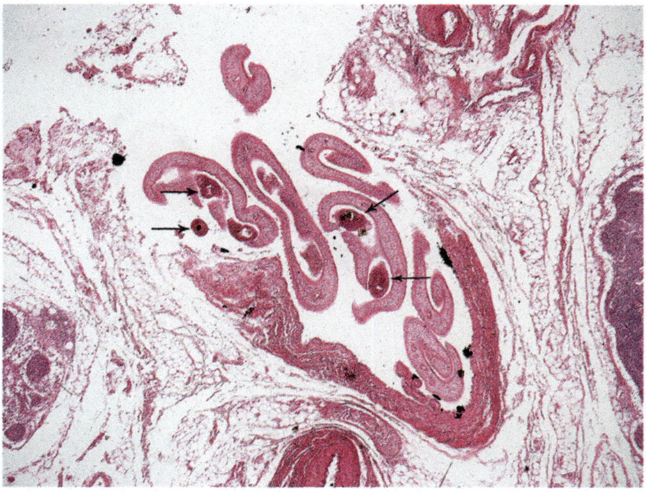

Fig. 5.29 Several copulating *S. mansoni* flukes within a mesenteric vein. Note cross-sections of female *S. mansoni* within the gynecophoral canals of males (*arrows*). H&E, 40× magnification

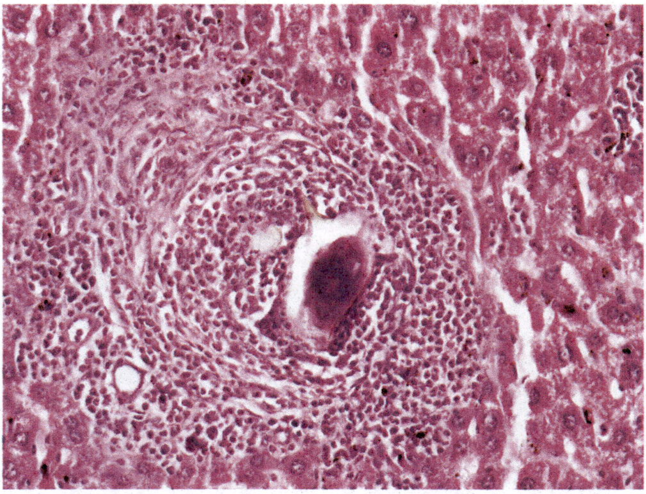

Fig. 5.30 While the colon is the primary site for migration of the eggs of *S. mansoni*, it is important to note that the eggs may be found in nearly any abdominal/pelvic location, with the liver, as seen here, another frequent destination. The prominent lateral spine in this image is diagnostic for *S. mansoni*. H&E, 400× magnification

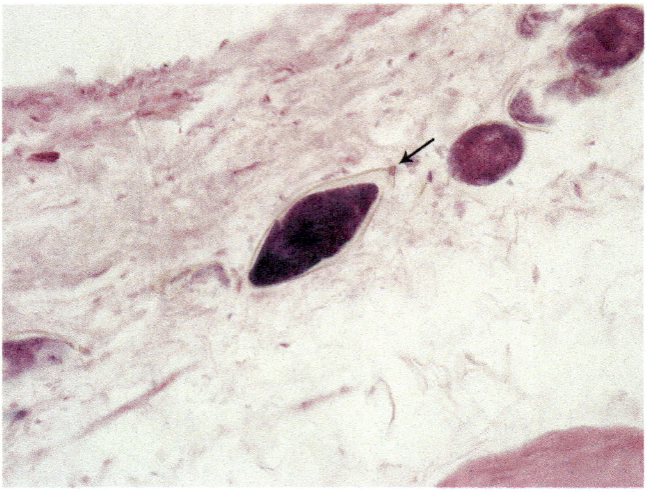

Fig. 5.31 In contrast to *S. mansoni*, *S. haematobium* is most frequently found within the urinary system, as the adults reside within the venous plexus surrounding the urinary bladder. Eggs of *S. haematobium* are more elongate than *S. mansoni* and feature a less prominent, terminal spine (*arrow*). H&E, 400× magnification

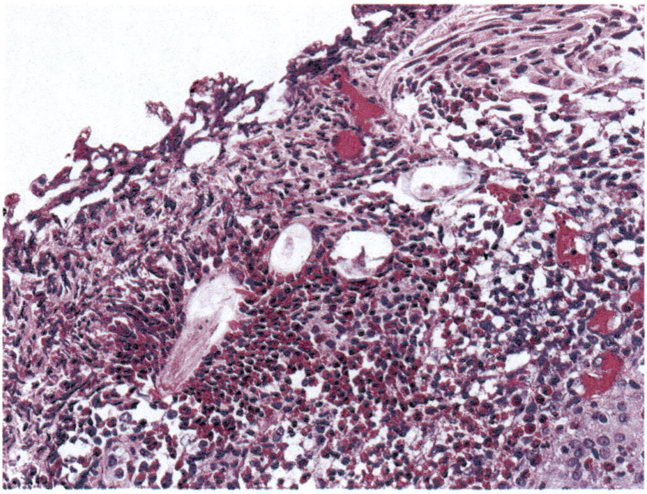

Fig. 5.32 *S. haematobium* eggs within the epithelium of the urinary bladder. The refractile shell of the eggs is readily apparent; however, the characteristic terminal spines are not. Note the elongate shape of the eggs and the location within the urinary bladder, which are good indicators of infection with *S. haematobium*. Note also a prominent eosinophilic inflammatory response, commonly seen with parasitic infections. H&E, 400× magnification

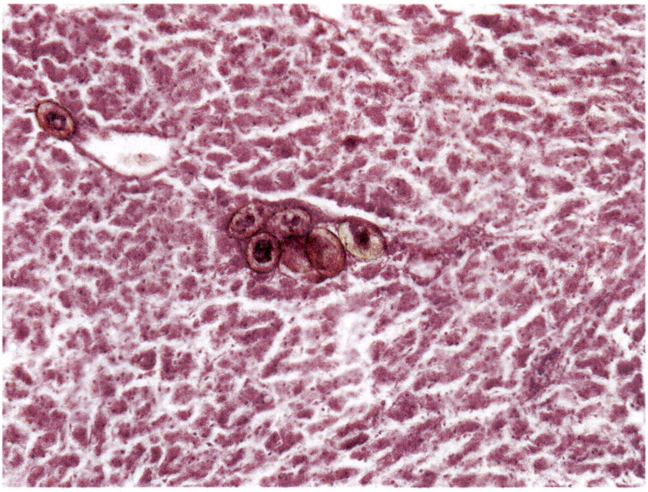

Fig. 5.33 *S. japonicum* seen in the liver. Like *S. mansoni*, the adult forms of *S. japonicum* usually reside in the mesenteric plexus and therefore, along with the colon, the liver is a frequent location where their eggs are identified. The eggs of *S. japonicum* are round to slightly oval and characteristically have a very small lateral spine, or nub, which is often unidentifiable. H&E, 200× magnification

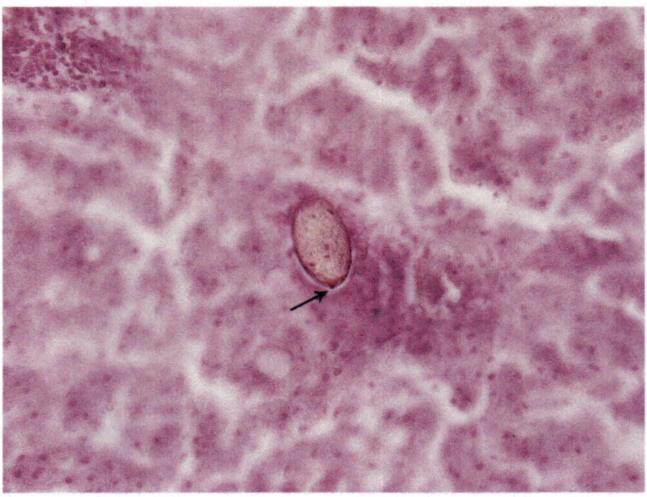

Fig. 5.34 The typical appearance of the small spine of *S. japonicum* eggs seen within a liver biopsy specimen (*arrow*). H&E, 400× magnification

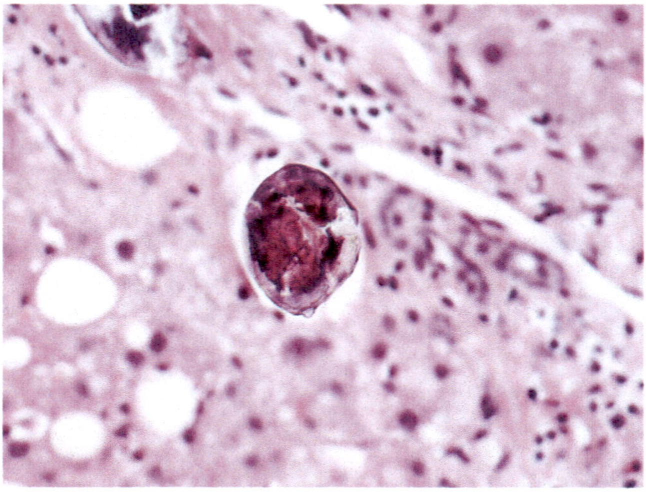

Fig. 5.35 A higher magnification image demonstrating the small lateral spine of *S. japonicum* in a partially calcified egg within the liver. Note that the liver tissue in the background is in a different plane of focus. Changing planes may be an important method to identify subtle features of infectious microorganisms. H&E, 600× magnification

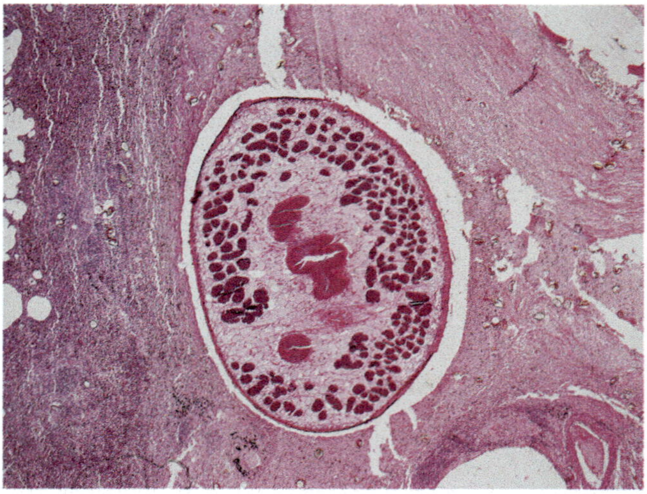

Fig. 5.36 *Paragonimus* species, also known as "lung flukes," are large trematodes that typically infect the pulmonary system following ingestion of undercooked crustaceans. While most commonly found in Asia, where *P. westermani* is most common, infections in North America with *P. kellicotti* have been documented. After entering the lung following migration from the intestines, the worm exhibits a chronic and granulomatous inflammatory response which, over time, creates a fibrous "capsule" around the organism. H&E, 40× magnification

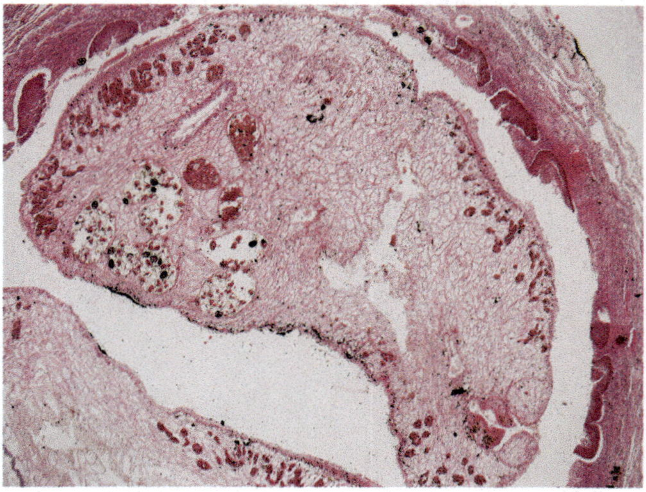

Fig. 5.37 Depending on where the fluke is sectioned, a significant perceived size variation may be noted, with the fluke appearing much larger if cut through the center. H&E, 40× magnification

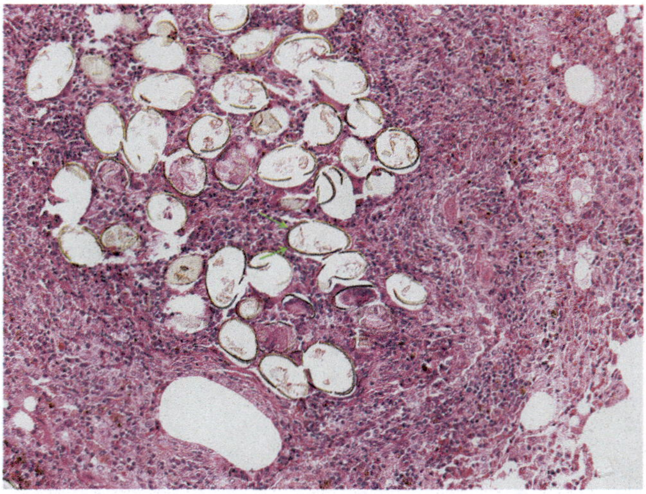

Fig. 5.38 The eggs of *Paragonimus* species are large, approximately 80–120 microns in length, and demonstrate a thick refractile shell. One end demonstrates a "shouldered" operculum having two tiny knobs on either side (*arrows*) and an opposite end that is slightly thickened. They may be identified within the fluke itself or scattered throughout the adjacent tissue, where they elicit a chronic and granulomatous inflammatory response. H&E, 200× magnification

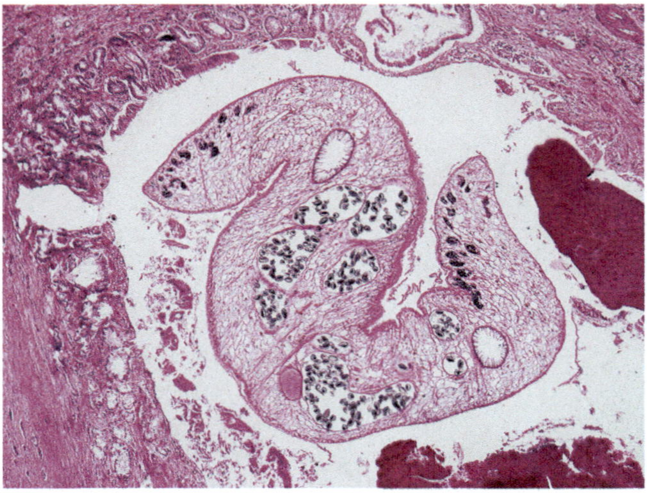

Fig. 5.39 *Clonorchis sinensis* within a bile duct. The liver flukes, *Clonorchis sinensis* and *Opisthorchis* species, are each small (10–15 mm in length) flukes that reside principally within the biliary duct system. Fibrosis and glandular hyperplasia are common features. *Fasciola* species reside within the hepatic biliary tree and are typically much larger (30–75 mm in length, depending on species). H&E, 100× magnification

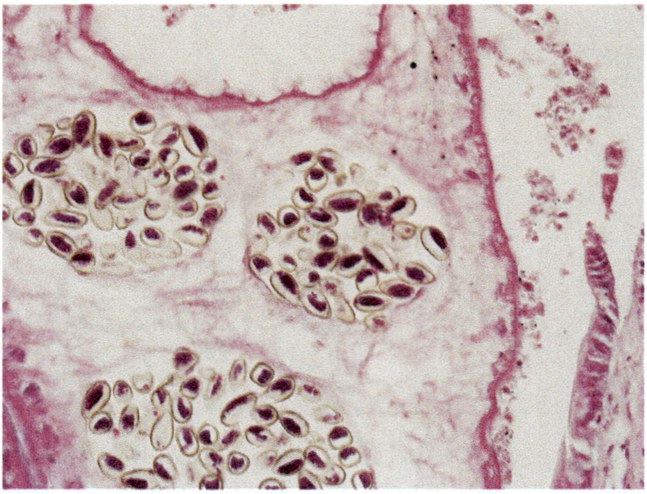

Fig. 5.40 At higher magnification, intrauterine clusters of eggs can be seen and may be helpful in making a diagnosis. H&E, 400× magnification

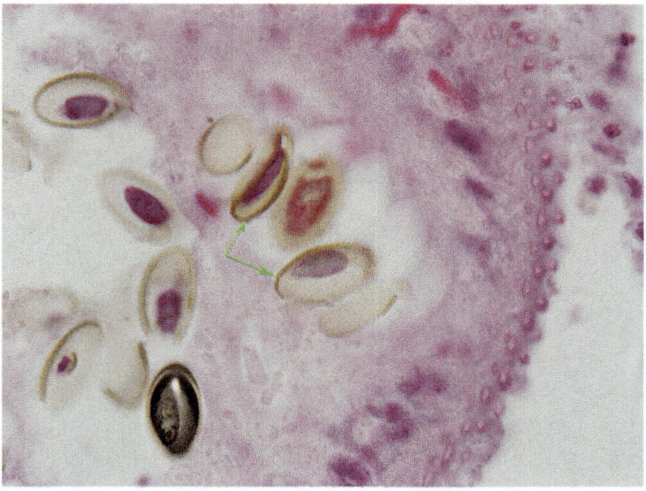

Fig. 5.41 The eggs of *Clonorchis* and *Opisthorchis* species are very similar in appearance and size (~25–35 μm long) and may be indistinguishable from each other. A "shouldered" (*arrows*) operculum is typically evident and a small abopercular knob may also be identified. The eggs are often described as being "urn-shaped."H&E, 1000× magnification

5.1.3 Nematode Infections

Nematodes are "roundworms" and are long and cylindrically shaped. They constitute the most common helminthic infections of humans, having a wide variety of members with humans as accidental, dead end, or definitive hosts, depending on the species. As such, they are associated with a wide variety of disease presentations (Figs. 5.42, 5.43, 5.44, 5.45, 5.46, 5.47, 5.48, 5.49, 5.50, 5.51, 5.52, 5.53, 5.54, 5.55, 5.56, 5.57, 5.58, 5.59, 5.60, 5.61, 5.62, 5.63, 5.64, 5.65, 5.66, 5.67 and 5.68).

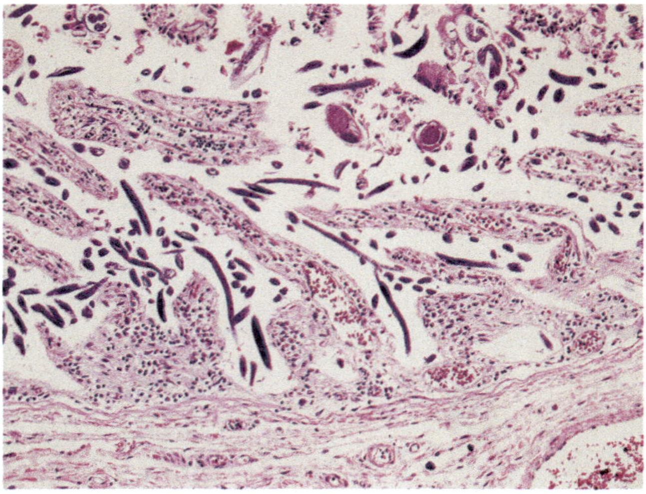

Fig. 5.42 *Strongyloides stercoralis,* also commonly known as "threadworm," most commonly causes an asymptomatic disease or mild gastrointestinal symptoms. Adult worms typically reside in the small intestine. However, the eggs they produce have the ability to hatch within the large intestine, producing rhabditiform larvae that may be excreted in the stool or mature into filariform larvae, which in turn migrate through the intestinal wall, through the bloodstream to the lungs, eventually returning to the small intestine where they can mature into adults, perpetuating the cycle known as "autoinfection." As a result of autoinfection, *Strongyloides* may persist in the gastrointestinal tract for the lifetime of the patient. While they usually cause asymptomatic or mild disease, patients who become immunocompromised may experience life-threatening "hyperinfection syndrome" in which high worm burdens migrate out of the gastrointestinal tract and throughout the body. As a result of mass migration though the intestinal wall, the first clinical manifestation of this disease is often bacteremia with enteric organisms. Small intestine demonstrating sections of many *Strongyloides* worms in a patient with hyperinfection syndrome. H&E, 200× magnification

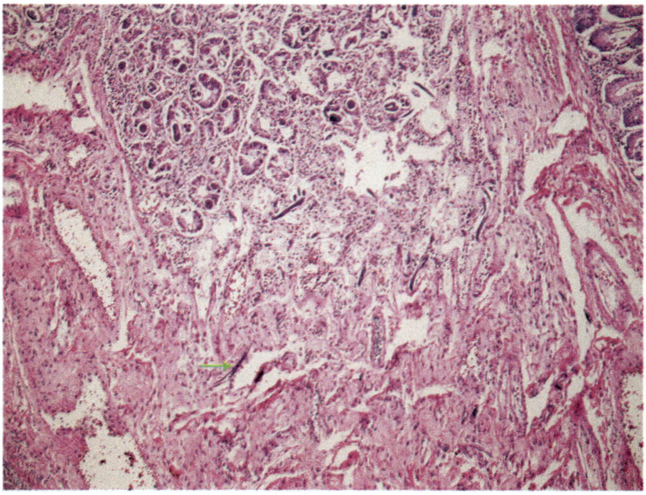

Fig. 5.43 In this image, several *Strongyloides* larvae (example at *arrow*) are seen migrating through the intestinal wall in a case of hyperinfection syndrome. H&E, 100× magnification

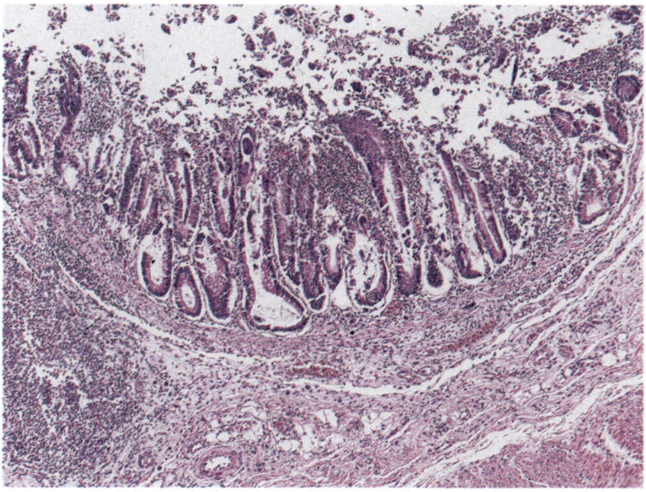

Fig. 5.44 Colon in a case of hyperinfection syndrome. Sections of migrating larvae are seen within the muscularis mucosa and submucosal layers. H&E, 100× magnification

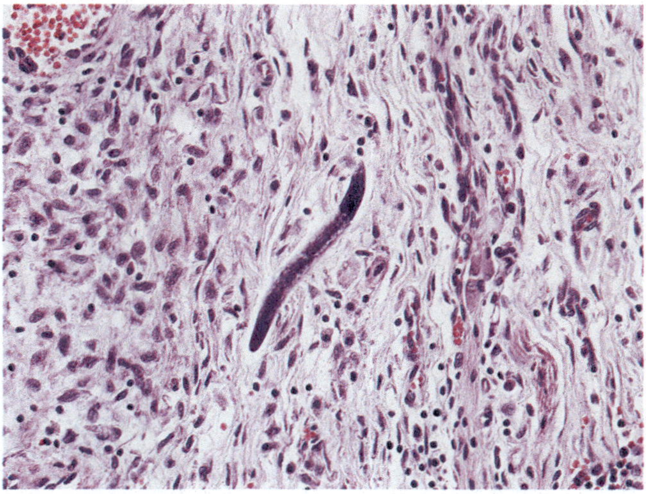

Fig. 5.45 High magnification image of migrating *Strongyloides* larva within the submucosa. H&E, 400× magnification

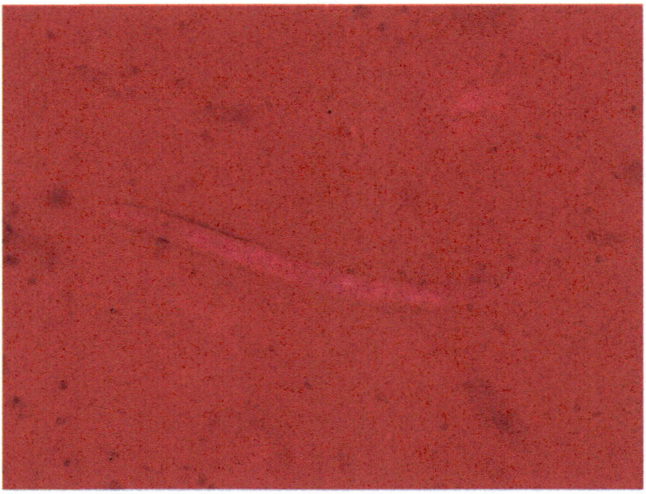

Fig. 5.46 Filariform larva of *S. stercoralis* from a bronchoalveolar lavage specimen. *S. stercoralis* migrating through the lungs may cause eosinophilic pneumonia (Loeffler syndrome). Gram stain, 400× magnification

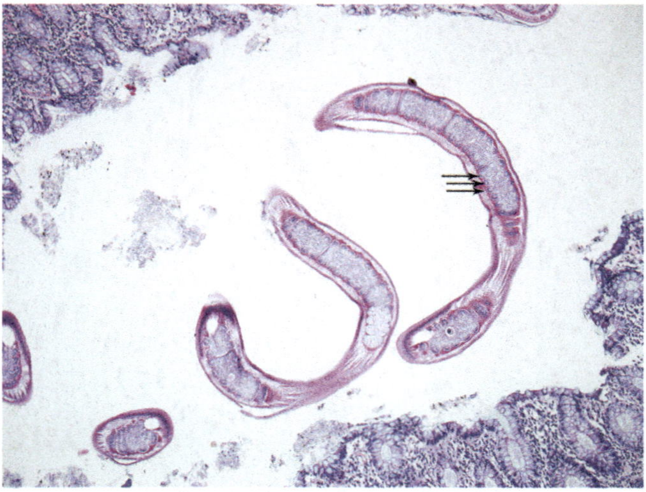

Fig. 5.47 *Trichuris trichiura* is commonly known as "whipworm" because of its body shape with a thin, threadlike anterior portion and a larger posterior portion resembling a handle. The adults typically reside in the colon, where the anterior portion of their body burrows into the intestinal mucosa. While occasionally retrieved whole at colonoscopy, usually only fragments of the organism are seen in anatomic pathology specimens and may appear to be floating above the tissue surface, with the embedded head often not represented in sections. Here, sections of the non-embedded anterior portion of *T. trichuria* are seen in a colon biopsy. The esophagus is encircled by prominent unicellular glandular structures called stichocytes (*arrows*), with the series of these structures being known as a stichosome. H&E, 100× magnification

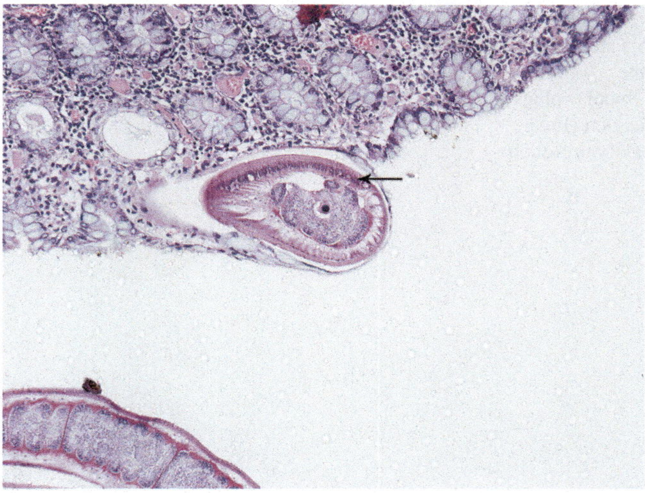

Fig. 5.48 A cross-section through a more anterior portion of the worm demonstrates the prominent nucleus of a stichocyte, along with a characteristic "bacillary band" (*arrow*), a basophilic staining row of columnar cells found in *Trichuris* and *Capillaria* species (not further discussed here). H&E, 200× magnification

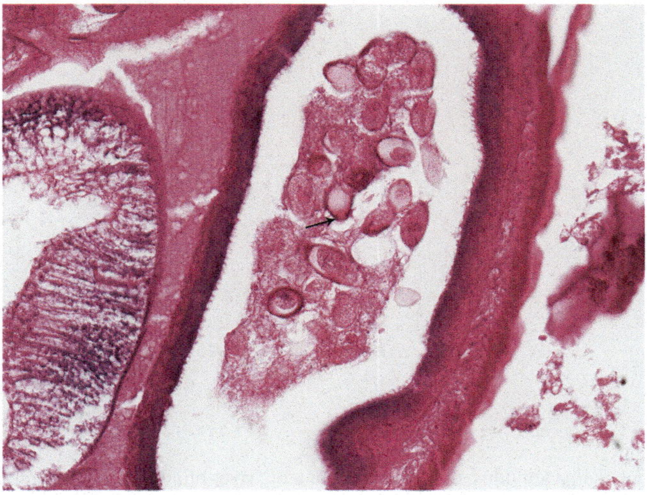

Fig. 5.49 Sections through the posterior end of gravid females may demonstrate characteristic oval eggs with "bipolar plugs" at each end. One of these plugs is demonstrated by the *arrow*. H&E, 400× magnification

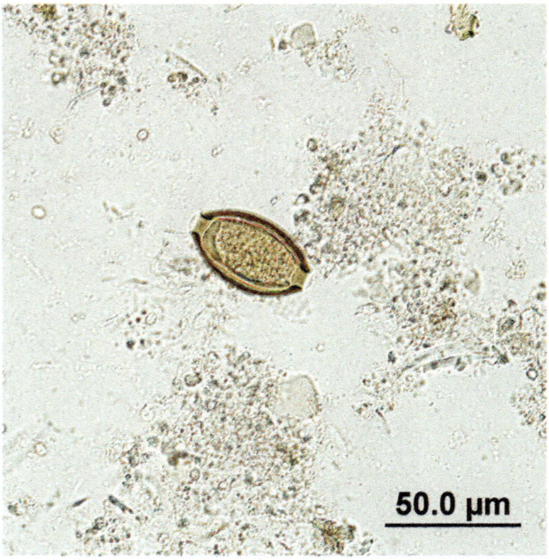

Fig. 5.50 Egg of *T. trichuria* obtained from a stool wet mount. Note the characteristic, bipolar plugs. 400× magnification (Image courtesy of Dr. Ryan Relich)

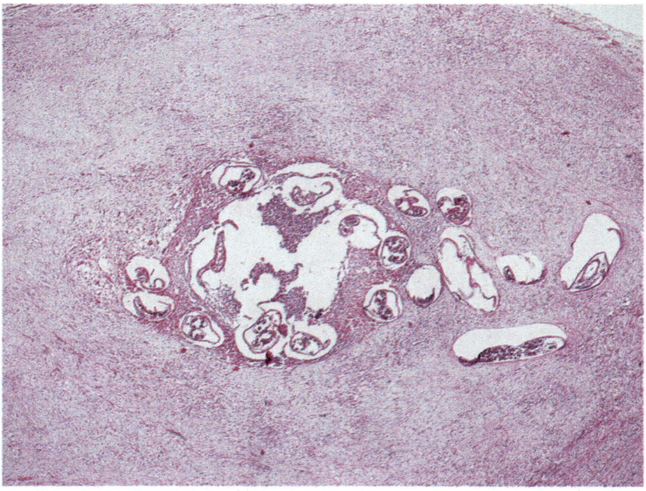

Fig. 5.51 Onchocerca volvulus, the causative agent of "river blindness," is transmitted by the bite of black flies of the genus *Simulium*. Adults typically reside in subcutaneous nodules along with the microfilarial forms. As such, microfilaria are not typically found in blood smears, which is the method of choice for the diagnosis of most other microfilarial infections. Instead, diagnosis is usually made by the examination of "skin snips" in which microfilaria can be found, or by histopathologic examination of subcutaneous nodules. Here is a subcutaneous nodule containing several adult worms. The adult worms induce a host fibroblastic reaction, leading to the formation of a fibrotic subcutaneous nodule. H&E, 40× magnification

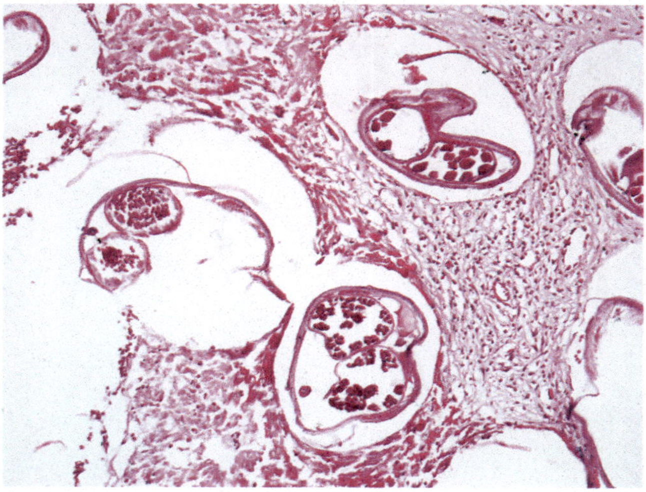

Fig. 5.52 Higher magnification image demonstrating cross-sections of microfilaria within the uteri of likely several adult females. H&E, 200× magnification

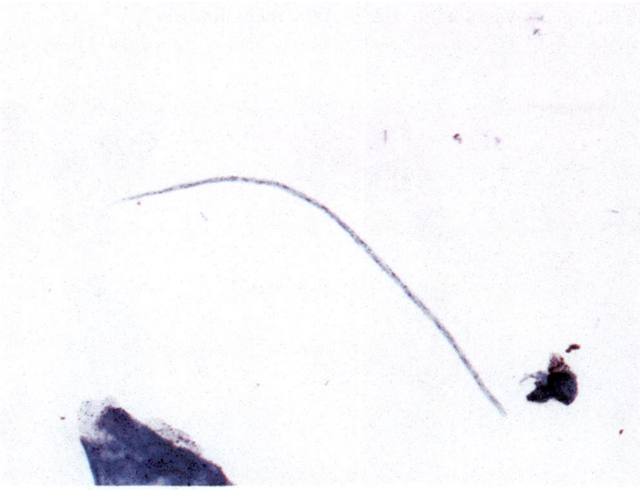

Fig. 5.53 A microfilaria of *O. volvulus*. Skin snips are typically placed in a physiologic solution such as saline, which causes the microfilaria to emerge, after which they can be examined microscopically. Giemsa stain, 500× magnification

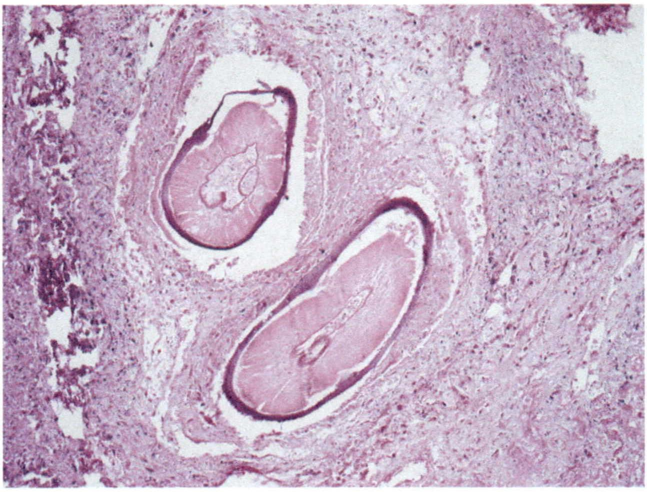

Fig. 5.54 *Dirofilaria* species typically infect carnivorous animals, particularly dogs and cats; however, humans are very rare hosts. While causing heartworm disease in most animals, in humans infection most often results in pulmonary infarcts caused by blockage of the pulmonary vessels. The species *D. repens* and *D. tenuis* have been implicated in subconjunctival lesions. A section of infarcted lung tissue caused by infection with *D. immitis*. Sections of the worm can be seen within the pulmonary vasculature. H&E, 200× magnification

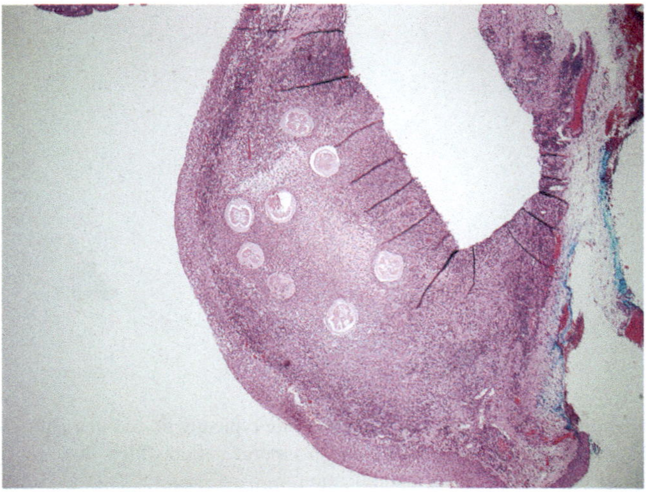

Fig. 5.55 Subconjunctival infection with *Dirofilaria* species. Note cross-sections of several worms surrounded by an intense inflammatory response. H&E, 40× magnification

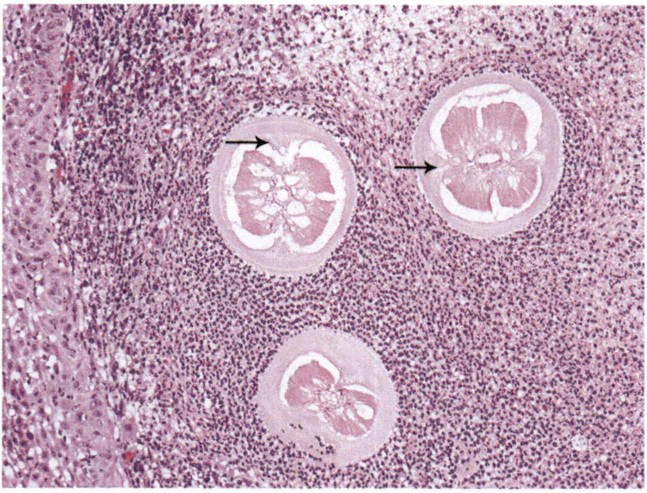

Fig. 5.56 Higher magnification image demonstrating prominent internal lateral ridges (*arrows*), a characteristic feature of this organism. Note also that within the primarily neutrophilic infiltrate, a few scattered eosinophils are seen, a common response to nematode infections. H&E, 200× magnification

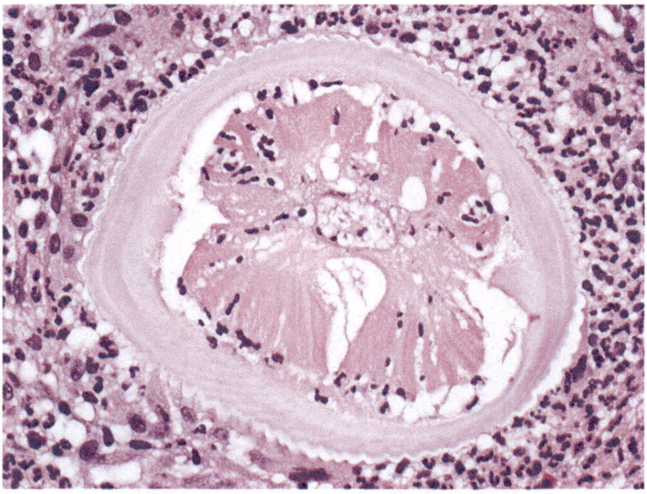

Fig. 5.57 High magnification image, again demonstrating prominent internal lateral ridges. In this particular example, neutrophils can be seen invading through the worms' internal musculature. Prominent ridging of the external cuticular surface can also be seen. H&E, 400× magnification

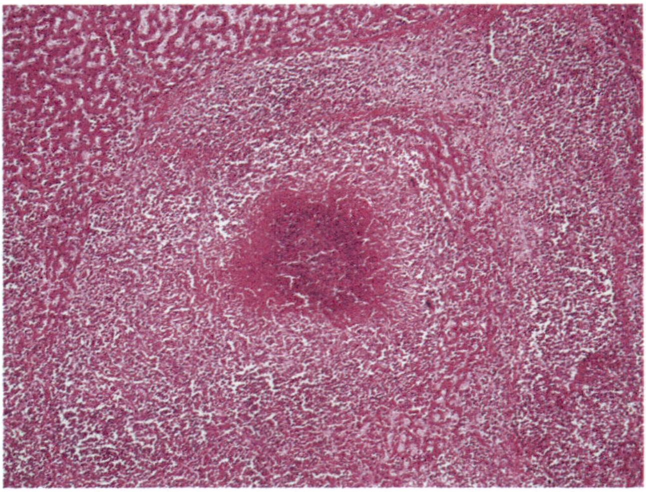

Fig. 5.58 Toxocariasis is caused by larval forms of nematodes of the *Toxocara* genus, most frequently *T. canis,* which primarily infects dogs and *T. felis,* which primarily infects cats. Humans become infected by ingestion of eggs, typically through contaminated soil. The eggs hatch in the intestine and the larvae migrate throughout the body, most typically the heart, brain, liver, lungs, and muscle (visceral larva migrans, VLM). However, they also may migrate to the eye. Visceral infections are usually accompanied by eosinophilia. As the worms are rarely identified in tissue, the mainstay of diagnosis relies on serology. A case of VLM involving the liver is shown. Classically migration of the organism causes the production of palisading granulomas containing eosinophils. The larvae themselves are not seen in this example. H&E, 100× magnification

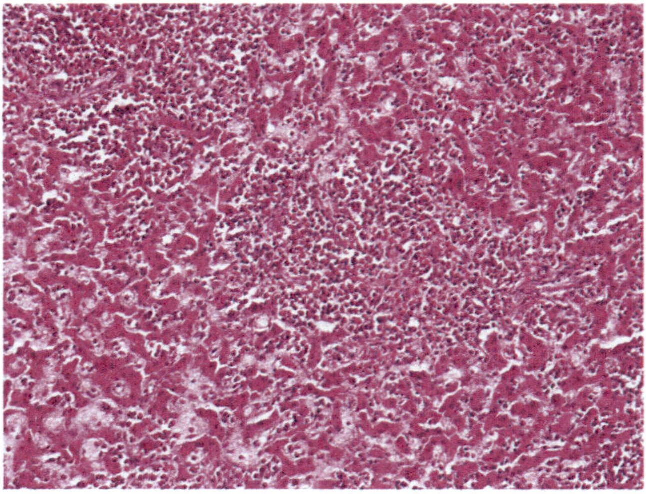

Fig. 5.59 Higher magnification image demonstrating a predominantly eosinophilic inflammatory response. H&E, 200× magnification

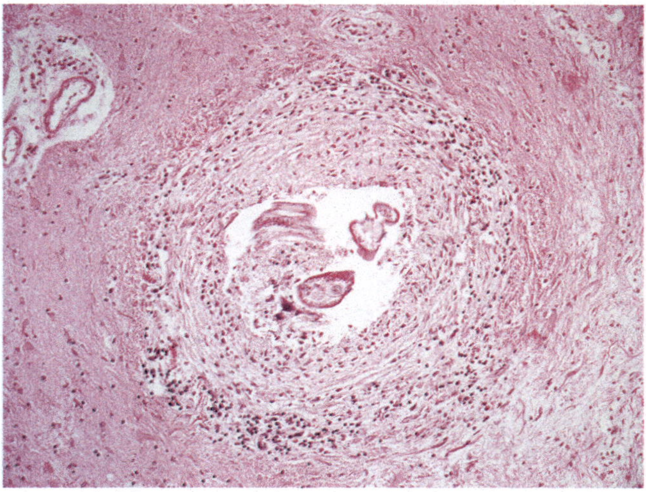

Fig. 5.60 *Baylisascaris procyonis* is the cause of baylisascariasis in humans. Primarily an intestinal nematode of raccoons and occasionally dogs, humans can come in contact with the eggs through environmental sources. Like toxocariasis, widespeard dissemination occurs, and both visceral and ocular larval migrans forms exist. However, the larval forms of *Baylisascaris* are larger, and do not readily die in human tissue and continue to mature. Because of this feature, infection of *Baylisascaris* tends to cause more severe disease. *Baylisascaris* migration also seems to prefer the central nervous system and ocular structures, which may result in permanent disability or death. *Baylisascaris* larvae in brain tissue. H&E, 200× magnification

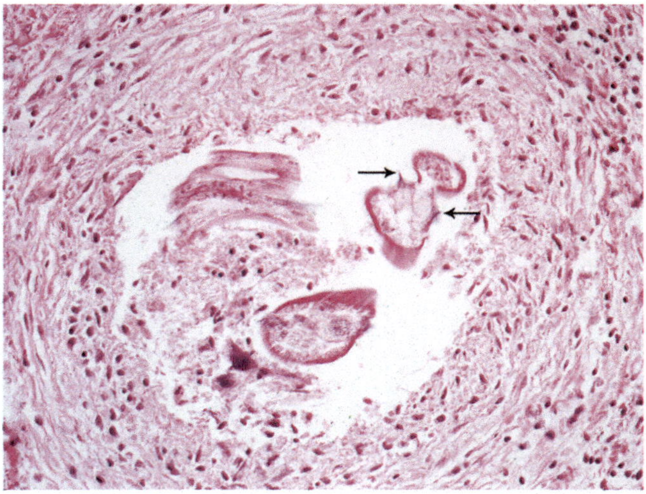

Fig. 5.61 Higher magnification image. Lateral alae or "wings" (*arrows*) are frequently identified in sections of the larvae of *Baylisascaris*. H&E, 400× magnification

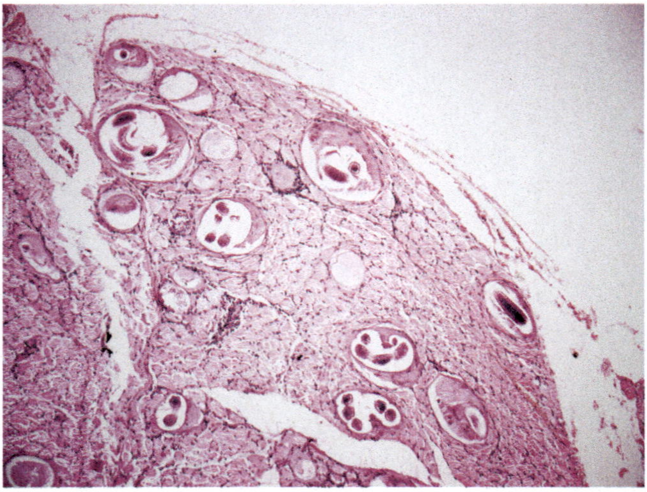

Fig. 5.62 Trichinosis is caused by nematodes of the species *Trichinella spiralis*. Sometimes referred to as the "pork worm," the infective form of the worm is also notably found in a variety of other animals, including bears and horses. Humans become infected by ingesting undercooked meat containing encysted larvae from these animals. When adult forms mature in the small intestinal mucosa, they release larvae that migrate to striated muscle, where they encyst. The cyst resides within a striated muscle cell often referred to as a "nurse cell." Several nurse cells containing encysted larval forms of *T. spirallis* are shown. Note the surrounding striated, skeletal muscle tissue. H&E, 100× magnification

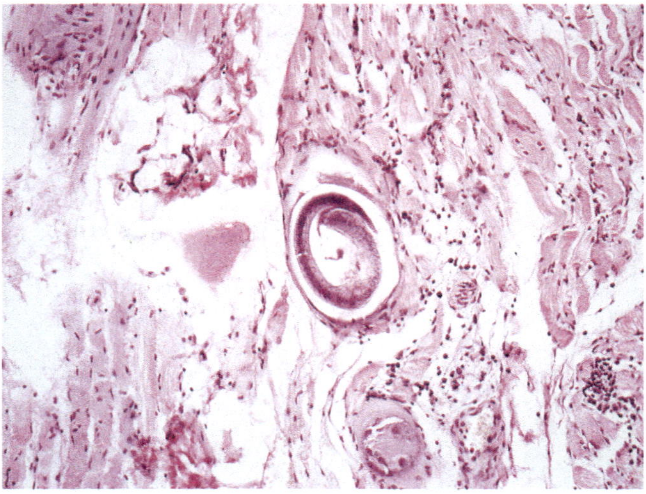

Fig. 5.63 Coiled *T. spiralis* larva within a nurse cell. H&E, 200× magnification

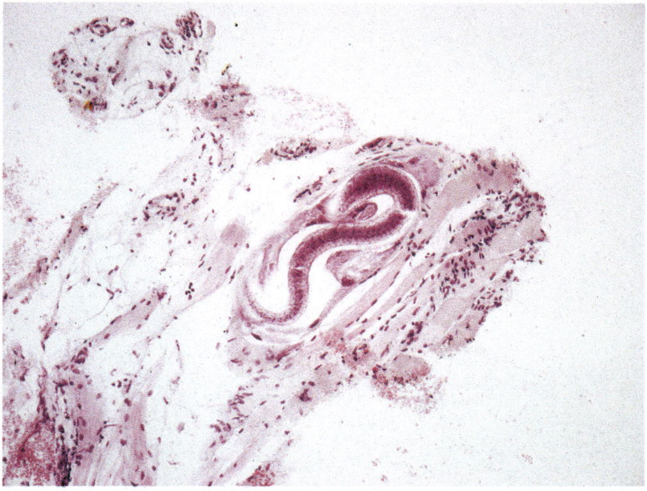

Fig. 5.64 While a tightly coiled larval form is the classic appearance of this parasite, this image demonstrates a larval form in a more relaxed state. H&E, 200× magnification

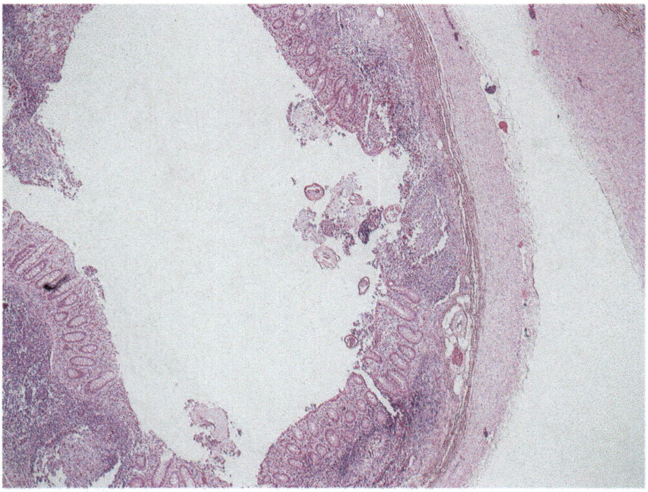

Fig. 5.65 *Enterobius vermicularis*, commonly referred to as "pinworm," is a common cause of pediatric perianal pruritus, worldwide. While most commonly identified by visualization of the eggs by the "scotch tape" method or variations thereof, the worms are occasionally seen in appendectomy specimens. In this location, they are usually considered an incidental finding but have rarely been implicated as a cause of appendicitis. Vermiform appendix demonstrating cross-sections of *E. vermicularis*. H&E, 40× magnification

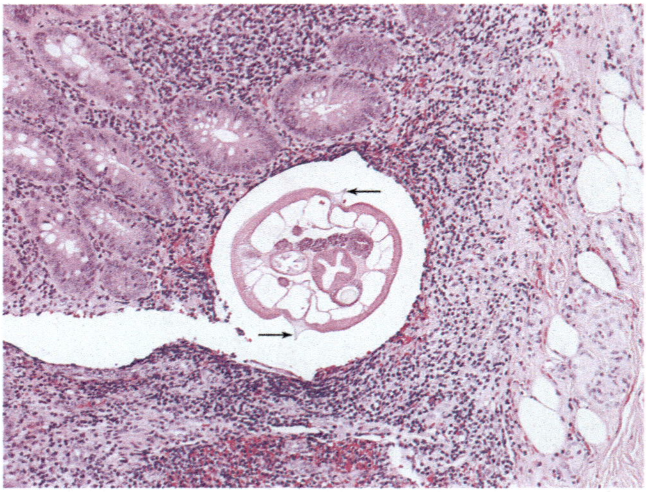

Fig. 5.66 Higher magnification image demonstrating prominent lateral alae (*arrows*). Note that a few more infrequently encountered nematodes, such as *Baylisascaris* species, also have lateral alae; however, the location in the appendix strongly indicates *E. vermicularis*. H&E, 200× magnification

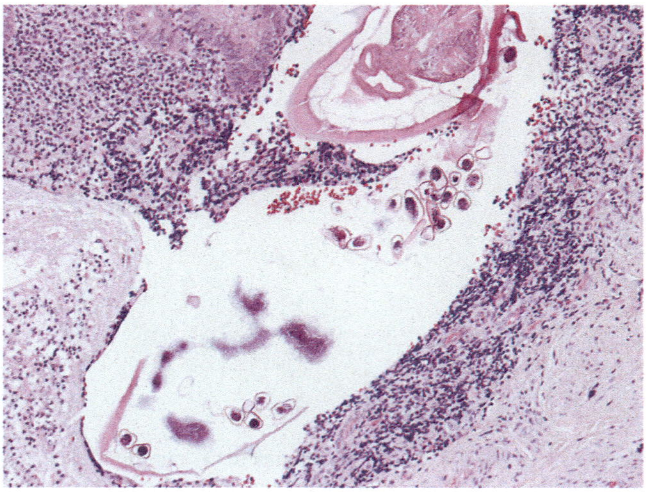

Fig. 5.67 Characteristic eggs of *E. vermicularis* which may be found inside the worms, or nearby, may also be helpful for identification. The eggs tend to be oval with a slightly flattened edge visible, depending on the plane of section. H&E, 200× magnification

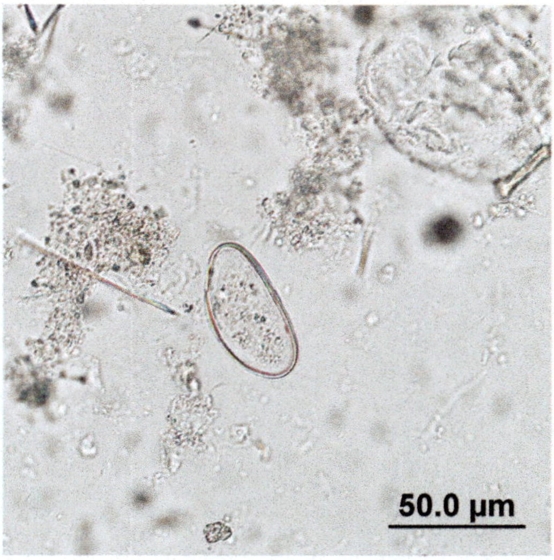

Fig. 5.68 An egg of *E. vermicularis* obtained from a wet mount. Note that it is slightly flattened on one side. 400× magnification (Image courtesy of Dr. Ryan Relich)

5.2 Protozoal Infections

The protozoa are a diverse group of unicellular eukaryotic organisms. Covered here are the most commonly identified members within anatomic pathology. Many protozoa are more frequently identified in blood or in stool specimens. As these specimen types are not generally the focus of anatomic pathology, they are only discussed as relevant to an anatomic pathology practice here.

5.2.1 Malaria

Cerebral malaria is the most severe complication of infection with *Plasmodium falciparum*, the most common and virulent species, and can lead to encephalopathy, seizures, coma, and death. Survivors often experience long-term neural sequelae. High parasitemia as well as the ability of *P. falciparum* infected cells to sequester in terminal blood vessels can lead to microinfarction of a variety of different organs. Some studies suggest that host response to the infection may also play a role in end organ damage (Figs. 5.69, 5.70, 5.71 and 5.72).

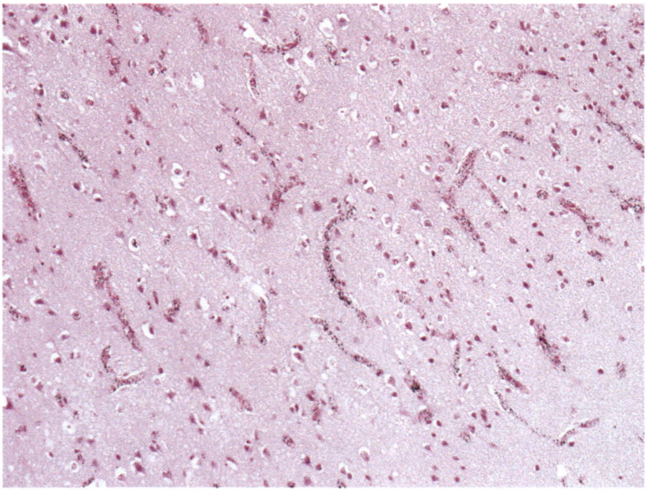

Fig. 5.69 Brain tissue demonstrating dilated blood vessels containing numerous red blood cells infected with late trophozoite stages of *P. falciparum*. Abundant dark malarial pigment is also characteristic. H&E, 200× magnification

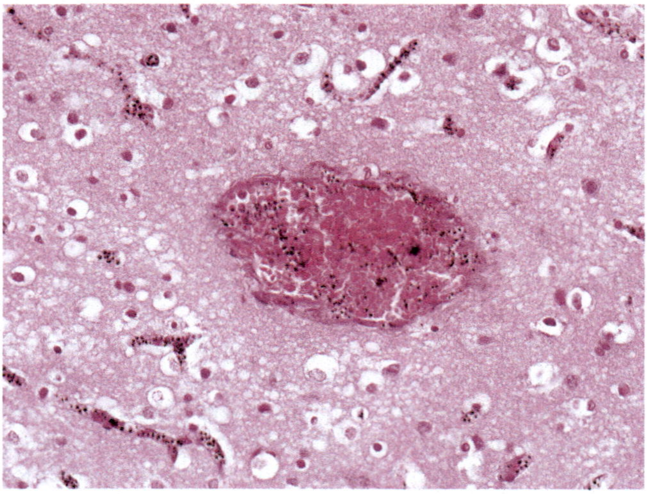

Fig. 5.70 Higher magnification image demonstrating congestion of a blood vessel in a case of cerebral malaria with abundant dark malarial pigment. H&E, 400× magnification

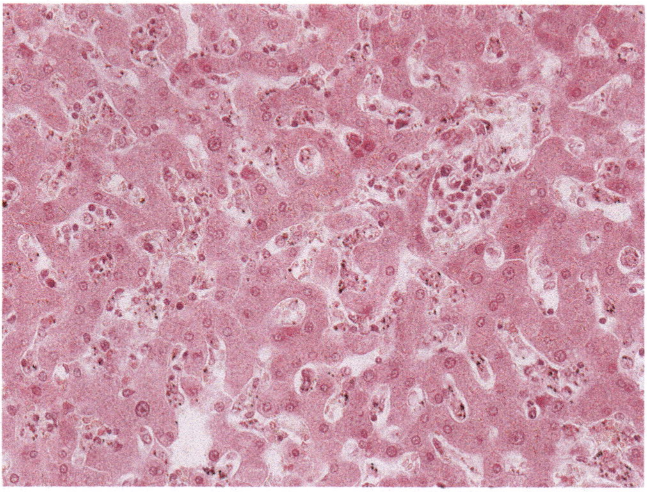

Fig. 5.71 Numerous parasitized and uninfected red blood cells within the sinusoids of the liver in a severe case of *P. falciparum* infection. Note expansion of the sinusoids and abundant malarial pigment. H&E, 400× magnification

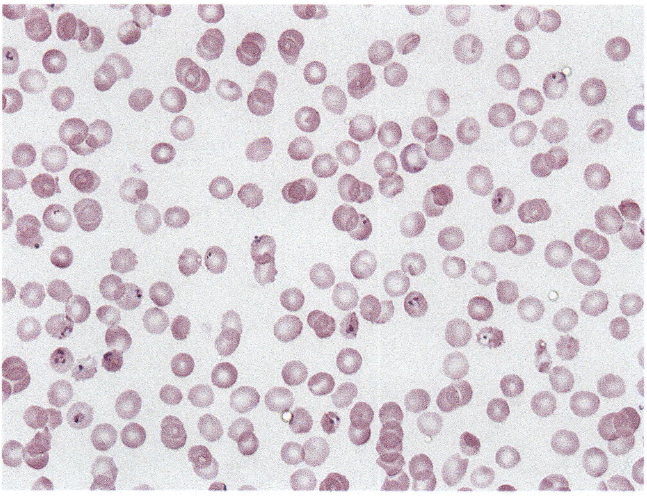

Fig. 5.72 Blood smear remains the mainstay of diagnosis for malaria. If histopathology is suggestive of organ infection with *Plasmodium*, blood smears or other diagnostic methods should be performed as part of the diagnostic workup. The infected red blood cells of the majority of *P. falciparum* infections, as seen here, demonstrate early trophozoite "ring" forms only, a feature that may be helpful for diagnosis. Rarely, banana-shaped gametocytes may also be seen. Giemsa stain, 1000× magnification

5.2.2 Toxoplasmosis

In human infections with *Toxoplasma gondii*, the organism will form cysts in a variety of organs, including the brain, skeletal muscle, heart, and eyes. The cysts contain the slowly reproducing, bradyzoite form of the parasite and persist for life, often being only an incidental finding at autopsy in patients who are not immunocompromised. Primary infection with or a reactivation of *T. gondii* infection in an immunocompromised host may be life threatening (Figs. 5.73, 5.74, 5.75 and 5.76).

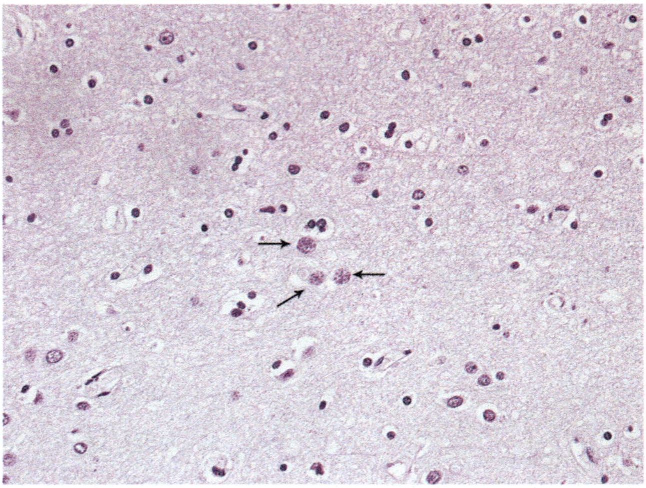

Fig. 5.73 Cysts containing bradyzoite forms of *T. gondii* in cerebral tissue (*arrows*). H&E, 400× magnification

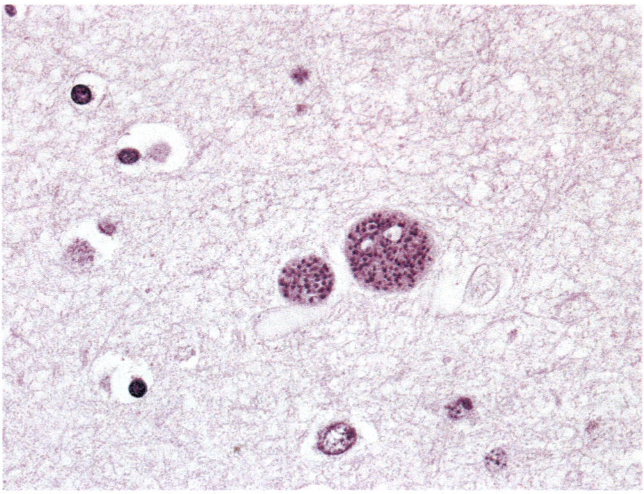

Fig. 5.74 Higher magnification image of *T. gondii* cysts in the brain containing numerous bradyzoite forms. H&E, 1000× magnification

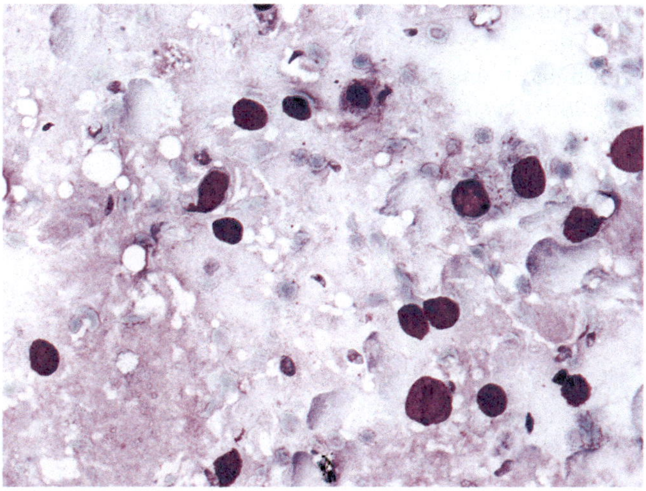

Fig. 5.75 The tachyzoite or rapidly reproducing form of *T. gondii* is seen in active infections. It is characteristically crescent-shaped, but several oval shaped forms are seen here as well. Brain biopsy tissue smear. Giemsa stain, 1000× magnification

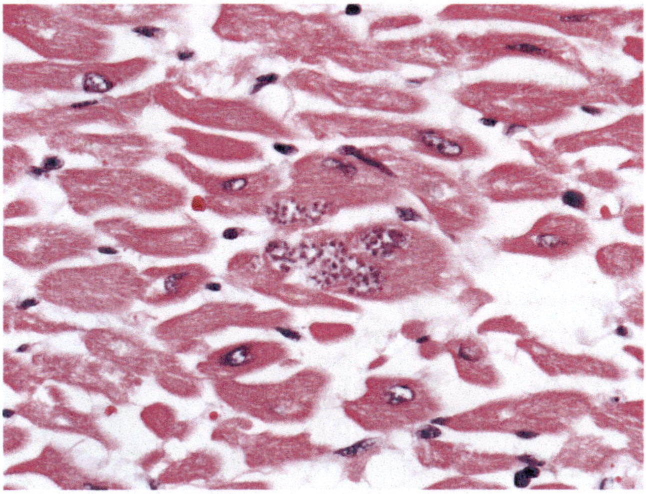

Fig. 5.76 Bradyzoites may be found in a wide variety of tissues. Seen here are cysts identified in cardiac muscle sampled during autopsy. H&E, 1000× magnification

5.2.3 Trypanosomiasis

Clusters of amastigote forms of *Trypanosoma cruzi* may appear microscopically similar to *Toxoplasma* cysts. They are more commonly found in cardiac muscle, which is a relatively rare location to find *Toxoplasma* species, the previous example not withstanding (Figs. 5.77 and 5.78).

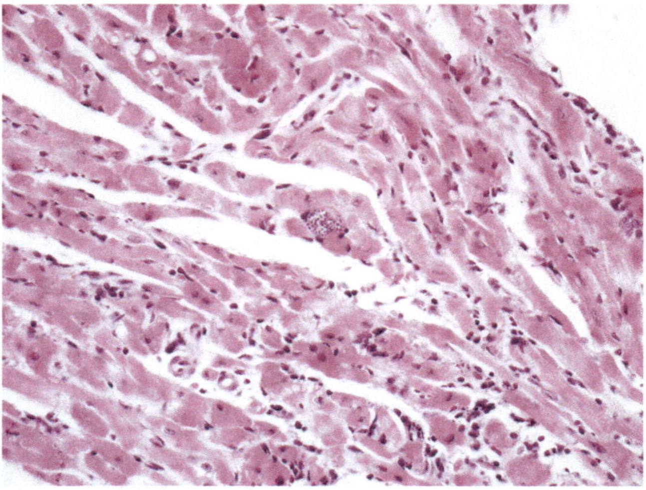

Fig. 5.77 *T. cruzi* amastigotes tend to cluster in looser aggregates, unlike the generally round, packed bradyzoite cyst forms of *Toxoplasma* species. H&E, 400× magnification

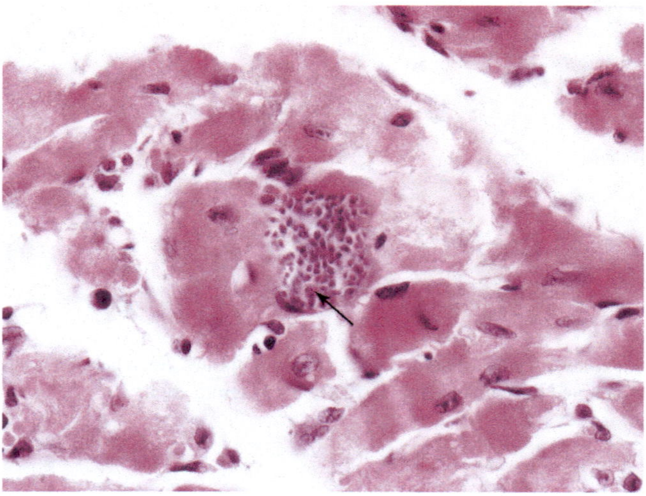

Fig. 5.78 At higher magnification, the loose aggregation of *T. cruzi* is more apparent. The organisms have a single nucleus and a bar shaped kinetoplast, which bradyzoites of *Toxoplasma* lack. The kinetoplast (*arrow*) is often very difficult to visualize on tissue sections. H&E, 1000× magnification

5.2.4 Leishmaniasis

Infection with *Leishmania* species can have several different forms, including cutaneous, mucocutaneous, and visceral leishmaniasis (kala-azar). The disease is endemic in areas where sandflies, the vector, are common. Cutaneous lesions manifest at the site of the initial bite, often appearing as a shallow, crater-like lesion, while visceral leishmaniasis manifests typically as fever accompanied by splenomegaly. Cutaneous manifestations may also occur following visceral leishmaniasis. Microscopically, the amastigotes of *Leishmania* species are indistinguishable from those of *T. cruzi*, a fact complicated by significant cross-reactivity of serologic assays, especially since they have overlapping endemicity in Central and South America. When organisms are found in the skin and bone marrow especially, the yeast forms of *Histoplasma capsulatum* may also enter the differential diagnosis. This is particularly important because both of these entities are commonly found in an intracellular location. Identification of the bar-shaped kinetoplast in *Leishmania* species can be helpful in determining a correct identification. Use of a Gomori methenamine silver stain may also be a useful method of ruling out *Histoplasma* since the yeast cells should stain black, while *Leishmania* do not stain (Figs. 5.79, 5.80, 5.81 and 5.82).

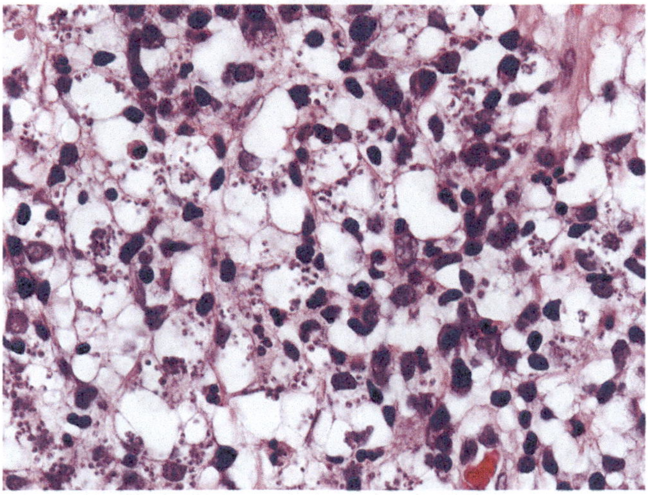

Fig. 5.79 Cutaneous lesion of leishmaniasis demonstrating many amastigotes within vacuolated appearing tissue. H&E, 500× magnification

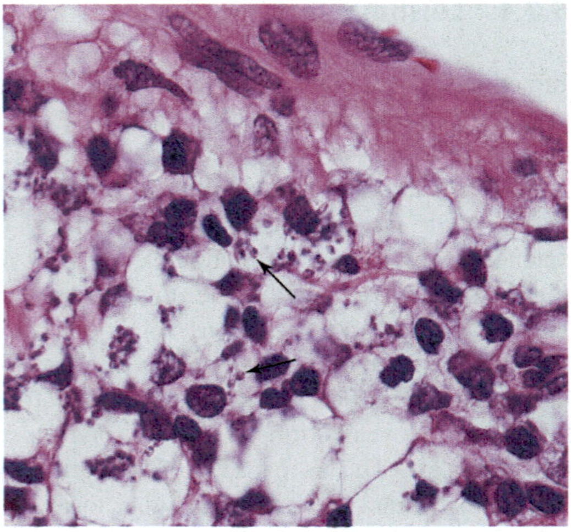

Fig. 5.80 At higher magnification, bar-shaped kinetoplasts can be identified in several of the amastigotes. H&E, 1000× magnification

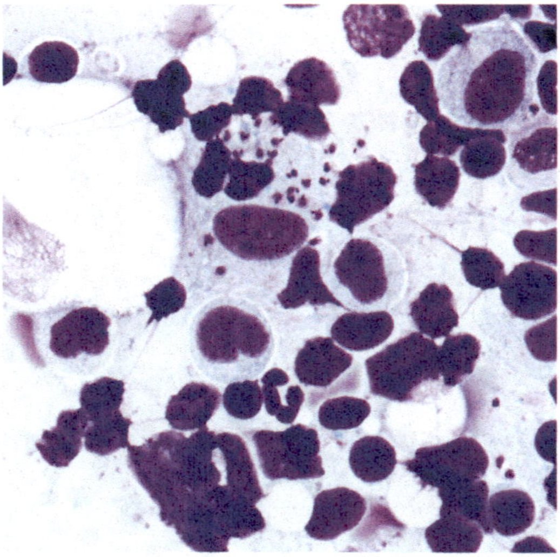

Fig. 5.81 Bone marrow aspirate remains the gold standard for the diagnosis of kala-azar. In some cases, splenic aspirates are performed, but this procedure is generally to be avoided if a bone marrow aspirate can be obtained, since it may carry significant risk to the patient. These methods also provide specimens for culture and further speciation of the organism by molecular methods. Bone marrow aspirate; note the presence of intracellular organisms. The kinetoplast is often much easier to visualize on cytologic/hematologic preparations. Diff-Quik stain, 1000× magnification

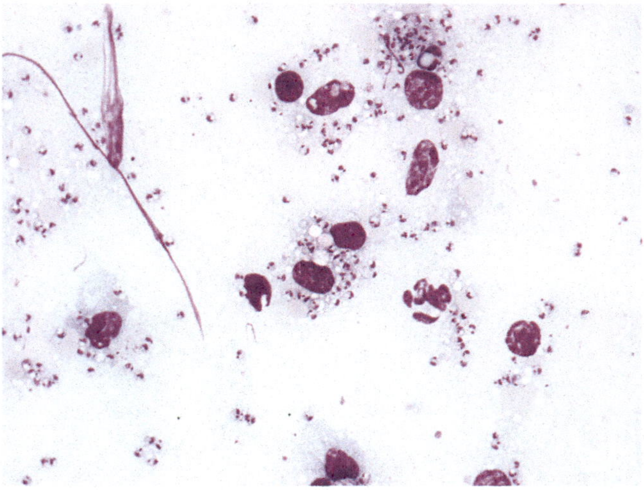

Fig. 5.82 Splenic aspirate. Again note the presence of intra- and extracellular organisms. Bar shaped kinetoplasts are clearly visible on this preparation. Giemsa stain, 1000× magnification

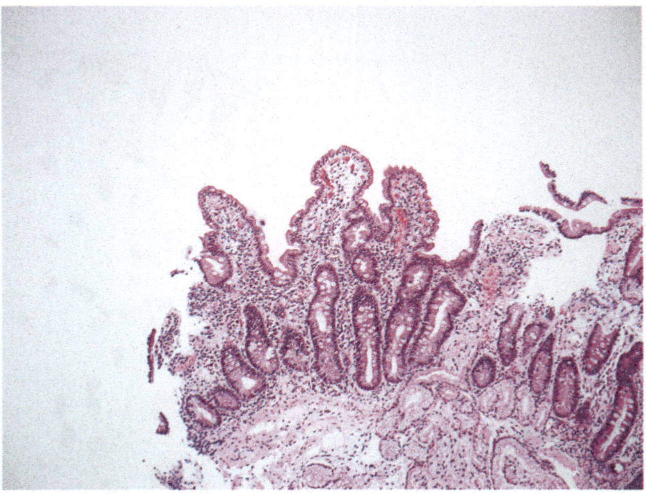

Fig. 5.83 Small intestine demonstrating villous blunting and a moderately increased inflammatory infiltrate in a case of cryptosporidiosis. H&E, 100× magnification

5.2.5 Cryptosporidiosis

This organism is a common but under-recognized cause of diarrhea, mostly within the pediatric population. Infection is through the fecal-oral route, by ingestion of the hardy oocyst form. While the organism can be identified by microscopic examination of stool, where the oocysts stain with modified acid-fast stains, and by direct fluorescent antibody stains, enzyme immunoassay (EIA) methods, or polymerase chain reaction (PCR) can also be used. The organism is also occasionally identified in gastrointestinal biopsy tissue (Figs. 5.83, 5.84 and 5.85).

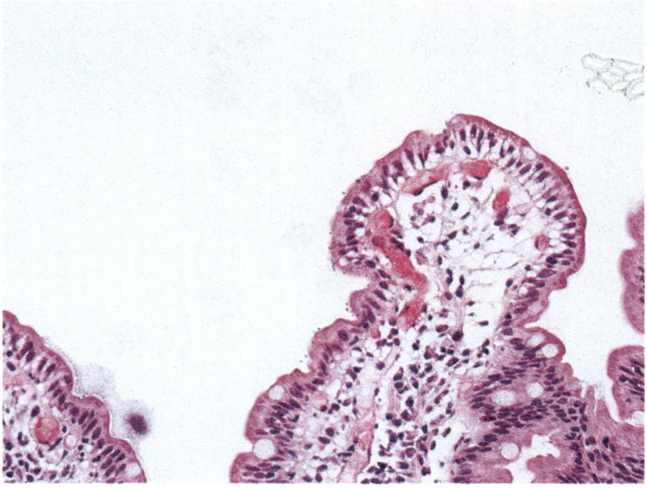

Fig. 5.84 On higher magnification, small (2–5 micron) basophilic, "blue bodies" are seen at the luminal surface. H&E, 400× magnification

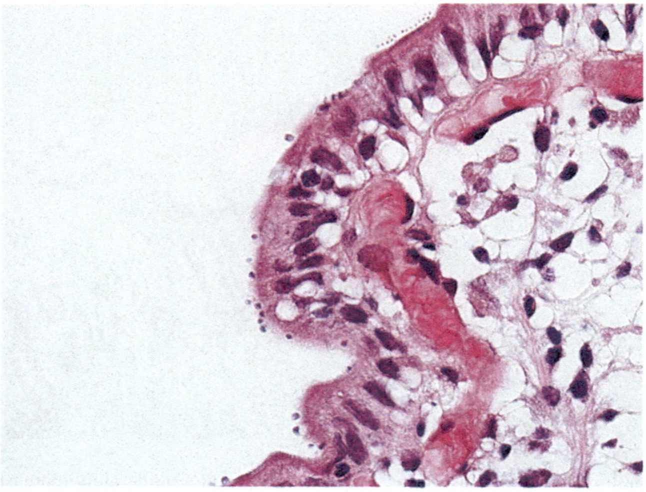

Fig. 5.85 Further magnification image demonstrating blue bodies at the luminal surface. While light microscopic examination suggests that the organisms are resting on the brush border of the small intestinal villi, they are in fact covered by a thin membrane and are intracellular. H&E, 1000× magnification

5.2.6 Giardiasis

Infection with *Giardia duodenalis* (syn. *G. lamblia, G. intestinalis*) typically demonstrates no to minimal villous blunting with minimal increase in inflammatory infiltrates. Diarrheal illness caused by infection with this organism is caused by malabsorption rather than toxin secretion or intestinal invasion. Also a common cause of parasitic diarrhea in the Western world (and indeed worldwide), *Giardia* is spread by ingestion of the cyst form of the organism (Figs. 5.86, 5.87 and 5.88).

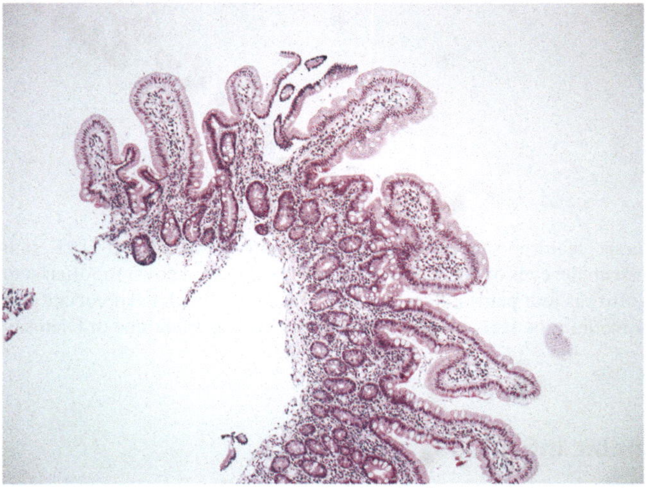

Fig. 5.86 Small intestine; note the minimal to absent villous blunting with no increase in typical inflammatory cell composition. H&E, 100× magnification

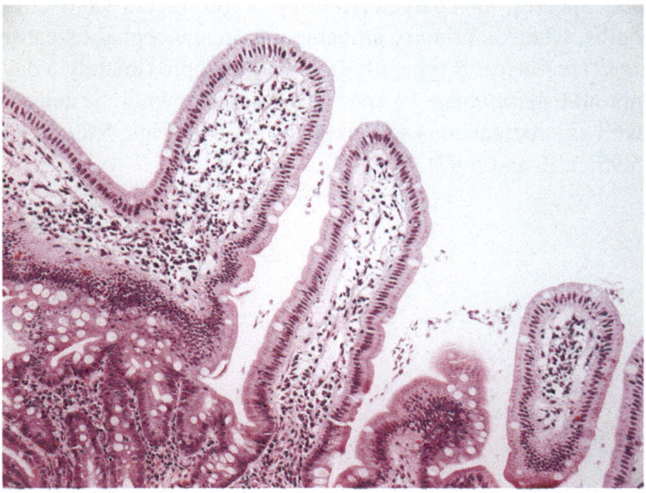

Fig. 5.87 At higher magnification, the organisms are more apparent and appear between the small intestinal villi. At first glace they may appear to be cellular debris. Importantly, they frequently do not appear in histopathologic section as the classic teardrop-shaped organisms with two prominent nuclei but are instead sectioned in multiple planes. H&E, 200× magnification

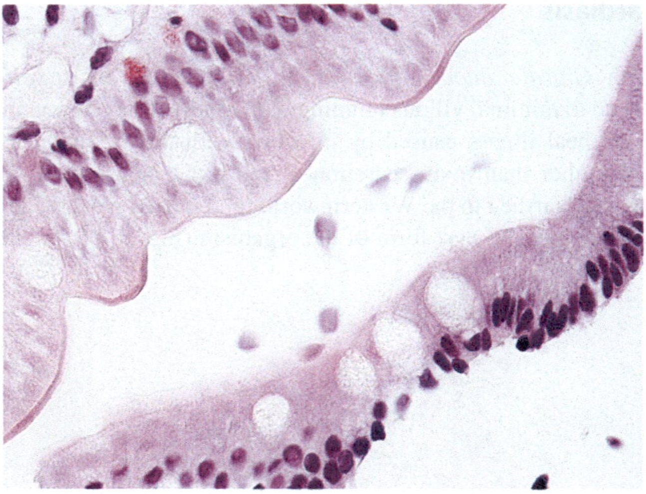

Fig. 5.88 Classic teardrop-shaped *Giardia* trophozoite. Note that on H&E staining, the two nuclei that make up the eyes of the "clown face" that *Giardia* is known for often stain very faintly. The organism also has four pairs of flagella that are usually difficult to appreciate on H&E staining, but they can sometimes be seen on other preparations such as trichrome or Giemsa. H&E, 1000× magnification

5.2.7 Amebic Infections

Amebic infections include amoebic colitis, soft tissue, and solid organ infections (most commonly liver) and are caused primarily by *Entamoeba histolytica*. Granulomatous amoebic encephalitis, caused by *Balamuthia mandrillaris* or by *Acanthamoeba* species, is characterized by a protracted course often lasting weeks to months, whereas primary amoebic meningoencephalitis caused by infection with *Naegleria fowleri* is typically fatal within approximately 5 days following onset of symptoms. *Acanthamoeba* species are also known to be causes of amoebic keratitis as well as subcutaneous soft-tissue infections (Figs. 5.89, 5.90, 5.91, 5.92, 5.93, 5.94, 5.95, 5.96 and 5.97).

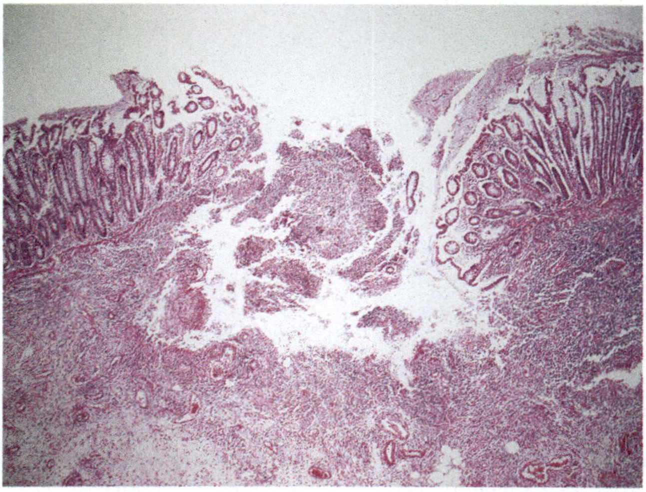

Fig. 5.89 Amebic colitis due to infection with *E. histolytica* classically demonstrates a "flask" shaped lesion with a relatively narrow opening through the mucosal surface and a widened base as the organisms progress deeper into the tissue. H&E, 40× magnification

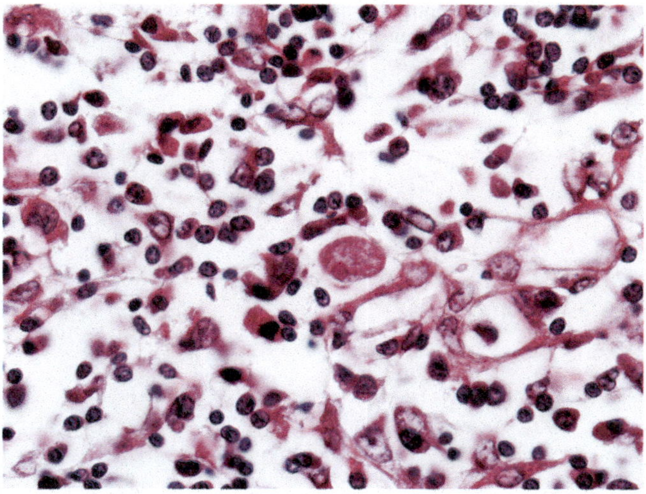

Fig. 5.90 *E. histolytica* trophozoites within colon tissue. The amoeba somewhat resembles a macrophage but has a well-circumscribed, round nucleus, with a centrally located, pinpoint karyosome. The karysome may be difficult to identify on H&E staining. The organisms are often easier to find at the edges of the lesion. H&E, 1000× magnification

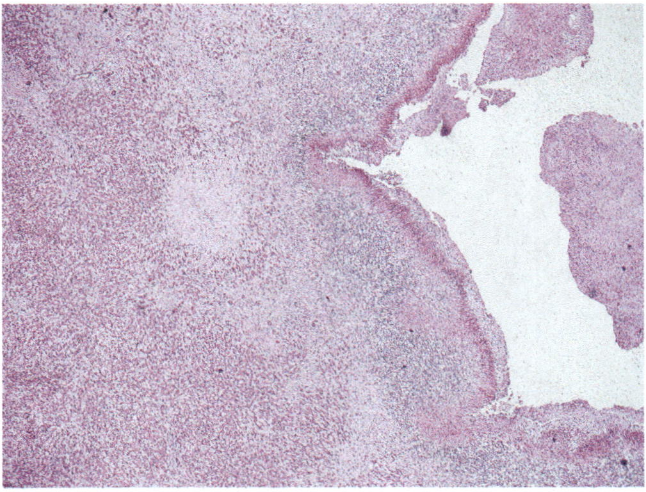

Fig. 5.91 Amoebic liver abscess caused by infection with *E. histolytica*. Grossly, these lesions may be filled with a reddish-brown fluid, often referred to as "anchovy paste." Aspiration of a suspected amoebic abscess for diagnostic purposes is generally not recommended. There is some risk that the abscess may leak post procedure resulting in amoebic peritonitis or that the needle tract may become seeded with organisms, worsening the problem. Additionally, organisms tend to congregate at the edge of lesions and are not likely to be properly sampled by a fine needle aspirate. Serologic testing in conjunction with radiologic findings is therefore the diagnostic method of choice. Most do not need to be removed surgically, but instead can be treated with amoebicidal drugs. Therapeutic aspiration is an option for large abscesses and may yield material for cytology, but organisms can be difficult to identify for the reasons stated above. Microscopically, resected lesions tend to have a "ragged" appearance, with more abundant organisms located at the edge. H&E, 40× magnification

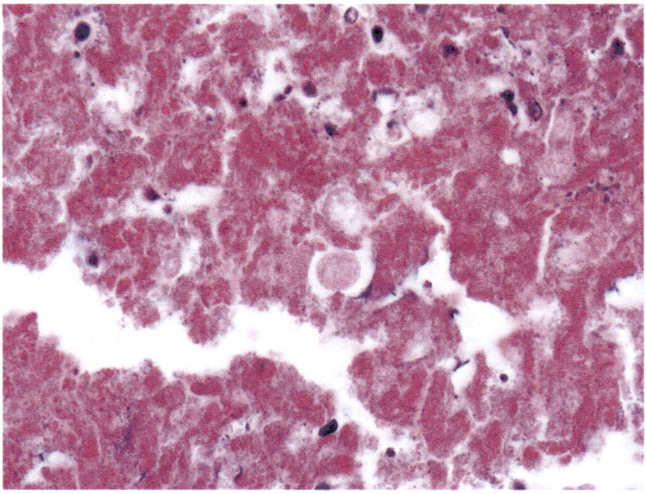

Fig. 5.92 *E. histolytica* trophozoite forms may be found within the necrotic tissue and at the edge of the lesion. In this particular example, the nucleus is only poorly visualized. H&E, 1000× magnification

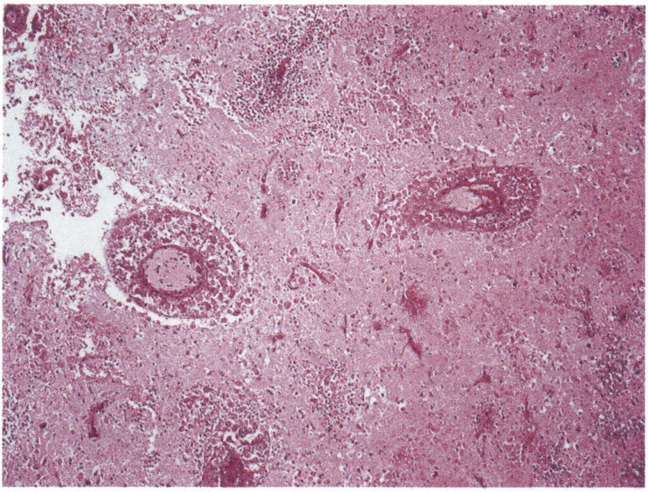

Fig. 5.93 Meningoencephalitis in a case of granulomatous amebic encephalitis (GAE). This entity is caused by either *Balamuthia mandrillaris* or *Acanthamoeba* species. As there is significant overlap in morphologic features between the two, differentiation by microscopy alone is not reliable. The causative agent in this case was later identified as *B. mandrillaris* by molecular identification methods. While presentations vary, a mixture of acute and granulomatous inflammation is typically seen. Note also the presence of many amoebae within the walls of the blood vessels. H&E, 200× magnification

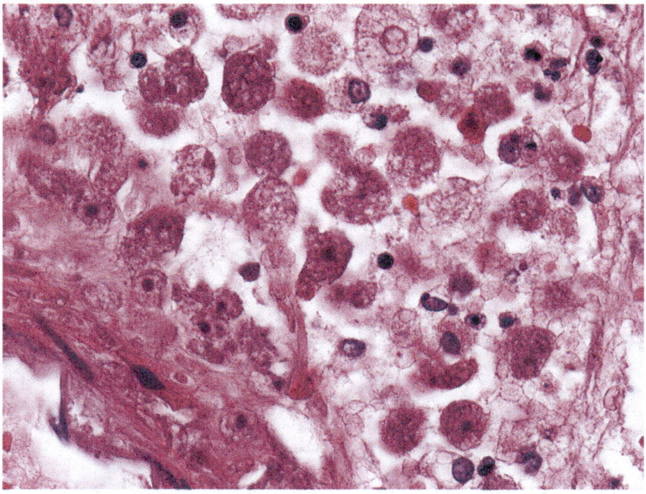

Fig. 5.94 At higher magnification, many trophozoite forms are evident within a blood vessel wall. Note that several of these organisms feature a prominent, large karyosome, a feature that is common in the free living amoebae, unlike the pinpoint karysome of *E. histolytica*. H&E, 1000× magnification

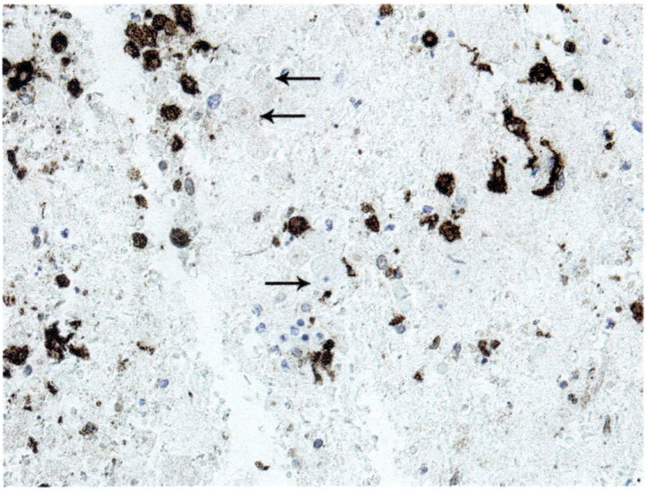

Fig. 5.95 The amoebae can be intermingled with macrophages, which being of the same approximate size and having a similar morphology, may present an additional diagnostic challenge. Immunohistochemical staining with CD68, which is expressed by monocytes and macrophages but not by amoebae, may be helpful in these cases. Note positive staining macrophages but also large nonstaining amoebae in the background (examples at *arrows*). CD68, 400× magnification

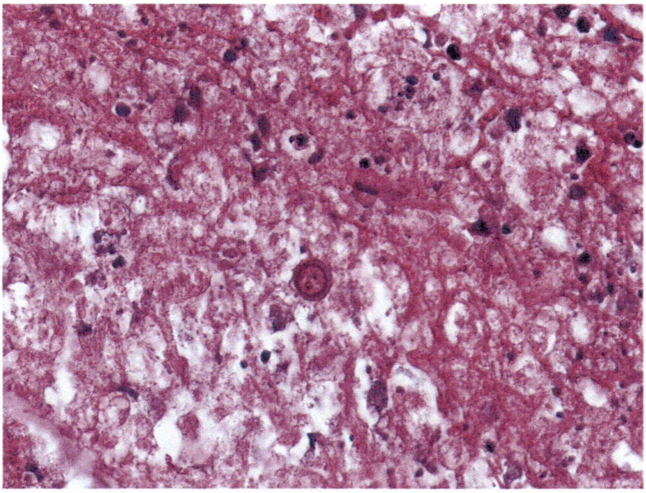

Fig. 5.96 Cyst forms of *B. mandrillaris* or *Acanthameoba* species are often seen in cases of GAE. The causative agent of primary amebic meningoencephalitis (PAM), *Naegleria fowleri,* does not produce cyst forms in human tissue. The clinical course of PAM is also notably more acute, differentiating it from GAE. H&E, 1000× magnification

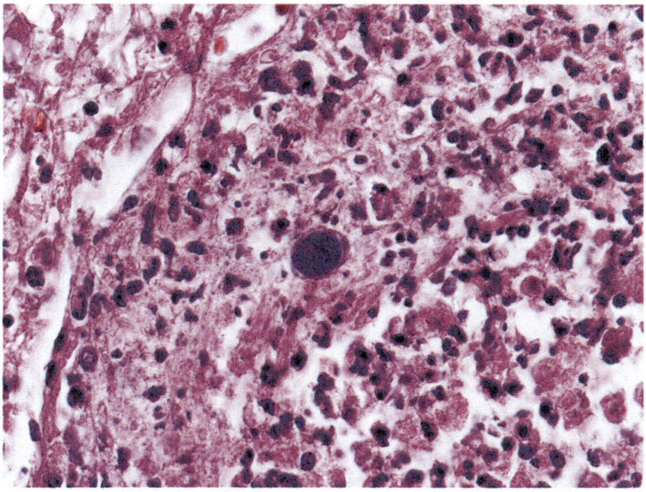

Fig. 5.97 Another example of a cyst form from the previously discussed case. The staining of the inner cyst (endocyst) with H&E can vary, appearing more basophilic in this example. Also note the characteristic "wrinkled" appearance of the outer wall (the exocyst). H&E, 1000× magnification

5.3 Ectoparasites

Ectoparasites, by definition, live on but not inside the body. From an anatomic pathology perspective the most frequently encountered of these will be arthropod adult or larval forms living within cutaneous or subcutaneous tissue. While most of the ectoparasites discussed here are better identified by submission to the microbiology laboratory, they are occasionally encountered within surgical specimens as incidental findings or because of initial misidentification. Ticks in particular may present grossly in many different ways, depending on stages of engorgement from a blood meal; they often appear as moles, seborrheic keratoses, or infarcted skin tags. While the ectoparasites of humans are extensive, this section concentrates on those that may most frequently wind up under the lens of the anatomic pathologist (Figs. 5.98, 5.99, 5.100, 5.101, 5.102, 5.103, 5.104, 5.105, 5.106, 5.107, 5.108 and 5.109).

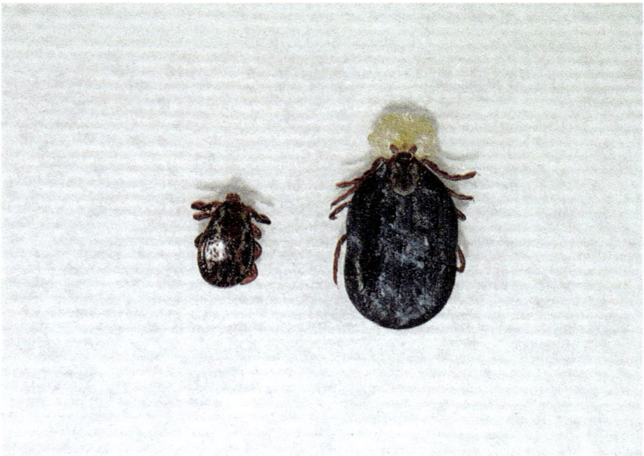

Fig. 5.98 Hard ticks, such as *Dermacentor variabilis* pictured here, have a hard exoskeleton containing chitin. These ticks additionally exhibit a backplate called a scutum, which in Latin means "shield." Males have a scutum that extends over their entire backs, while females feature a scutum that extends only approximately 1/3 of the way down the back. The shorter scutum allows for females, which take much larger blood meals, to expand. As females tend to feed for much longer, often several days, they are the more likely of the two sexes to be biopsied or otherwise removed and submitted to surgical pathology. Soft ticks, as the name suggests, have a membranous outer surface and are more frequently parasites of animals, seldom encountered in human anatomic pathology. In male *D. variabilis* (*left*), note the ornate scutum which extends fully over the back. In a partially engorged female *D. variabilis* (*right*), note the smaller scutum and the significant overall increase in size and deformity in shape, leading to misidentification as a variety of cutaneous growths. A fragment of skin remains attached to the mouthparts

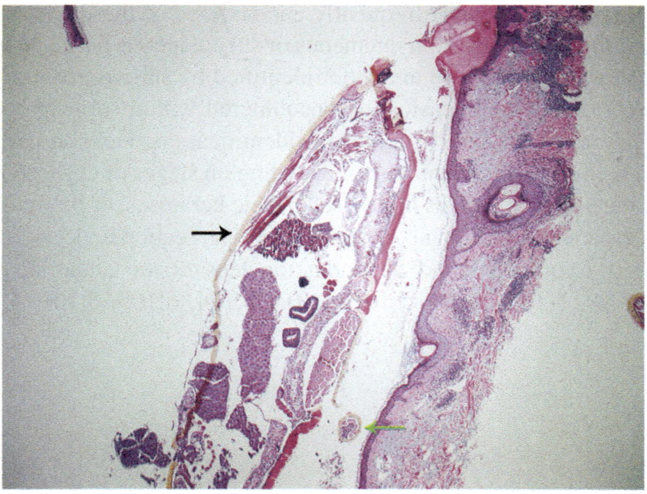

Fig. 5.99 Skin biopsy demonstrating sections through a hard tick. Note that speciation at this point is nearly impossible. If recognized as a tick, submission to microbiology of the whole arthropod, or its remaining parts for identification is preferable, as the species will dictate which diseases it may possibly transmit to the human host. A chitinous scutum is evident and appears yellow on H&E staining (*black arrow*). A thick, eosinophilic cuticle is seen as well. Internally, muscle fibers and various organ structures are noted. A cross-section of a leg demonstrating skeletal muscle is also seen (*green arrow*). H&E, 40× magnification

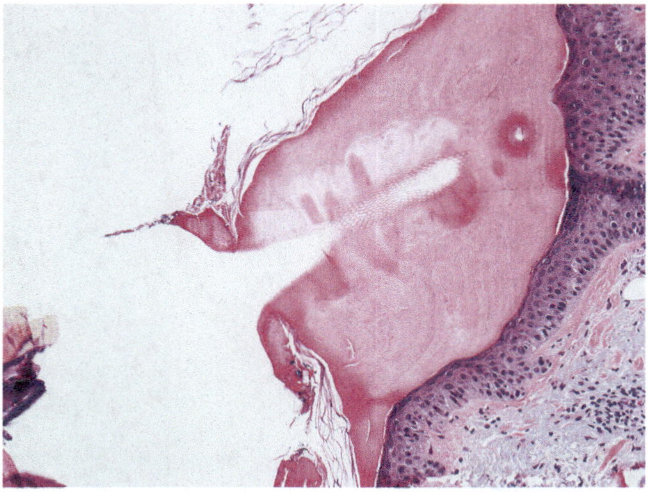

Fig. 5.100 Ticks feed by means of a hypostome, often described as a needle-like structure which penetrates the skin allowing access to the hosts blood. The hypostome of most ticks features recurved barbs that serve to further anchor the tick in place during feeding. Its hold is so strong that it, along with other mouthparts and the head of the tick, is often retained in the host after removal is attempted. Shown here is a fortuitous section demonstrating an embedded hypostome with prominent barbs. H&E, 200× magnification

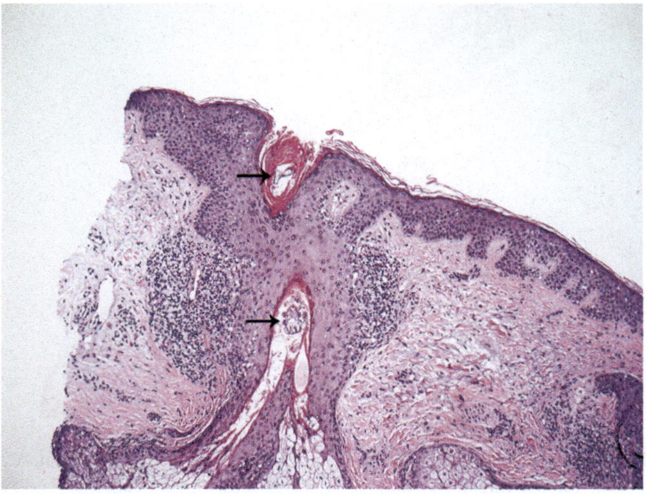

Fig. 5.101 *Demodex* mites are very common findings in skin biopsy sections and are usually considered to be commensal organisms of cutaneous pilosebaceous structures. They have, however, been implicated as a cause of folliculitis, blepharitis, and rosacea among other conditions. *Demodex* has an elongate appearance with a head, a thorax that contains four pairs of rudimentary legs, and a long, tail-like abdomen. While it is generally not important to differentiate between the two primary species that infect humans, *D. folliculorum* tends to reside within hair follicles, and the shorter *D. brevis* usually inhabits the sebaceous glands. Note fragments of mite parts within the hair shaft (*arrows*) in a case of perifolliculitis associated with *D. folliculorum*. H&E, 100× magnification

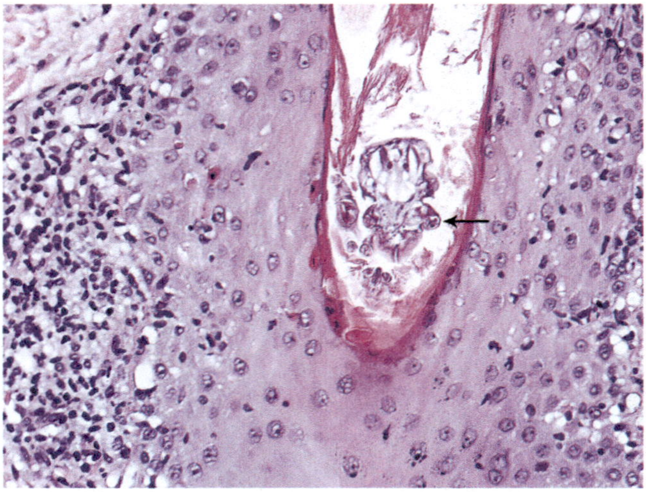

Fig. 5.102 Higher magnification image demonstrating the head and thorax of *D. folliculorum*. The arrow highlights an example of the rudimentary legs extending from the thorax that can sometimes be seen. H&E, 400× magnification

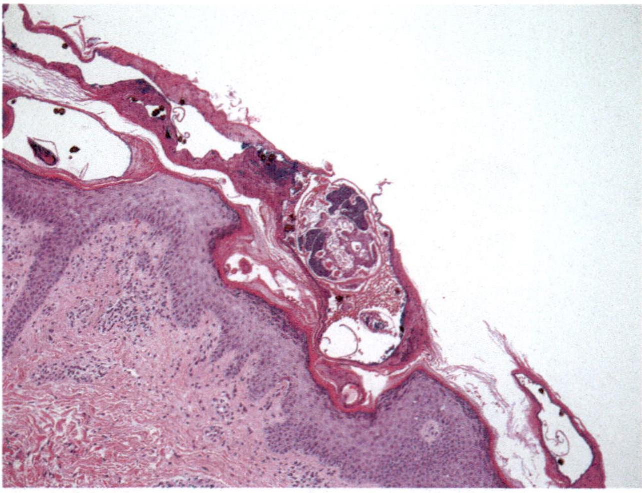

Fig. 5.103 Infestations by *Sarcoptes scabiei* can be found in a variety of cutaneous locations, with a predilection for the finger webs, wrists, axillae, and genital regions. The rash caused by scabies is usually very pruritic and may also result in the formation of papules or pustules. On biopsy, arthropod parts, eggs, and scybala, the yellowish-brown fecal pellets seen in this image, may be noted in the subcorneal region. The inflammatory response immediately surrounding the mites tends to be neutrophilic with a lymphocytic and eosinophilic component within the underlying dermis. H&E, 100× magnification

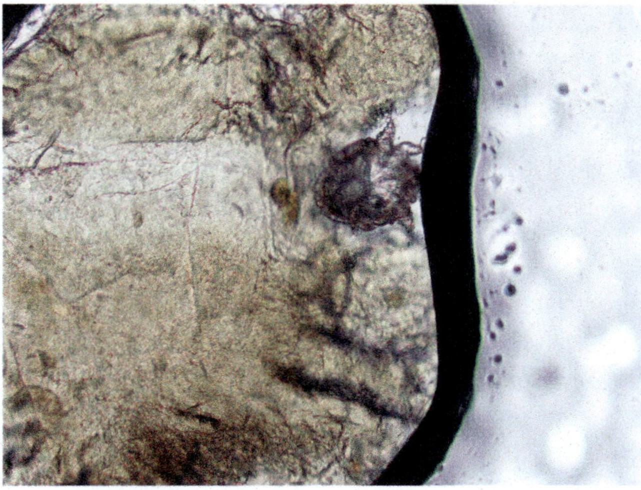

Fig. 5.104 Seen here is a whole *Sarcoptes scabiei* mite obtained from skin scrapings and placed onto a slide with a few drops of mineral oil, the preferred collection method for identifying scabies in the microbiology laboratory. A second slide can then be placed on top, sealing the specimens inside for later observation under the microscope. 100× magnification (Image courtesy of Jeremy Koehlinger)

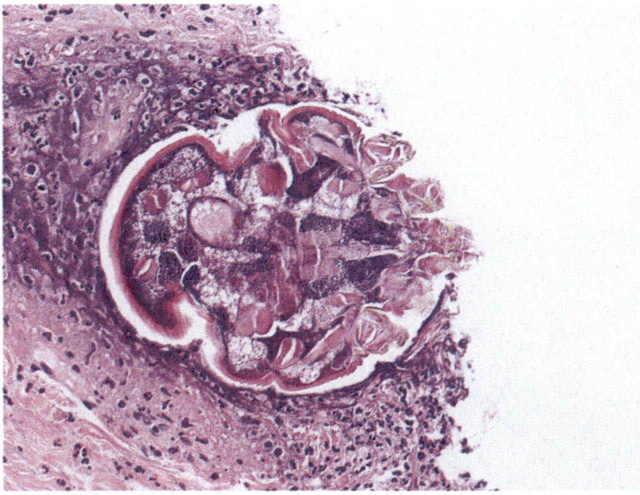

Fig. 5.105 A near perfect coronal section through a *S. scabiei* mite. Compare to Fig. 5.104. H&E, 400× magnification

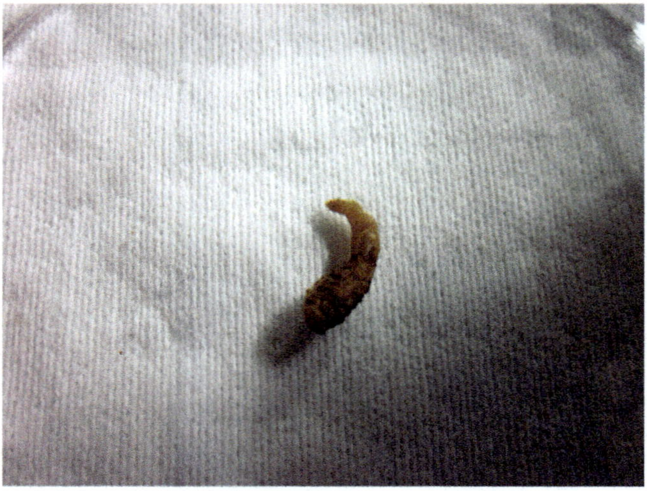

Fig. 5.106 Larva of *Dermatobia hominis*, more commonly known as the human botfly. Full grown larvae measure between 15 and 20 mm in length. Note the rows of dark cuticular spines which ring the body. Other causes of myiasis, such as *Cordylobia anthropophaga,* more commonly known as the tumbu fly, can have a similar gross appearance, although the spines tend to be more randomly distributed. As such, evaluation by a parasitologist or thorough examination utilizing one of many excellent medical parasitology atlases may be required for definitive identification. A history of travel to certain parts of the world (botflies are found in Mexico as well as Central and South America, while tumbu flies are found in tropical Africa) may also be helpful. Specimens that are surgically resected are found in a subdermal cavity, where the larva feeds on surrounding tissues

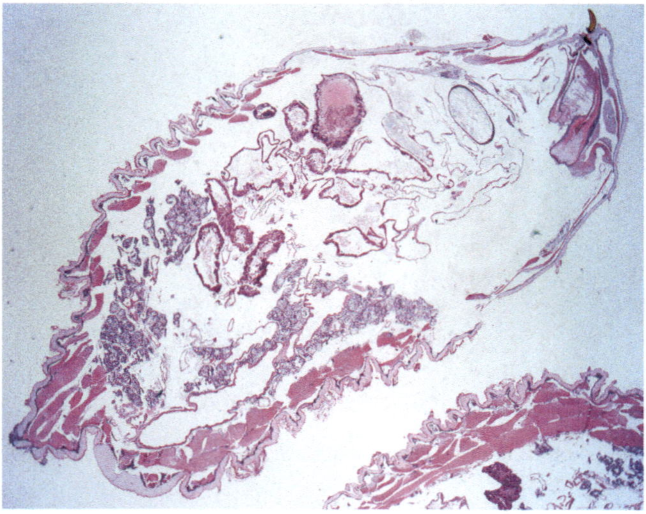

Fig. 5.107 Sections of *D. hominis* larvae that were submitted for surgical pathology. Note the presence of many triangular cuticular spines as well as internal muscle fibers and various organ structures. A refractile, yellow-appearing portion of the curved mandibles of the larvae is also seen in the upper right portion of the section. H&E, 20× magnification

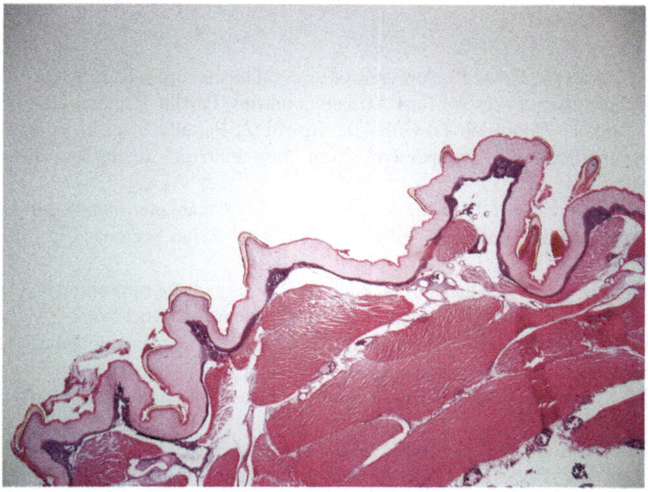

Fig. 5.108 Higher magnification image demonstrating sections through the cuticular spines. The spines appear yellow and refractile on H&E staining, having a vaguely triangular appearance. Note also bands of muscle fibers just below the cuticle. H&E, 100× magnification

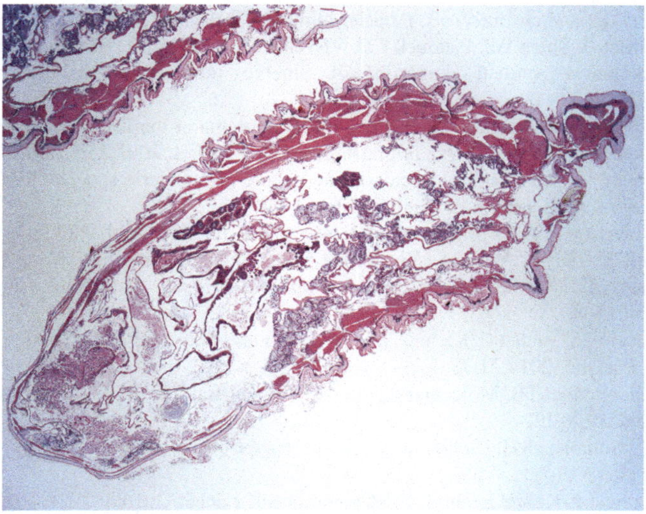

Fig. 5.109 Sections of *C. anthropophaga* larva determined by travel history. Note the similarity in microscopic appearance to the botfly larvae discussed above. Definitive identification is very difficult by histopathology alone and is best accomplished by gross examination of the larvae by an experienced parasitologist and correlation with the patient's travel history. H&E, 20× magnification

Suggested Reading

Al-Salem W, Herricks JR, Hotez PJ. A review of visceral leishmaniasis during the conflict in South Sudan and the consequences for East African countries. Parasit Vectors. 2016;9:460.

Angheben A, Boix L, Buonfrate D, Gobbi F, Bisoffi Z, Pupella S, et al. Chagas disease and transfusion medicine: a perspective from non-endemic countries. Blood Transfus. 2015;13:540–50.

Belizario Jr V, Delos Trinos JP, Garcia NB, Reyes M. Cutaneous manifestations of selected parasitic infections in Western Pacific and Southeast Asian regions. Curr Infect Dis Rep. 2016;18:30.

Bowen LN, Smith B, Reich D, Quezado M, Nath A. HIV-associated opportunistic CNS infections: pathophysiology, diagnosis and treatment. Nat Rev Neurol. 2016;12:662–74.

Cama VA, Mathison BA. Infections by intestinal Coccidia and Giardia duodenalis. Clin Lab Med. 2015;35:423–44.

Del Brutto OH, García HH. Taenia solium cysticercosis—the lessons of history. J Neurol Sci. 2015;359:392–5.

DuPont HL. Persistent diarrhea: a clinical review. JAMA. 2016;315:2712–23.

Faccini-Martínez ÁA, Pérez-Díaz CE, Botero-García CA, Benítez-Baracaldo FC, Rodríguez-López AE, Rodríguez-Morales AJ. Role of the blood smear in febrile returning travelers: beyond malaria. Travel Med Infect Dis. 2016;14:515–6.

Feldman DM, Keller R, Borgida AF. Toxoplasmosis, parvovirus, and cytomegalovirus in pregnancy. Clin Lab Med. 2016;36:407–19.

Gajurel K, Dhakal R, Deresinski S. Leishmaniasis in solid organ and hematopoietic stem cell transplant recipients. Clin Transplant. 2016; doi:10.1111/ctr.12867. [Epub ahead of print.]

Gonzales I, Rivera JT. Garcia HH; cysticercosis working group in Peru. Pathogenesis of Taenia solium taeniasis and cysticercosis. Parasite Immunol. 2016;38:136–46.

Guarner J, Bartlett J, Shieh WJ, Paddock CD, Visvesvara GS, Zaki SR. Histopathologic spectrum and immunohistochemical diagnosis of amebic meningoencephalitis. Mod Pathol. 2007;20:1230–7.

Kaplan KJ, Goodman ZD, Ishak KG. Eosinophilic granuloma of the liver: a characteristic lesion with relationship to visceral larva migrans. Am J Surg Pathol. 2001;25:1316–21.

Lala S, Upadhyay V. Enterobius vermicularis and its role in paediatric appendicitis: protection or predisposition? ANZ J Surg. 2016;86:717–9.

Lamps LW. Infectious causes of appendicitis. Infect Dis Clin N Am. 2010;24:995–1018.

Lobo SA, Patil K, Jain S, Marks S, Visvesvara GS, Tenner M, Braun A, Wang G, El Khoury MY. Diagnostic challenges in *Balamuthia mandrillaris* infections. Parasitol Res. 2013;112:4015–9.

Massolo A, Liccioli S, Budke C, Klein C. *Echinococcus multilocularis* in North America: the great unknown. Parasite. 2014;21:73.

O'Connell EM, Nutman TB. Molecular diagnostics for soil-transmitted helminths. AmJTrop Med Hyg. 2016;95:508–13.

Othman AA, Soliman RH. Schistosomiasis in Egypt: a never-ending story? Acta Trop. 2015;148:179–90.

Qian MB, Utzinger J, Keiser J, Zhou XN. Clonorchiasis. Lancet. 2016;387:800–10; doi:10.1099/jmmcr.0.005011.

Roiko MS, Schmitt BH, Relich RF, Meyer TL, Zhang S, Davis TE. An unusual presentation of leishmaniasis in a human immunodeficiency virus-positive individual. J Med Microbiol Case Rep. 2016; doi: 10.1099/jmmcr.0.005011. (ePub May 2, 2016).

Shimoni Z, Froom P. Uncertainties in diagnosis, treatment and prevention of trichinellosis. Expert Rev Anti-Infect Ther. 2015;13:1279–88.

Soares R, Tasca T. Giardiasis: an update review on sensitivity and specificity of methods for laboratorial diagnosis. J Microbiol Methods. 2016;129:98–102.

Starr MC, Montgomery SP. Soil-transmitted helminthiasis in the United States: a systematic review—1940–2010. Am J Trop Med Hyg. 2011;85:680–4.
Visvesvara GS. Amebic meningoencephalitides and keratitis: challenges in diagnosis and treatment. Curr Opin Infect Dis. 2010;23:590–4.
Wilhelm CL, Yarovinsky F. Apicomplexan infections in the gut. Parasite Immunol. 2014;36:409–20.
Yan C, Liang LJ, Zheng KY, Zhu XQ. Impact of environmental factors on the emergence, transmission and distribution of *Toxoplasma gondii*. Parasit Vectors. 2016;9:137.
Yoder JS, Eddy BA, Visvesvara GS, Capewell L, Beach MJ. The epidemiology of primary amoebic meningoencephalitis in the USA, 1962-2008. Epidemiol Infect. 2010;138:968–75.

Mimics and Artifacts

6

Bryan H. Schmitt

Discussed in this chapter are commonly seen artifacts and mimics that may resemble infectious agents. Initial hematoxylin and eosin (H&E) or cytologic stains such as Giemsa or Diff-Quik may highlight a variety of different structures that can be of concern for the presence of microorganisms. While this is not an exhaustive list, many of the common situations in which this may occur are presented here.

Additionally, certain stains, in particular, Gomori methenamine silver (GMS) and its variants, may be very nonspecific or prone to the production of artifactual changes that may mimic infectious microorganisms. Special attention will therefore be paid to commonly seen artifacts associated with silver staining methods.

6.1 Common Artifacts and General Considerations in Cytology Specimens

This section details common findings and considerations that can be seen in tissues and cytology specimens regardless of stains used (Figs. 6.1, 6.2, 6.3, 6.4, 6.5, 6.6, 6.7, 6.8 and 6.9).

B.H. Schmitt (✉)
Department of Pathology and Laboratory Medicine, Indiana University School of Medicine, Indianapolis, IN, USA
e-mail: bhschmit@iupui.edu

B.H. Schmitt (ed.), *Atlas of Infectious Disease Pathology*,
Atlas of Anatomic Pathology, DOI 10.1007/978-3-319-54702-2_6

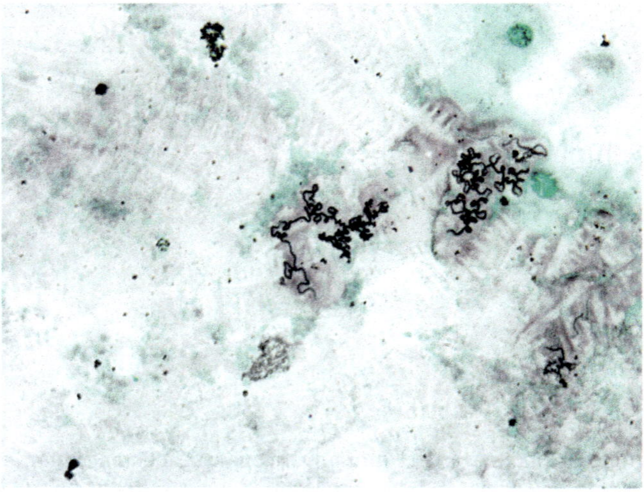

Fig. 6.1 Curschmann's spirals will manifest on a variety of stains from deep respiratory cytology specimens. Most commonly seen in bronchoalveolar lavage fluids, they are occasionally identified on less invasively obtained specimens. While they are most frequently associated with asthmatic patients or patients with chronic obstructive pulmonary disease, these structures can be found in a variety of chronic lung diseases and represent inspissated mucous plugs dislodged from bronchioles. Seen here is the general appearance of a Curschmann's spiral on Gomori methenamine silver staining (GMS). Note that from an infectious disease pathology standpoint, the appearance may resemble a coiled worm. The size of the spirals can vary greatly. GMS, 1000× magnification

6.2 Control Contamination

It is common practice in many institutions to place special stain controls on the same slide as the specimen. While this practice saves on the cost of glass slides and provides ease for control comparison by the microscopist, it may also be problematic because microorganisms can become detached and wash over the patient tissue during processing; this will give the impression that the control organism is present within the patient specimen (Figs. 6.10 and 6.11).

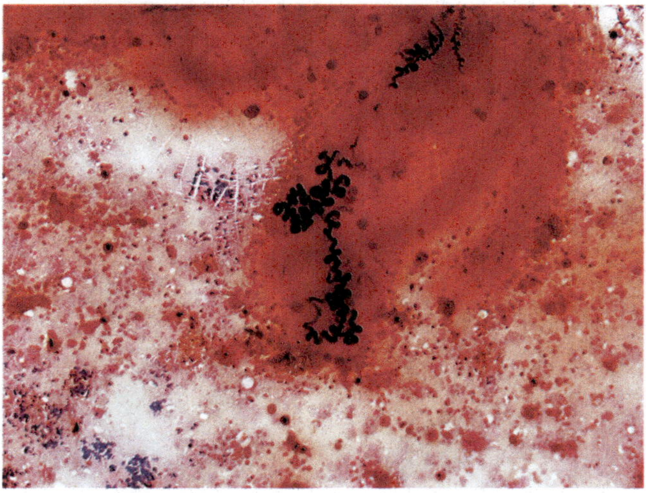

Fig. 6.2 Curschmann's spiral on Gram stain. Note the significant variation in size as this image was obtained at 200× magnification compared to Fig. 6.1, which was obtained at 1000× magnification. Curschmann's spirals tend to retain crystal violet on Gram staining, appearing *dark* or *purple*. Gram stain, 200× magnification

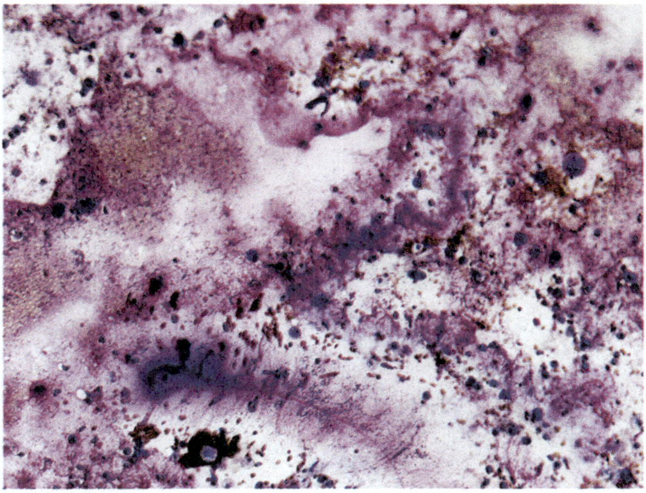

Fig. 6.3 Curschmann's spirals seen on Romanowsky stains tends to have a much less defined appearance, instead appearing with a "smudged" or diffuse staining pattern rather than a distinct spiral. Giemsa stain, 200× magnification

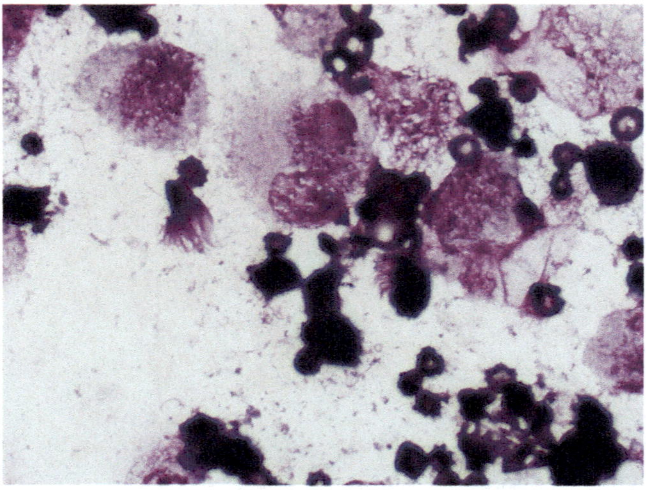

Fig. 6.4 Ciliocytophthoria, detached ciliary tufts from ciliated respiratory epithelial cells in a bronchoalveolar lavage specimen. Ciliocytophthoria may be found in specimens obtained from any anatomic site with cells demonstrating cilia, and it may be mistaken for ciliated protozoa. Of note, the only known ciliated protozoan parasite of humans is the relatively rarely encountered *Balantidium coli* (not further discussed in this text) which is much larger and is typically found only within gastrointestinal tract specimens. Diff-Quik, 1000× magnification

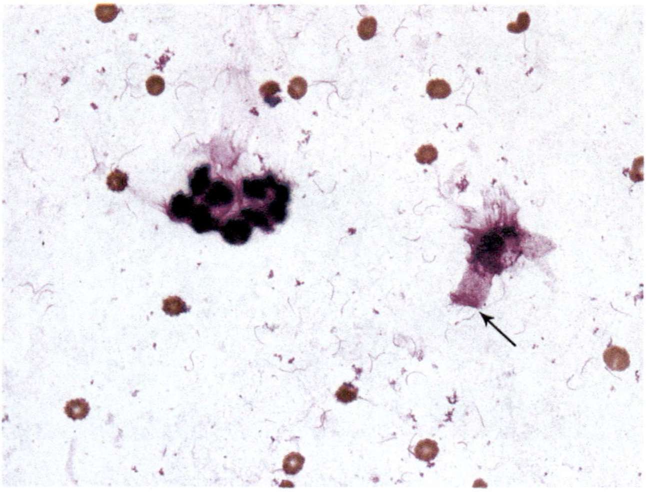

Fig. 6.5 Individual cilia may also become detached from their cells, particularly in cytospun or centrifuged specimens. The detached cilia may be confused with long, thin bacilli. Note also in this image, a degenerating respiratory epithelial cell that demonstrates a terminal bar (*arrow*) without attached cilia. Giemsa stain, 1000× magnification

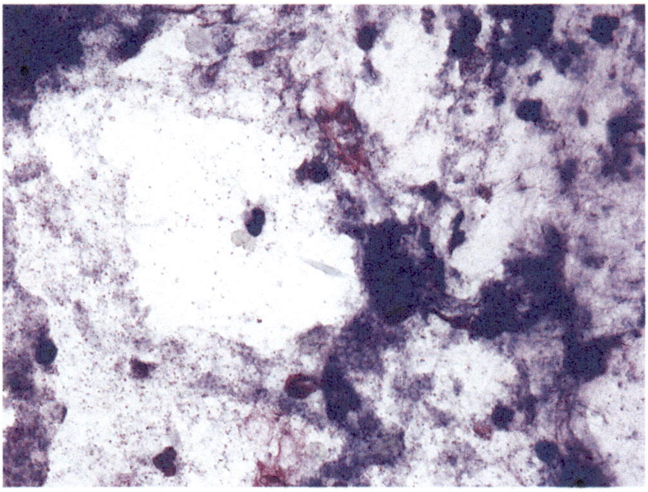

Fig. 6.6 Charcot-Leyden crystals are elongate, *needle-shaped* structures consisting of lysophospholipase and produced by the breakdown of eosinophils. Often found in respiratory specimens of patients with asthma, they are also found at the sites of infection with parasites or certain fungi. While large Charcot-Leyden crystals may be reminiscent of eggs or possibly fungal structures, they more significantly serve as an indicator that there has been an eosinophilic response at the specimen site. While often appearing *red* in color, on Romanowsy stains, such as the Giemsa stain shown here, they are colorless. 1000× magnification

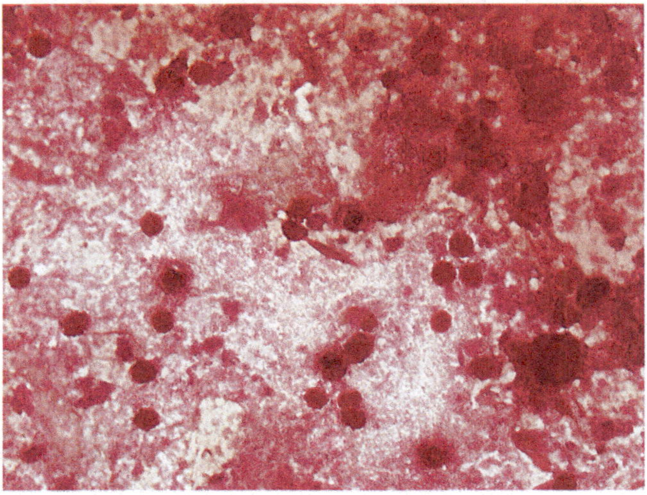

Fig. 6.7 The appearance of Charcot-Leyden crystals on Gram stain. The crystals retain the safranin stain, appearing *red*. 1000× magnification

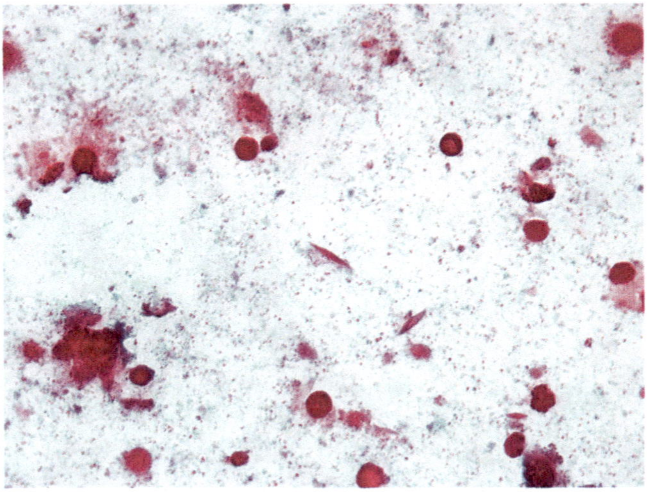

Fig. 6.8 Classic appearance of Charcot-Leyden crystals on a trichrome stained stool wet mount. This stain is commonly performed as part of ova and parasite stool examinations in parasitology laboratories and is not routinely performed in anatomic pathology. 1000× magnification

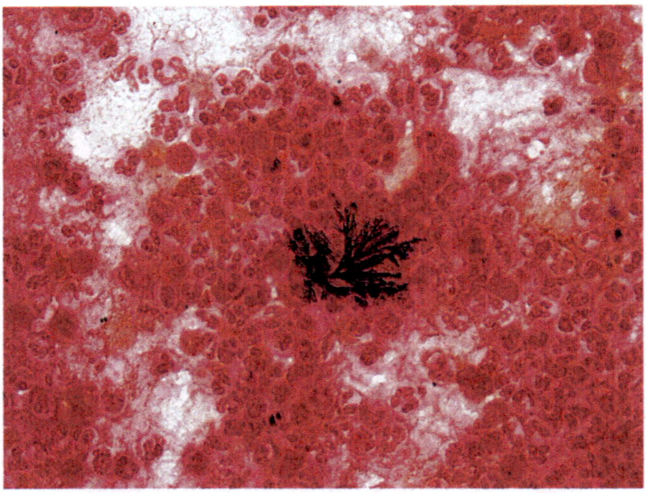

Fig. 6.9 Precipitation of crystal violet may be seen on Gram-stained fluids, in this case from a bronchoalveolar lavage specimen. While close observation should reveal that the precipitate appears to be forming crystalline structures, at first glance it may appear to be clusters of hyphae or filamentous bacteria. Crystal violet precipitate is often birefringent under polarized light. 1000× magnification

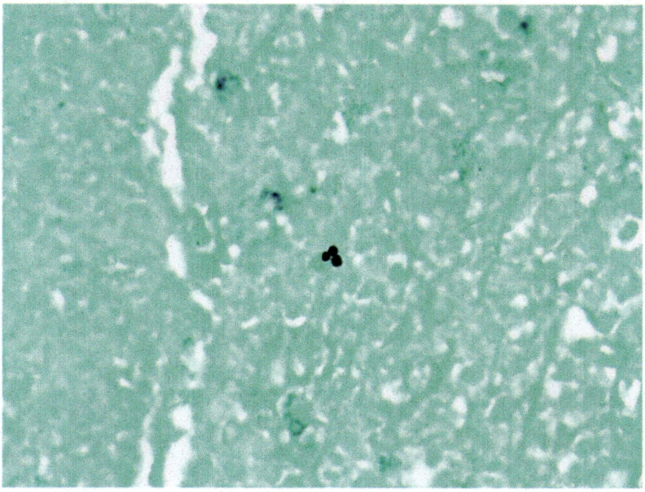

Fig. 6.10 This case was brought to us for suspicion of yeast in a lymph node. Several clusters of "yeast-like" structures, as shown here, were seen. Clinical suspicion of a fungal infection was low. No surrounding inflammatory response was seen. Note also that the Gomori methenamine silver (GMS) positive structures are significantly out of the plane of focus when compared to the background. GMS, 1000× magnification

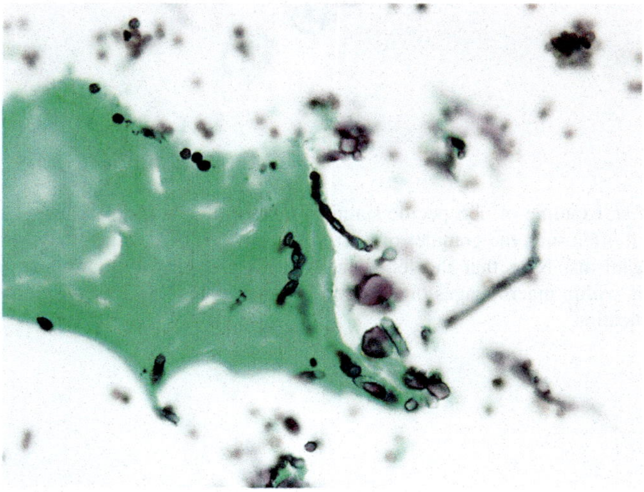

Fig. 6.11 On further examination, a control *Aspergillus* species was noted to have been placed on the same slide. Note the similarity of staining pattern observed with the conidia. Contamination from the control was strongly suspected. Upon restaining of the patient's specimen alone, no Gomori methenamine silver (GMS) positive structures were noted. GMS, 1000× magnification

6.3 Artifacts and Obstacles When Interpreting Silver Staining Methods

Silver staining methods such as GMS are perhaps the most difficult to interpret correctly. While they are very helpful in identifying fungi in particular, they are very nonspecific, both creating artifact and staining other structures that may result in false-positive interpretations (Figs. 6.12, 6.13, 6.14, 6.15, 6.16 and 6.17).

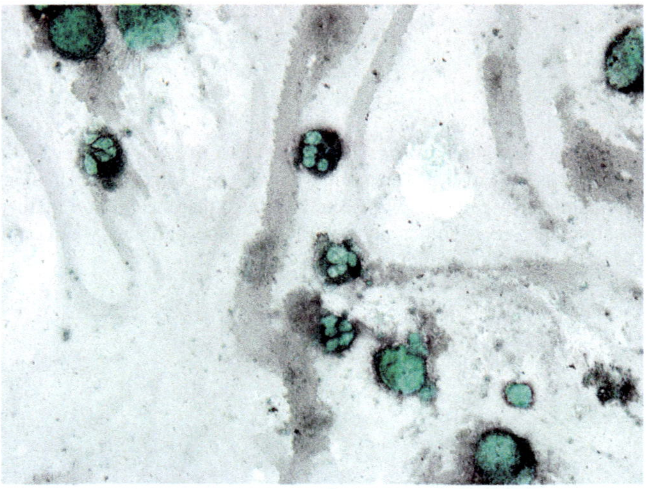

Fig. 6.12 As an example of nonspecific staining, Gomori methenamine silver stain in a heavy application will often stain the granules of neutrophils, as seen here, which may suggest intracellular microorganisms. Note that the lobed nuclei characteristic of neutrophils are also seen. Ingested debris within macrophages or even red blood cells may be stained with silver as well. 1000× magnification

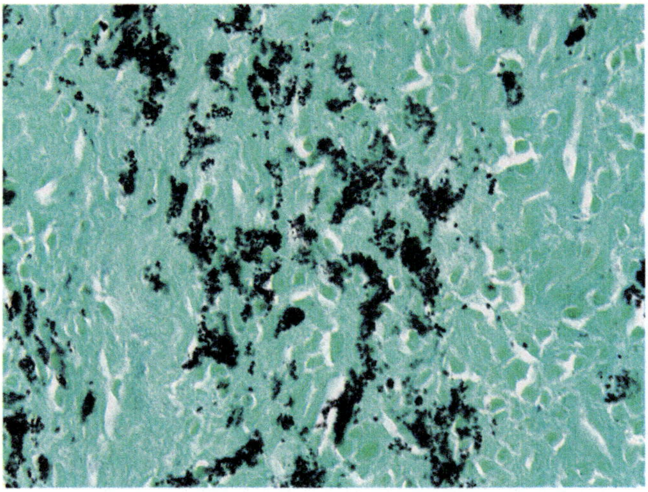

Fig. 6.13 Anthracotic pigment may be seen in the lungs and regional lymph nodes of patients who smoke or live in urban environments where carbon is heavily found in the air. Appearing *black* on a variety of stains, the presence of anthracotic pigment may particularly present a conundrum on the examination of silver stains for fungus, where fungal elements are expected to appear *black* on microscopy. Examination reveals that the *black* staining granules have significant variability in size, are generally smaller than most yeasts, and have a "chunky" non-uniform appearance. Gomori methenamine silver stain, 1000× magnification

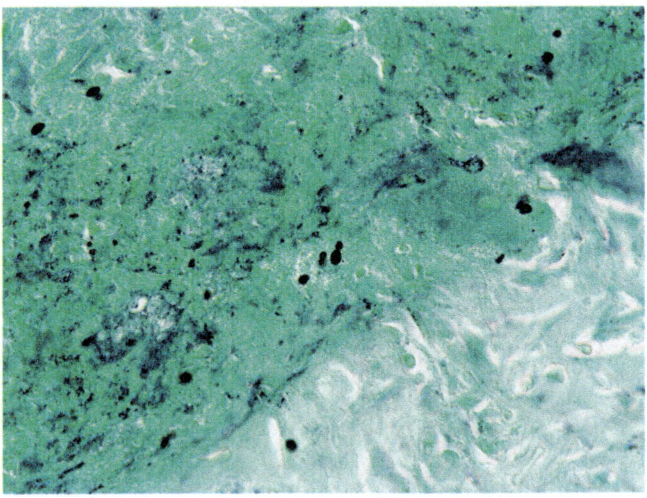

Fig. 6.14 Contrast the appearance of *H. capsulatum* to the anthracotic pigment shown in Fig. 6.13. Note that true yeast forms tend to have consistent staining and smooth, uniform walls. This field is adjacent to that shown in Fig. 6.13, illustrating that, in particular with pulmonary specimens and regional anatomic structures including lymph nodes, the presence of *black*-appearing anthracotic pigment must be taken into account when considering fungal etiologies on silver stains. Note also scattered anthracotic granules in the background. Gomori methenamine silver stain, 1000× magnification

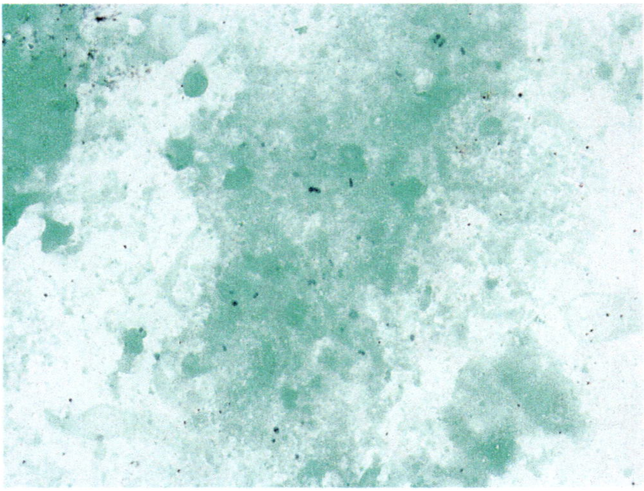

Fig. 6.15 Many bacteria, in particular, Gram-positives, including the mycobacteria, also stain with silver deposition stains such as Gomori methenamine silver stain (GMS). In general, they will still measure less than one micron in width, but it is important to note that GMS stains the outside of microorganisms. This feature may make bacteria appear slightly larger than on other methods, such as the commonly performed Gram stain. Gram-positive cocci from a bronchoalveolar lavage, later identified from culture as *S. aureus* is shown here. GMS stain, 1000× magnification

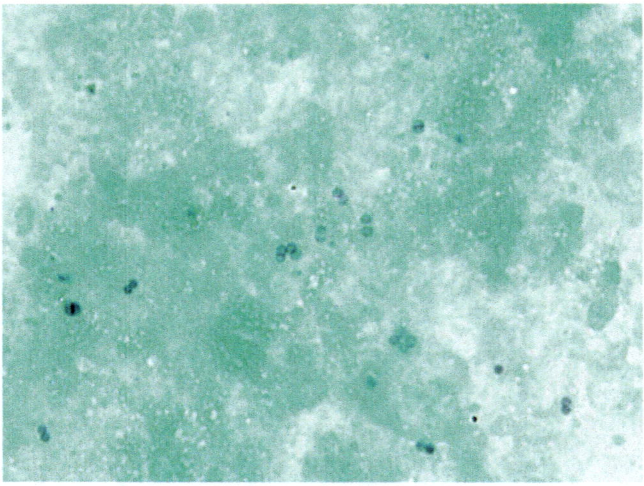

Fig. 6.16 In this enlarged image taken from Fig. 6.15, the staining pattern of the Gram-positive cocci is more evident. Again, note that the outside of the bacterial cells are stained with Gomori methenamine silver stain, which may make them appear larger than expected. The size and appearance may raise suspicion for the presence of small yeast or conidia

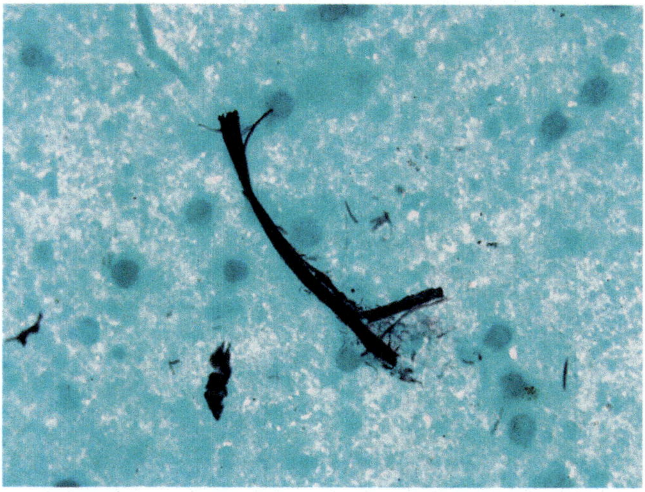

Fig. 6.17 Silver stains can stain a variety of noninfectious structures such as textile fibers that may be introduced during specimen collection or the preparation of slides. Particularly if "branching" is present, the appearance may raise suspicion for fungal organisms. Note the relative nonregularity and general "frayed" appearance, particularly at the ends, features not usually present in true fungal hyphae. Gomori methenamine silver stain, 1000× magnification

6.4 Other Findings That May Be Interpreted as Parasites or Fungi (Figs. 6.18, 6.19, 6.20, 6.21, 6.22, 6.23, 6.24, 6.25, 6.26 and 6.27)

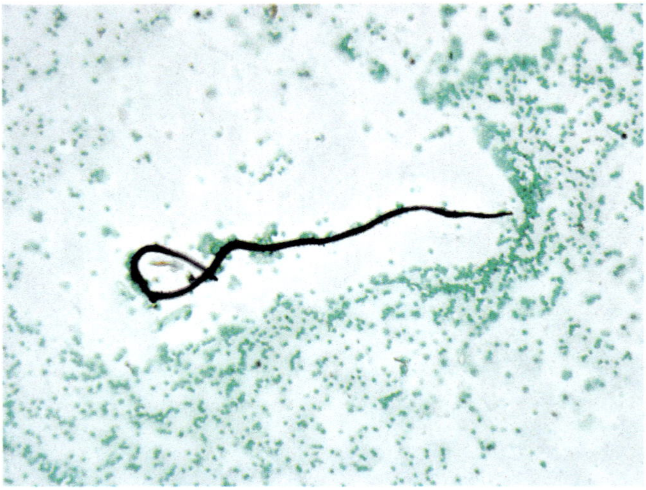

Fig. 6.18 While most often artifactual staining with Gomori methenamine silver stain (GMS) and other silver stains suggest fungal organisms, structures resembling parasites may also be seen, such as in this example of a "worm-like" textile fiber. In this particular case, it should also be stated that parasites, with rare exceptions, such as some amoebic cysts, will not stain with silver stains such as GMS. GMS, 200× magnification

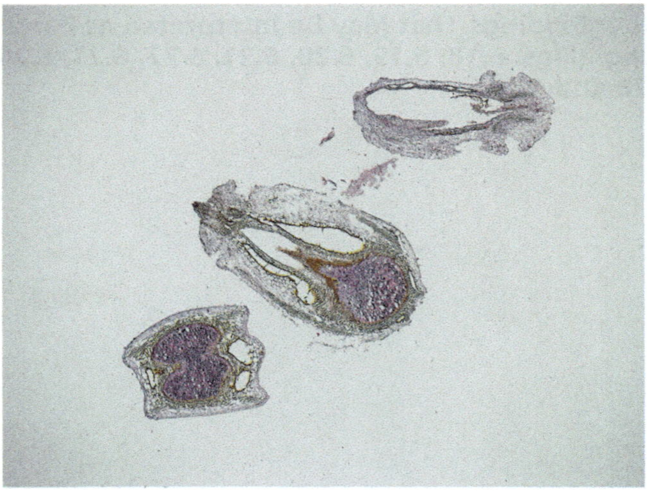

Fig. 6.19 An infrequently encountered specimen, plant seeds may resemble very large eggs or the relatively complex structures of nematodes and trematodes. Note the presence of eosinophilic granules within honeycomb-like structures and rough-appearing walls. The internal structures commonly seen in parasitic worms such as the gastrointestinal tract, reproductive organs, and muscle fibers are not seen. Seeds are mostly commonly encountered as part of the luminal material accompanying gastrointestinal tract specimens, but larger seeds may at times be mistaken for polyps or other lesions and biopsied. H&E, 40× magnification

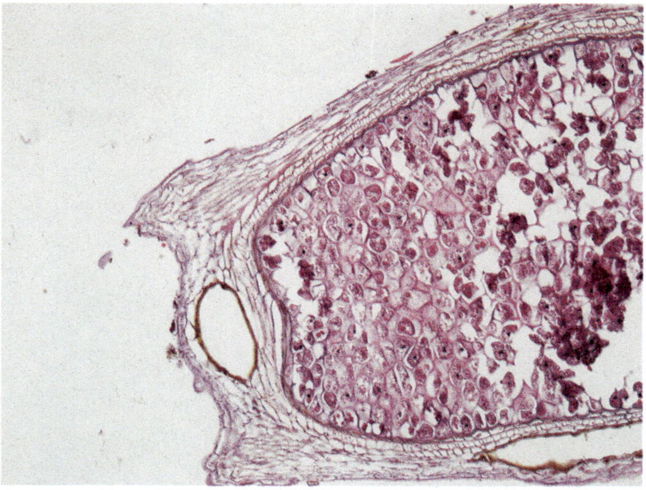

Fig. 6.20 A higher magnification image of a plant, in this case tomato, seed demonstrating eosinophilic granules within a honeycomb-like structure. H&E, 200× magnification

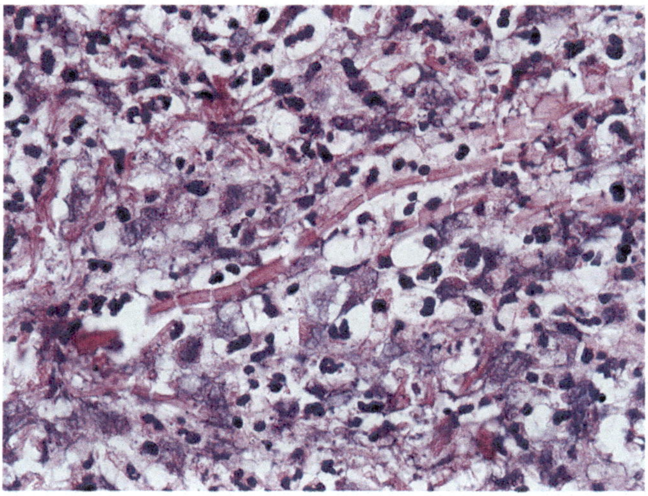

Fig. 6.21 Calcifications within a subcutaneous thigh lesion in a patient with suspected calciphylaxis. Calcifications may be round and mimic yeast, but they are particularly troublesome in that they may also be elongated, mimicking fungal hyphae. Fractures in these thin, hyphae-like elements may resemble septations. These structures can also be associated with tissue or fat necrosis, further raising suspicion for a fungal infection. While often basophilic staining, they can also appear more eosinophilic as shown here. H&E, 1000× magnification

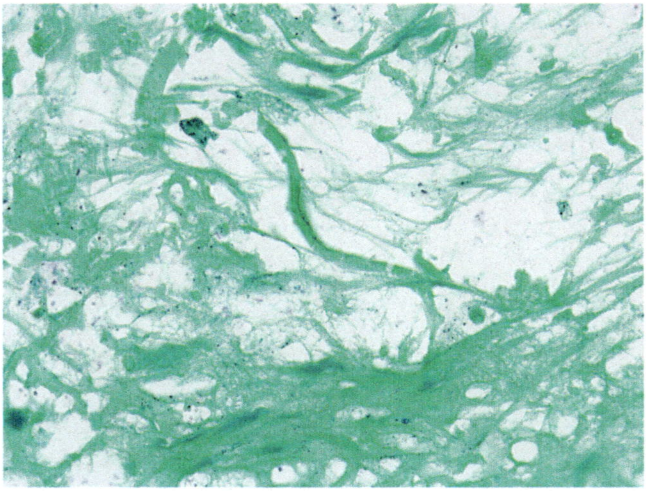

Fig. 6.22 A negative Gomori methenamine silver stain in light of properly staining controls may help to confirm that these structures are, in fact, nonfungal in origin. 1000× magnification

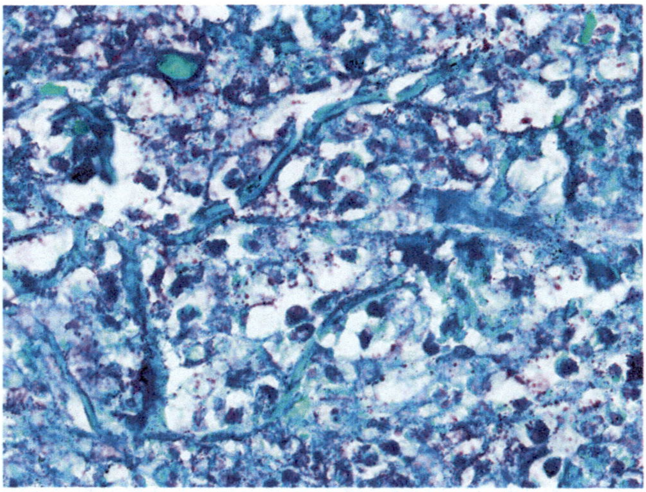

Fig. 6.23 This case also demonstrated negative staining with periodic acid–Schiff stain for fungus. 1000× magnification

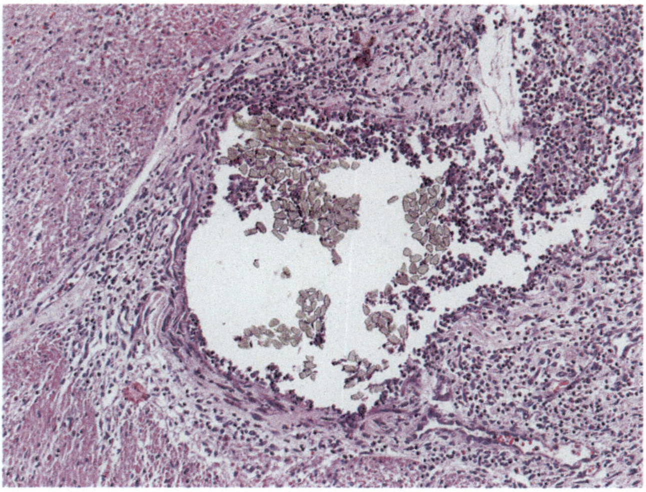

Fig. 6.24 Suture material is commonly encountered in surgical pathology specimens but does appear in a variety of different forms. Inflammatory responses can vary, depending on the type of material used and length of time it was in place prior to resection, with long standing material usually exhibiting a chronic inflammatory foreign body type reaction. The appearance of suture material, particularly with larger width fibers, may sometimes raise suspicion for parasitic worms or eggs. Note here that the cross-sections through suture fibers demonstrate a somewhat refractile, homogeneous cut surface without evidence of internal structures. H&E, 200× magnification

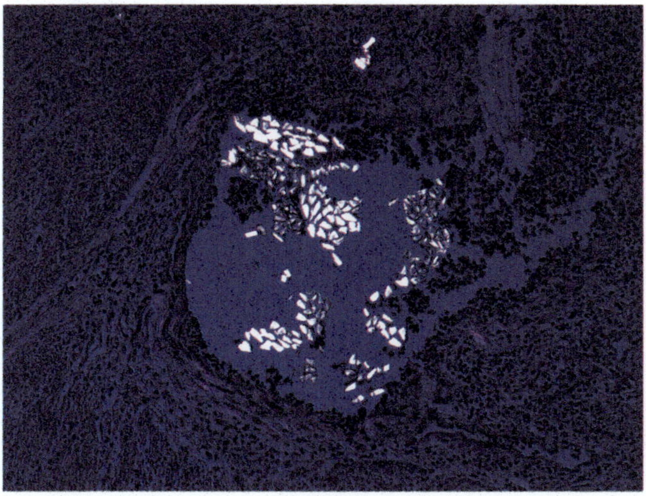

Fig. 6.25 Suture material is usually strongly birefringent under polarized light, while for the most part, parasite eggs or structures, with the exception of cestode hooklets, do not display this property. H&E, 200× magnification

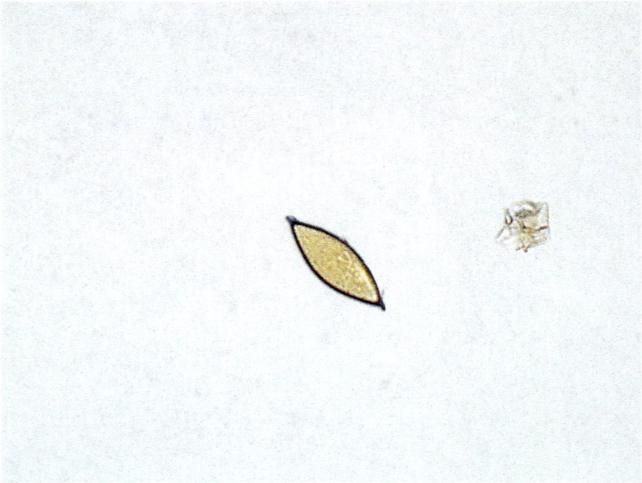

Fig. 6.26 Uric acid crystals may bear a strong resemblance to the eggs of *Schistosoma haematobium*. As *S. haematobium* is also most frequently found in the urine, it is important to recognize the differences. Uric acid crystals usually demonstrate significant variability in size and in general are smaller than the eggs of *S. haematobium*, which typically measure 150–170 μm in length. Uric acid crystals are also tapered at both ends to a triangular point, whereas the single terminal spine of *S. haematobium* eggs has a "pinched-off" appearance. The eggs of *S. haematobium* also demonstrate internal structures, whereas uric acid crystals do not. Urine, Papanicolaou stain, 400× magnification (Image courtesy of Dr. Ryan Relich)

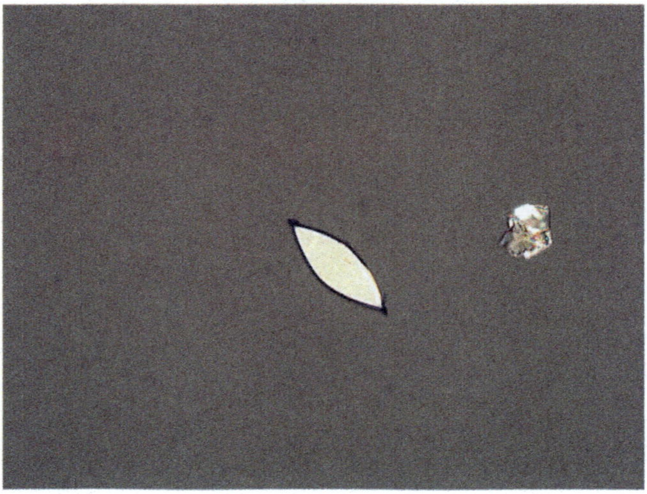

Fig. 6.27 Uric acid crystals are strongly birefringent under polarized light, whereas *S. haematobium* eggs tend to demonstrate much weaker or no birefringence. 400× magnification (Image courtesy of Dr. Ryan Relich)

Suggested Reading

Ash LR, Orihel TC. Pseudoparasites and artifacts. In: Atlas of human parasitology. 5th ed. Chicago: American Society for Clinical Pathology; 2015. p. 384–415.

Baird JK, Lack EE. Artifacts and false parasites. In: Connor DH, Chandler FW, Schwartz DA, Manz HJ, Lack EE, editors. Pathology of infectious diseases, vol. II. Stamford: Appleton & Lange; 1997. p. 1591–600.

Garcia LS. Artifacts that can be confused with parasitic organisms. In: Diagnostic medical parasitology. 5th ed. Washington, DC: ASM Press; 2007. p. 947–59.

Hadziyannis E, Yen-Lieberman B, Hall G, Proco GW. Ciliocytophthoria in clinical virology. Arch Pathol Lab Med. 2000;124:1220–3.

Marler LM, Siders JA, Allen SD. Artifacts. In: Direct smear atlas: a monograph of gram-stained preparations of clinical specimens. Baltimore: Lippincott Williams & Wilkins; 2001. p. 19–42.

Pritt BS, Elhosseiny A. Artifacts and pitfalls in infectious disease pathology. In: Procop GW, Pritt BS, editors. Pathology of infectious diseases. Philadelphia: W.B. Saunders; 2015. p. 647–88.

Rastogi V, Puri N, Arora S, Kaur G, Yadav L, Sharma R. Artefacts: a diagnostic dilemma – a review. J Clin Diagn Res. 2013;7:2408–13.

Relich RF, Faught PR, McCoy MH, Alexander RE, Pritt BS. Photo quiz: an unexpected colonoscopic finding in a 13-year-old boy. J Clin Microbiol. 2014;52:2749.

Vila M, Thompson K, Erdem G. Motile ciliary microorganisms in peritoneal fluid. Diagn Cytopathol. 2011;39:606–7.

Index

B.H. Schmitt (ed.), *Atlas of Infectious Disease Pathology*,
Atlas of Anatomic Pathology, DOI 10.1007/978-3-319-54702-2

Printed by Printforce, the Netherlands